High-Risk Localized and Locally Advanced Prostate Cancer

High-Risk Localized and Locally Advanced Prostate Cancer

Editor

Kouji Izumi

MDPI • Basel • Beijing • Wuhan • Barcelona • Belgrade • Manchester • Tokyo • Cluj • Tianjin

Editor
Kouji Izumi
Kanazawa University
Graduate School of Medical
Science
Kanazawa, Japan

Editorial Office
MDPI
St. Alban-Anlage 66
4052 Basel, Switzerland

This is a reprint of articles from the Special Issue published online in the open access journal *Cancers* (ISSN 2072-6694) (available at: https://www.mdpi.com/journal/cancers/special_issues/High-Risk_Localized_Locally_Advanced_Prostate_Cancer).

For citation purposes, cite each article independently as indicated on the article page online and as indicated below:

LastName, A.A.; LastName, B.B.; LastName, C.C. Article Title. *Journal Name* **Year**, *Volume Number*, Page Range.

ISBN 978-3-0365-8168-2 (Hbk)
ISBN 978-3-0365-8169-9 (PDF)

Contents

About the Editor

Kouji Izumi

Kouji Izumi, MD, Ph.D, Associate professor, Department of Integrative Cancer Therapy and Urology, Kanazawa University Graduate School of Medical Science. Japanese Urological Association Board Certified Urologist; Japanese Society of Medical Oncology Diplomate and Subspeciality Board of Medical Oncology.

cancers

Editorial

Editorial for the Special Issue on High-Risk Localized and Locally Advanced Prostate Cancer

Kouji Izumi

Department of Integrative Cancer Therapy and Urology, Kanazawa University Graduate School of Medical Science, 13-1 Takara-machi, Kanazawa 920-8641, Ishikawa, Japan; azuizu2003@yahoo.co.jp

The recent development of imaging modalities, such as diffusion-weighted whole-body imaging with background suppression (DWIBS) and positron emission tomography of prostate-specific membrane antigen (PSMA-PET) with a radioactive diagnostic agent, has enabled the detection of minute metastases in patients diagnosed with high-risk localized and locally advanced prostate cancer by conventional modalities. The impact of imaging developments on prognosis has not been fully assessed. However, the increasing prevalence of cutting-edge imaging modalities may soon change the definitions of high-risk localized and locally advanced prostate cancer. Even now, around 20–30% of nonmetastatic prostate cancer patients have high-risk localized disease requiring curative treatment. The best treatment for high-risk localized disease is also still unclear, and the reliability of the definition of "high-risk" may need to be validated first. Although recent advances in radiotherapy for prostate cancer have yielded excellent long-term results, even in high-risk localized disease, there are no studies directly comparing it with local treatment options, such as prostatectomy. To address current challenges in high-risk localized and locally advanced prostate cancer, 12 original and 3 review articles covering aspects from basic research to clinical trials are published in this Special Issue.

Cancer aggressiveness

Ottman et al. investigated the factors involved in prostate cancer aggressiveness and racial disparity with miRNA expression studies and suggest a role for some miRNAs in prostate cancer diagnosis, prognosis, and the elimination of health disparities [1]. Diop et al. report that intraductal carcinoma of the prostate, an aggressive histological subtype, showed a reduced number of infiltrated immune cells compared to the surrounding tissues and it provided different survival [2]. Samarija et al. showed that amino acid metabolism-related gene expression is aberrant in prostate cancer. The expression of SERINC3 and CSAD genes strongly differentiated between better and worse prognosis for high and low Gleason scores, respectively [3]. Bui et al. examined the endogenous CCL2 functions in murine bone marrow-derived mesenchymal stem cells. They discovered that CCL2 plays a crucial role in prostate cancer growth within the tumor microenvironment [4]. Baba et al. reviewed 557 prostate cancer patients who underwent radical prostatectomy and found that a tumor volume over 2.8 cc was an independent predictive factor for biochemical recurrence. They also established a novel risk assessment model based on tumor volume and location [5].

Regional lymph node invasion

Di Pierro et al. evaluated the accuracy of the four most used nomograms for predicting lymph node invasion. Comparing them in high-risk prostate cancer patients, the predictive performance of the four nomograms was virtually the same, as was their ability to avoid unnecessary extended pelvic lymph node dissection. [6]. Yamashita et al. conducted a prospective study in high-risk prostate cancer patients. They aimed to assess the impact of lymphatic invasion on biochemical recurrence in patients who underwent robot-assisted radical prostatectomy and extended lymph node dissection. They found that lymphatic invasion in the primary site was a significant independent predictor of biochemical recurrence [7].

Citation: Izumi, K. Editorial for the Special Issue on High-Risk Localized and Locally Advanced Prostate Cancer. *Cancers* **2023**, *15*, 3153. https://doi.org/10.3390/cancers15123153

Received: 20 May 2023
Revised: 5 June 2023
Accepted: 7 June 2023
Published: 11 June 2023

Radiotherapy

Faccenda et al. investigated the dosimetric impact on the target, and organs at risk, of intrafraction prostate motion and interfraction anatomical changes in dose-escalated linac-based stereotactic body radiation therapy [8]. Francolini et al. conducted the STARR trial and reported early toxicity and biochemical outcomes after stereotactic salvage radiotherapy for macroscopic recurrence within the prostate bed after radical prostatectomy. They demonstrated an optimal tolerability profile and promising oncologic outcomes [9]. Yamazaki et al. contributed to this Special Issue by providing two brachytherapy studies. They report a lower biochemical control rate and distant metastasis-free survival rate in patients with both T3b–4 and Gleason score 9–10, than in those with a single risk factor. They also evaluated the different role of brachytherapy boost according to each risk group [10,11]. Shih et al. compared intensity-modulated radiotherapy plus antiandrogen therapy and radical prostatectomy in relatively young patients (aged $\leq$ 65 years). Although both had similar oncological outcomes, radical prostatectomy showed a greater reduction in the risk of biochemical failure [12].

Reviews

Gogola et al. provide a synopsis of the transcription factors and signaling pathways involved in epithelial-to-non-epithelial ("mesenchymal") transition prostate cancer progression [13]. Iwamoto et al. discuss the position, indications, complications, and prospects of androgen deprivation therapy for high-risk localized and locally advanced prostate cancer [14]. Finally, Makino et al. review the current literature with a focus on the definition of very high-risk prostate cancer, the role of modern imaging, and its treatment options [15].

I am very proud of this Special Issue; the papers are excellent, and I would like to thank all the authors. I would also like to acknowledge the reviewers for their time and careful appraisals of the manuscripts for this Special Issue. I believe that this publication will help physicians and academics involved in prostate cancer care and research, to better understand the essentials of "High-risk Localized and Locally Advanced Prostate Cancer."

Conflicts of Interest: The author declares no conflict of interest.

References

1. Ottman, R.; Ganapathy, K.; Lin, H.Y.; Osterman, C.D.; Dutil, J.; Matta, J.; Ruiz-Deya, G.; Wang, L.; Yamoah, K.; Park, J.Y.; et al. Differential Expression of miRNAs Contributes to Tumor Aggressiveness and Racial Disparity in African American Men with Prostate Cancer. *Cancers* **2023**, *15*, 2331. [CrossRef] [PubMed]
2. Diop, M.K.; Molina, O.E.; Birlea, M.; LaRue, H.; Hovington, H.; Têtu, B.; Lacombe, L.; Bergeron, A.; Fradet, Y.; Trudel, D. Leukocytic Infiltration of Intraductal Carcinoma of the Prostate: An Exploratory Study. *Cancers* **2023**, *15*, 2217. [CrossRef] [PubMed]
3. Samaržija, I.; Trošelj, K.G.; Konjevoda, P. Prognostic Significance of Amino Acid Metabolism-Related Genes in Prostate Cancer Retrieved by Machine Learning. *Cancers* **2023**, *15*, 1309. [CrossRef] [PubMed]
4. Bui, Q.T.; Lee, K.D.; Fan, Y.C.; Lewis, B.S.; Deng, L.W.; Tsai, Y.C. Disruption of CCL2 in Mesenchymal Stem Cells as an Anti-Tumor Approach against Prostate Cancer. *Cancers* **2023**, *15*, 441. [CrossRef] [PubMed]
5. Baba, H.; Sakamoto, S.; Zhao, X.; Yamada, Y.; Rii, J.; Fujimoto, A.; Kanesaka, M.; Takeuchi, N.; Sazuka, T.; Ichikawa, T.; et al. Tumor Location and a Tumor Volume over 2.8 cc Predict the Prognosis for Japanese Localized Prostate Cancer. *Cancers* **2022**, *14*, 5823. [CrossRef] [PubMed]
6. Di Pierro, G.B.; Salciccia, S.; Frisenda, M.; Tufano, A.; Sciarra, A.; Scarrone, E.; Del Giudice, F.; Asero, V.; Bevilacqua, G.; Canale, V.; et al. Comparison of Four Validated Nomograms (Memorial Sloan Kettering Cancer Center, Briganti 2012, 2017, and 2019) Predicting Lymph Node Invasion in Patients with High-Risk Prostate Cancer Candidates for Radical Prostatectomy and Extended Pelvic Lymph Node Dissection: Clinical Experience and Review of the Literature. *Cancers* **2023**, *15*, 1683. [CrossRef] [PubMed]
7. Yamashita, S.; Muraoka, S.; Wakamiya, T.; Kikkawa, K.; Kohjimoto, Y.; Hara, I. Prognostic Impact of Lymphatic Invasion in Patients with High-Risk Prostate Cancer after Robot-Assisted Radical Prostatectomy and Extended Lymph Node Dissection: A Single-Institution Prospective Cohort Study. *Cancers* **2022**, *14*, 3466. [CrossRef] [PubMed]
8. Faccenda, V.; Panizza, D.; Daniotti, M.C.; Pellegrini, R.; Trivellato, S.; Caricato, P.; Lucchini, R.; De Ponti, E.; Arcangeli, S. Dosimetric Impact of Intrafraction Prostate Motion and Interfraction Anatomical Changes in Dose-Escalated Linac-Based SBRT. *Cancers* **2023**, *15*, 1153. [CrossRef] [PubMed]
9. Francolini, G.; Garlatti, P.; Di Cataldo, V.; Detti, B.; Loi, M.; Greto, D.; Simontacchi, G.; Morelli, I.; Burchini, L.; Livi, L.; et al. Three Months' PSA and Toxicity from a Prospective Trial Investigating STereotactic sAlvage Radiotherapy for Macroscopic Prostate Bed Recurrence after Prostatectomy—STARR (NCT05455736). *Cancers* **2023**, *15*, 992. [CrossRef] [PubMed]

10. Yamazaki, H.; Suzuki, G.; Masui, K.; Aibe, N.; Shimizu, D.; Kimoto, T.; Yamada, K.; Shiraishi, T.; Fujihara, A.; Okabe, H.; et al. Novel Prognostic Index of High-Risk Prostate Cancer Using Simple Summation of Very High-Risk Factors. *Cancers* **2021**, *13*, 3486. [CrossRef] [PubMed]
11. Yamazaki, H.; Suzuki, G.; Masui, K.; Aibe, N.; Shimizu, D.; Kimoto, T.; Yamada, K.; Okihara, K.; Ueda, T.; Okabe, H.; et al. Role of Brachytherapy Boost in Clinically Localized Intermediate and High-Risk Prostate Cancer: Lack of Benefit in Patients with Very High-Risk Factors T3b–4 and/or Gleason 9–10. *Cancers* **2022**, *14*, 2976. [CrossRef] [PubMed]
12. Shih, H.J.; Chang, S.C.; Hsu, C.H.; Lin, Y.C.; Hung, C.H.; Wu, S.Y. Comparison of clinical outcomes of radical prostatectomy versus IMRT with long-term hormone therapy for relatively young patients with high-to very high-risk localized prostate cancer. *Cancers* **2021**, *13*, 5986. [CrossRef] [PubMed]
13. Gogola, S.; Rejzer, M.; Bahmad, H.F.; Abou-Kheir, W.; Omarzai, Y.; Poppiti, R. Epithelial-to-Mesenchymal Transition-Related Markers in Prostate Cancer: From Bench to Bedside. *Cancers* **2023**, *15*, 2309. [CrossRef] [PubMed]
14. Iwamoto, H.; Izumi, K.; Makino, T.; Mizokami, A. Androgen deprivation therapy in high-risk localized and locally advanced prostate cancer. *Cancers* **2022**, *14*, 1803. [CrossRef] [PubMed]
15. Makino, T.; Izumi, K.; Iwamoto, H.; Mizokami, A. Treatment strategies for high-risk localized and locally advanced and oligometastatic prostate cancer. *Cancers* **2021**, *13*, 4470. [CrossRef] [PubMed]

cancers

MDPI

Article

Differential Expression of miRNAs Contributes to Tumor Aggressiveness and Racial Disparity in African American Men with Prostate Cancer

Richard Ottman [1], Kavya Ganapathy [1], Hui-Yi Lin [2], Carlos Diaz Osterman [3], Julie Dutil [3], Jaime Matta [3], Gilberto Ruiz-Deya [3], Liang Wang [4], Kosj Yamoah [5], Anders Berglund [6], Ratna Chakrabarti [1,*] and Jong Y. Park [7,*]

1 Burnett School of Biomedical Sciences, University of Central Florida, Orlando, FL 32816, USA; rjottman@gmail.com (R.O.); kaganapathy@knights.ucf.edu (K.G.)
2 Biostatistics Program, School of Public Health, Louisiana State University Health Sciences Center, New Orleans, LA 70112, USA; hlin1@lsuhsc.edu
3 Department of Basic Sciences, Ponce Research Institute, School of Medicine, Ponce Health Sciences University, Ponce, PR 00716, USA; cjdiaz@psm.edu (C.D.O.); jdutil@psm.edu (J.D.); jmatta@psm.edu (J.M.); gruiz@psm.edu (G.R.-D.)
4 Department of Tumor Biology, H. Lee Moffitt Cancer Center, Tampa, FL 33612, USA; liang.wang@moffitt.org
5 Department of Radiation Oncology, H. Lee Moffitt Cancer Center, Tampa, FL 33612, USA; kosj.yamoah@moffitt.org
6 Department of Biostatistics and Bioinformatics, H. Lee Moffitt Cancer Center, Tampa, FL 33612, USA; anders.berglund@moffitt.org
7 Department of Cancer Epidemiology, H. Lee Moffitt Cancer Center, Tampa, FL 33612, USA
* Correspondence: ratna.chakrabarti@ucf.edu (R.C.); jong.park@moffitt.org (J.Y.P.)

Simple Summary: Prostate cancer (PCa) is the leading cancer in incidence and second leading cause of cancer mortality in US men. Recent data showed a 3% increase in PCa incidence rate each year from 2014 through 2019. African American (AA) men have 1.6-fold higher incidence and 2.2-fold higher PC mortality rates than European American (EA) men. Growing evidence shows that miRNAs are closely associated with aggressiveness and racial disparity in prostate cancer and might facilitate the prediction of prognosis and a treatment plan. In this study, we identified differentially expressed miRNAs, which are significantly correlated with the aggressiveness and health disparity of prostate cancer. These findings may assist personalized medicine, suggesting miRNAs as promising biomarkers for prostate cancer, especially in African American men.

Abstract: Prostate cancer is the leading cancer in incidence and second leading cause of cancer mortality in US men. African American men have significantly higher incidence and mortality rates from prostate cancer than European American men. Previous studies reported that the disparity in prostate cancer survival or mortality can be explained by different biological backgrounds. microRNAs (miRNAs) regulate gene expression of their cognate mRNAs in many cancers. Therefore, miRNAs may be a potentially promising diagnostic tool. The role of miRNAs in prostate cancer aggressiveness and racial disparity has not been fully established. The goal of this study is to identify miRNAs associated with aggressiveness and racial disparity in prostate cancer. Here we report miRNAs that are associated with tumor status and aggressiveness in prostate cancer using a profiling approach. Further, downregulated miRNAs in African American tissues were confirmed by qRT-PCR. These miRNAs have also been shown to negatively regulate the expression of the androgen receptor in prostate cancer cells. This report provides a novel insight into understanding tumor aggressiveness and racial disparities of prostate cancer.

Keywords: prostate cancer; miRNA; health disparity; aggressiveness

Citation: Ottman, R.; Ganapathy, K.; Lin, H.-Y.; Osterman, C.D.; Dutil, J.; Matta, J.; Ruiz-Deya, G.; Wang, L.; Yamoah, K.; Berglund, A.; et al. Differential Expression of miRNAs Contributes to Tumor Aggressiveness and Racial Disparity in African American Men with Prostate Cancer. *Cancers* **2023**, *15*, 2331. https://doi.org/10.3390/cancers15082331

Academic Editor: Alfonso Urbanucci

Received: 10 March 2023
Accepted: 15 April 2023
Published: 17 April 2023

1. Introduction

Prostate cancer (PCa) is the leading cancer in incidence and second leading cause of cancer mortality in US men [1]. In 2023, new prostate cancer cases and deaths expected in the US are 288,000 and 34,700, respectively. In addition, recent data showed a 3% increase in PCa incidence rate each year from 2014 through 2019 [2]. African American (AA) men have 1.6-fold higher incidence and 2.2-fold higher PC mortality rates than European American (EA) men [3]. Previous studies have reported that PCa survival or mortality disparities cannot be fully explained by different socioeconomic status [4,5]. These results suggest that biological background accounts for a significant portion of PCa disparity with regard to mortality, incidence, and progression in AA men compared to EA men. However, further investigation is required to uncover the mechanisms underlying abnormal gene regulation and racial disparity. Also, there is an unmet need to develop prognostic biomarkers that enable the reduction of AA PCa racial disparities.

MiRNAs are endogenous, short (19–24 nucleotides) non-protein-coding RNAs that regulate gene expression at the posttranscriptional level via binding to 3′-untranslated regions of protein-coding transcripts [6]. MiRNAs are pleiotropic in terms of functions; they regulate the expression of a broad range of genes involved in cancer [7]. MicroRNAs (miRNAs) are involved in gene silencing through inhibition of translation and destabilization of mRNAs, and thereby regulation of a variety of signaling pathways [8]. Dysregulated expression of miRNAs contributes to the abnormal expression of mRNAs which mediates phenotypic changes in various cancers [9]. Recently, several studies were reported on the role of miRNAs in risk, progression, and prognosis of prostate cancer. miR-5100, miR-199b-3p, miR-26b-5p, and miR-98-5p were associated with the risk of prostate cancer [10–12]. In addition, miR-26b-5p, miR-4732-3p, miR-181A, miR-205, miR-3195, and miR-4417 were suggested as potential biomarkers for differentiating advanced cases from an early stage of prostate cancer [11,13,14]. miRNA-532-5p, miR-17-5p, and miR-199b-3p were proposed as biomarkers for prognosis [12,15,16]. However, the role of miRNA-mediated gene expression regulation in the biological contribution to the observed racial disparities in prostate cancer has not been established. Thus, the goal of this study is to identify miRNAs involved in the racial disparities of PCa. Additionally, these miRNAs may be a risk factor for poor prognosis among AA patients. Thus, regulation of these miRNAs may offer a preventative and therapeutic approach for men at risk of PCa in the AA population.

2. Materials and Methods

2.1. Patient Selection and Procurement of Human Prostate Tissues

Prostate tissues obtained by radical prostatectomies were procured in the Cooperative Human Tissue Network (Southern division) at the University of Alabama at Birmingham (UAB) in accordance with an approved IRB protocol. Formalin-fixed and paraffin-embedded (FFPE) tissues from 25 PCa patients, including 10 AA patients, were evaluated by a pathologist, and tumor and adjacent non-involved areas were macro-dissected for RNA extraction followed by qRT-PCR for the expression of candidate miRNAs in patient tissues, as described previously [17,18]. Cases were selected based on the Cancer of the Prostate Risk Assessment (CAPRA)-S score, a prognostic tool for predicting a patient's risk for biochemical failure following radical prostatectomy [19].

2.2. RNA Extraction and cDNA Synthesis

RNA extraction from FFPE tissue sections was conducted using the RecoverAll kit (Life Technologies, Carlsbad, CA, USA). Before RNA was extracted, the tissue sections were evaluated for the presence of tumor lesions. Adjacent non-involved tissue blocks were used for the control group. The non-involved tissue sections were evaluated for the presence of tumor lesions by a pathologist. If tumor cells were observed in more than 10% of the section, additional sections were evaluated in a similar manner. Total RNA was isolated from 20 μm thick sections from tissue blocks and used for subsequent cDNA synthesis using the QuantiMir RT kit (System Biosciences, Palo Alto, CA, USA). Poly-A tail synthesis was first conducted using PolyA polymerase, and oligo dT anchor was annealed to the RNAs. RNA samples were next used for reverse transcription and quantitative RT-PCR (qRT-PCR).

2.3. Quantitative Real-Time PCR

The expression of mature miRNAs from FFPE tissues was determined by using the miRNome miRNA Profiling Kit (System Biosciences). The kit provides specific primers for 1,113 mature miRNAs and includes primers for 3 internal control RNAs (U6 snRNA, RNU43 snoRNA, RNU1A snRNA). MiRNA IDs listed in the text are based on Sanger miRBase identifiers. Primers were designed to maintain uniform amplification efficiencies. qRT-PCR reaction mixtures were prepared using 2X Maxima SYBR Green/ROX qPCR Master Mix (Thermo Fisher Scientific, Waltham, MA, USA). For profiling and validation, qRT-PCR was conducted using the 7900HT thermal cycler (Applied Biosystems Inc., Foster City, CA, USA). The data were initially analyzed using the SDS v2.3 software (ABI). DNA concentrations were reported through SYBR Green fluorescence and normalized to that of the passive reference dye, ROX. Ct values calculated by the SDS 2.3 software were transferred to the miRNome analysis software (SBI) to derive ΔΔCt values. The miRNome analysis software calculates the ΔCt values based on the mean of the reference genes. The individual ΔCt values are then compared across samples to generate the ΔΔCt values for each miRNA. miRNAs that showed significant changes in expression were then subject to further analysis. The statistical analysis of the qRT-PCR data is described below. We used macro-dissected prostate tumor tissues and corresponding adjacent uninvolved areas to monitor the expression of mature miRNAs. Patients were selected based on specific criteria including no prior treatments, Gleason scores, pre-surgical prostate-specific antigen (PSA), local invasion, and CAPRA-S score [19] stratified into low, medium, and high risk of biochemical recurrence (Table 1). We used a profiling approach with miRNome miRNA profiling kit (System Biosciences) to identify miRNA expression patterns for each patient's tumor and associated adjacent uninvolved prostate tissue.

Table 1. Selected characteristics of patients.

Patient ID	Age	Race	PSA	Gleason Score	SM [1]	ECE [2]	LN Invasion	SVI [3]	Stage	CAPRA-S Score	Risk
1	78	White	14.3	3 + 2 = 5	Neg	Neg	Neg	Neg	PT3NOMO	2	low
2	43	Hispanic	5.9	3 + 3 = 6	Pos	Neg	Neg	Neg	PT2CNXMX	2	low
3	53	Black	4.3	3 + 3 = 6	Pos	Neg	Neg	Neg	T2cR1NXMX	2	low
4	69	White	8.2	3 + 4 = 7	Neg	Neg	Neg	Neg	PT2CNOMX	2	low
5	62	White	7.8	3 + 4 = 7	Neg	Neg	Neg	Neg	PT2CNOMX	2	low
6	40	Black	8.8	3 + 4 = 7	Neg	Neg	Neg	Neg	PT2CNXMX	2	low
7	58	White	6.6	3 + 4 = 7	Neg	Neg	Neg	Neg	PT2CNXMX	2	low
8	61	White	3.7	3 + 4 = 7	Neg	Pos	Neg	Neg	PT3ANOMX	2	low
9	69	Black	23.3	3 + 3 = 6	Neg	Neg	Neg	Neg	PT2NOMX	3	med
10	60	NA	6.3	3 + 4 = 7	Pos	Neg	Neg	Neg	PT3BNOMX(IV)	3	med
11	67	White	6.2	3 + 4 = 7	Pos	Neg	Neg	Neg	PT2CR1NXMX	3	med
12	72	Black	4.7	3 + 4 = 7	Neg	Neg	Neg	Pos	T3bN0MX	3	med
13	61	UK [4]	5.1	3 + 3 = 6	Pos	Neg	Neg	Pos	PT3BNOMX	4	med
14	54	Black	87.4	3 + 3 = 6	Neg	Pos	Neg	Neg	PT3aN0MX	4	med
15	61	Black	9.8	3 + 4 = 7	Pos	Neg	Neg	Neg	PT3AR1NOMX	4	med
16	48	Black	9.4	3 + 4 = 7	Pos	Neg	Neg	Neg	PT2CNOMX	4	med

Table 1. *Cont.*

Patient ID	Age	Race	PSA	Gleason Score	SM [1]	ECE [2]	LN Invasion	SVI [3]	Stage	CAPRA-S Score	Risk
17	65	Black	8.8	3 + 4 = 7	Pos	Neg	Neg	Neg	PT2cNXMX	4	med
18	61	White	5.4	4 + 3 = 7	Neg	Neg	Neg	Pos	PT3BNOMX	4	med
19	48	Black	6.5	3 + 4 = 7	Pos	Pos	Neg	Neg	T1cNXMX	5	med
20	53	White	8.5	3 + 4 = 7	Pos	Pos	Neg	Neg	PT3aR1NXMX	5	med
21	63	White	4.8	3 + 4 = 7	Pos	Pos	Pos	Pos	PT3BR1N1MX	7	high
22	62	Black	14.9	3 + 4 = 7	Pos	Neg	Neg	Pos	pT3bN0MX	7	high
23	54	White	13.9	4 + 3 = 7	Pos	Pos	Neg	Neg	PT3bR1N0MX	7	high
24	60	White	5.6	4 + 3 = 7	Pos	Pos	Pos	Pos	PT3bN1MX	8	high
25	64	White	51.8	4 + 5 = 9	Pos	Pos	Neg	Neg	NA	9	high

[1.] SM: surgical margin [2.] ECE: extra-capsular extension [3.] SVI: seminal vesicle invasion [4.] UK: unknown.

The analysis of miRNA expressions stratified by CAPRA-S score identified patterns consistent with our hypothesis and previous reports [10,11].

2.4. Data Analysis

Normalization of qRT-PCR expression values was further refined using the qBasePlus software 2.0 (Biogazelle: Zwijnaarde, Oost-Vlaanderen, Belgium). Using the Genorm functionality included with the qBasePlus software, 7 additional stably expressed miRNAs were identified. The ΔCt value for each miRNA was then re-calculated utilizing the 7 additional miRNAs plus the 3 original controls. Following normalization, the expression of the reference miRNAs was re-evaluated to ensure their stability across samples was maintained. For the fold change, values were calculated next to determine expression differences between paired adjacent uninvolved and tumor tissues. After normalization, the software assigned relative expression values where the mean expression of the reference genes is determined to be a value of 1. The expression of each miRNA is then assigned a relative expression value with respect to the geometric mean of the controls. The geometric means were compared using the formula:

$$\Delta\text{Ct control} = 2^{-(\text{GMc-GMr})} \quad (1)$$

where GMc is the geo-mean of the control sample and GMr is the geo-mean of the reference sample. The fold change or ΔΔCt, for each miRNA was then calculated using the formula:

$$\Delta\Delta\text{Ct} = 2^{-(\text{CtR-CtC})} \times (\Delta\text{Ct control}) \quad (2)$$

where CtR = Reference sample miRNA Ct value, and CtC = Control sample miRNA Ct value.

Additional analysis was conducted using Cluster 3.0 software. For cluster analysis, log2 transformed normalized Ct values for each miRNA in each tumor, and uninvolved samples were used in an expression matrix where each miRNA is presented in rows and samples are presented in columns. For hierarchical clustering, we used a gene-centric (miRNA) approach to analyze and display the expression pattern upon centering; which, shows the relative up–down expression pattern for a particular miRNA across the samples based on its median expression value in shades of red (up) and green (down). The results of cluster analysis are displayed as heat maps generated by Java TreeView software. Heatmaps of differentially expressed miRNAs are created for viewing similar miRNA groups in a dataset using Pearson correlation with Average Linkage.

2.5. Statistical Analysis

Statistical analysis of the expression data was performed using log2 transformed Ct values using GraphPad Prizm. The *p*-values were calculated by the Mann–Whitney U test to estimate the statistical significance between the two groups.

3. Results

3.1. miRNA Expressions Deregulated in Human Prostate Tumors

Normalized relative expression values were used for Cluster analysis. Hierarchical clustering of the normalized and log2-transformed expression data showed four distinct clusters of miRNAs (Figure 1).

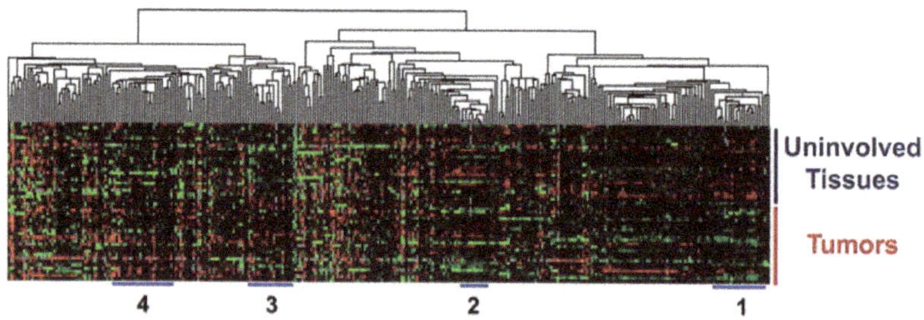

Figure 1. Clustering of miRNA expressions in tumor tissues and uninvolved prostate tissues. Hierarchal clustering of log2-transformed relative expression values of miRNAs in uninvolved prostate and tumor tissues.

Clusters 1 and 3 identified miRNAs distinctly expressed between malignant and uninvolved tissues (Figure 2A). The Log2-transformed relative expression values were extracted from each cluster and the average expression of each miRNA was calculated for both uninvolved tissue and tumor tissue samples. The average relative expression for individual miRNAs (unidentified) in both uninvolved and tumor groups is presented in Figure 2B,C for clusters 1 and 3, respectively. The jittered strip chart displays the distribution of average miRNA expression values for both groups including the average of all miRNAs in the cluster (black bars) ± 1 SD. In cluster 1 (Figure 2B), we identified 24 miRNAs (average values) that displayed downregulation in tumor tissues compared to uninvolved tissues. Examination of this cluster distinguished six miRNAs (miR-143. -133a, -133b, -204, -221, -222) with on average greater than 2-fold downregulation ($p = 0.0002$, 1.68×10^{-5}, 0.005, 0.0009, 1.17×10^{-5}, 0.0005, respectively) in expression in malignant tissues. Alternatively, the trend of average miRNA expression presented in cluster 3 identified 17 miRNAs with increased expression in tumor tissues compared to uninvolved tissues (Figure 2C). Cluster 3 also contained a subset of six miRNAs that displayed on average a change in expression greater than 2-fold. These six miRNAs (miR-375, -183, -93, -96, -127-5p, and -380) expressed higher levels in malignant tissues compared to uninvolved tissue samples ($p = 0.06$, 0.0003, 0.0002, 0.032, 0.012, 0.013, respectively).

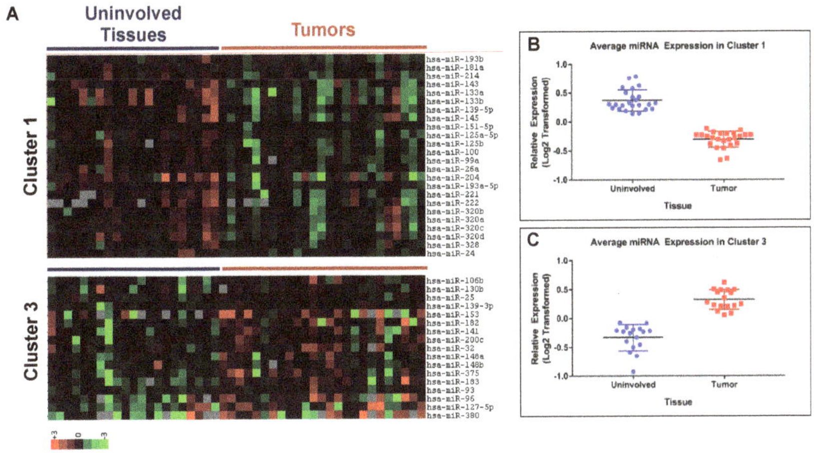

Figure 2. Analysis of clusters 1 and 3 identified from miRNA profiling of prostate tissues. (**A**) Heat maps of expression data for miRNAs in clusters 1 and 3; uninvolved tissue samples grouped under the blue line (left side) and tumor samples grouped under the red line (right side). (**B**,**C**) The average expression value of each miRNA was calculated for uninvolved tissue samples (blue circles) and tumor samples (red squares). These values were used to generate dot plots for cluster 1 (**B**) ($p = 4.83 \times 10^{-18}$) and cluster 3 (**C**) ($p = 1.70 \times 10^{-10}$).

3.2. Deregulation of miRNA Expressions Associated with Aggressiveness of Prostate Tumors

Initial analysis of clusters 2 and 4, identified from miRNA array expression analysis (Figure 1), did not show the visibly unique expression patterns between tumor and uninvolved prostate tissues, as identified in clusters 1 and 3. The cluster 2 heat map (Figure 1) depicts similar levels of expressions for all miRNAs (miR-103, -107, -29a/b/c, -199a/b-3p, and let-7a/b/d/e/g/i) within individual patient tissue; while, miRNAs display heterogeneous expression across samples. Further interrogation of the cluster revealed a correlation of miRNA expression profiles with the patient's CAPRA-S score (Figure 3C). Fifty percent (9/18) of tumor tissues from low- and medium-risk patients (CAPRA-S score 0–5) expressed cluster-specific miRNA averages below the average expression observed in all benign samples. However, 83% (5/6) of tumor tissues from high-risk patients (CAPRA-S score $\geq$6) expressed cluster-specific miRNA averages below the average expression observed in all benign samples (Figure 3A,C). When the cluster was dissected into individual miRNAs, there was a 2-fold change in expression ($\pm$0.2) for nine of 13 miRNAs in cluster 2, while there was no significant reduction observed in low- and medium-risk patient tumors. In cluster 4, the trend of increasing miRNA expression correlates positively with increasing risk of disease recurrence as predicted by CAPRA-S score groups: low risk (CAPRA-S: 0–2), medium risk (CAPRA-S: 3–5), and high risk (CAPRA-S: $\geq$6) (Figure 3B,D). Based on the fold change in the expression of miRNAs stratified by CAPRA-S risk groups, and have identified the top 60 miRNAs with >1.5-fold changes in expression in high-risk groups (30 upregulated and 30 downregulated).

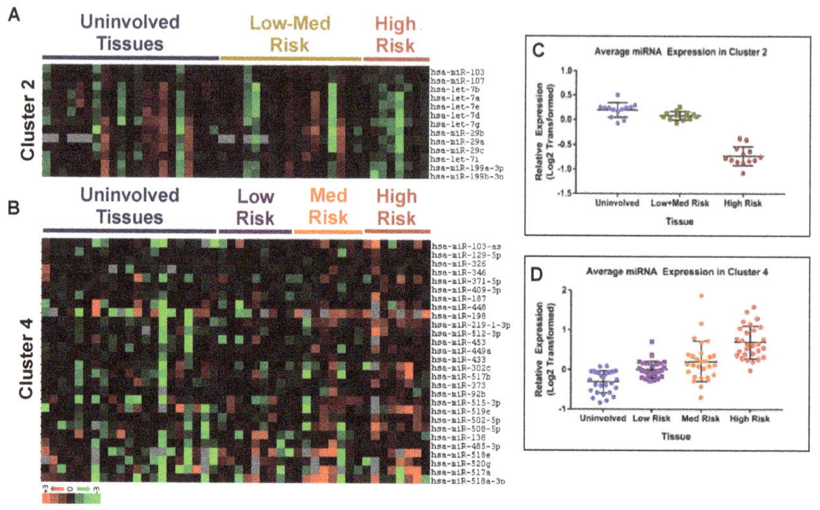

Figure 3. Analysis of clusters 2 and 4 identified from miRNA profiling of prostate tissues. Correlation of miRNA expressions with CAPRA-S risk group. (**A**,**B**) Heat maps of expression data for miRNAs in clusters 2 (**A**) and 4 (**B**). (**A**) Uninvolved tissue samples (U) grouped under the blue line, low- and medium-risk (L+M) patient tumor samples grouped under the gold line, and high-risk (H) patient tumor samples grouped under the red line. (**B**) Uninvolved tissue samples appear under the blue line, low-risk patient tumor samples are grouped under the purple line, medium are grouped under the orange line, and high-risk patient tumor samples are grouped under the red line. (**C**,**D**) The average expression value of each miRNA was calculated for uninvolved tissues and tumor tissues grouped by CAPRA-S risk. Values were used to generate dot plots for cluster 2 (**C**) ($p = 0.024$ U vs. L+M, 2.14×10^{-12} U vs. H, 1.57×10^{-10} L+M vs. H) and cluster 4 (**D**) ($p = 1.46 \times 10^{-5}$ U vs. L, 2.60×10^{-5} U vs. M, 2.51×10^{-14} U vs. H, 0.06 L vs. M, 1.01×10^{-9} L vs. H, 0.0002, M vs. H).

3.3. *Differential Expression of miRNAs in Prostate Tumors from African American and European American Patients*

Next, we sought to identify miRNA expression profiles differentially expressed in malignant prostate tissues from AA men, specifically. From the data generated in our miRNA profiling study, we compared the relative expression of miRNAs in prostate tumor tissues from AA and European American (EA) men. Our analysis identified miRNAs that, on average, exhibited a >2-fold difference in expression (increased and decreased) in AA compared to EA men. Expressions of some miRNAs, miR-541, -34c-5p, -135b, -299-3p, -491-5p, and -30e, were reduced in the tumors of AA men compared to EA men. These miRNAs also have been shown to negatively regulate the expression of the androgen receptor in PCa [20]. To better understand how these miRNAs are regulated, we examined the fold change in expression of these miRNAs in patient-specific tumor tissues compared with matched benign prostate tissue. The patients were grouped by race and subdivided by CAPRA-S score (0–3 or ≥4). This analysis highlighted the consistent pattern of down-regulation of these six miRNAs in AA men. In comparison, EA patients displayed a much broader distribution in expression. No significant difference in expression was noted in samples with a CAPRA-S score lower than or equal to 3 (Figure 4A); while, a significant difference in expression of five miRNAs at a 5% level and one at a 10% level was noted in AA tumors with a CAPRA-S score ≥4 compared to EA tumors (Figure 4B).

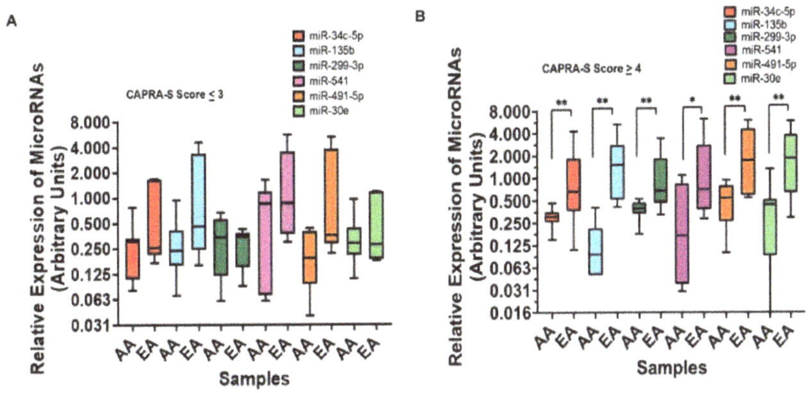

Figure 4. Top miRNAs with differential regulation between European American (EA) and African American (AA) men: (**A**,**B**) the fold change in expression of AR-regulating miRNAs grouped by race. Patients with CAPRA-S scores lower than 3 (**A**) and greater than 3 (**B**) are presented (*p* values: * < 0.07, ** < 0.05.

4. Discussion

African American (AA) men are at a 2.2-fold increased risk of prostate-cancer-specific (PCa) mortality compared with European American (EA) men. However, the relationship between this observation and miRNAs, and how this relationship explains PCa racial disparities, is not well established. This study represents an ongoing effort to investigate miRNAs in AA men with PCa. We observed that several differentially expressed miRNAs were found in tumor tissue from AA PCa patients. Our findings may help us to understand potential mechanisms for tumor aggressiveness and racial disparity. Once we identify these unique miRNA profiles at diagnosis, this information may provide biomarkers to determine treatment strategies for men with aggressive PCa. In this study, we identified miRNAs associated with PCa, aggressiveness, and potential health disparities among AA men.

4.1. miRNAs Associated with Tumor Status

Several miRNAs showed at least a 2-fold difference in expression between the tumor and adjacent uninvolved tissues. These miRNAs are miR-375, -183, -93, -96, -127-5p, -380, -143, -133a, -133b, -204, -221, and -222. Among these miRNAs, several miRNAs have been extensively investigated in previous studies.

For example, miR-375 was identified as a biomarker with a high-level sensitivity and specificity in PCa detection [21]. Several studies have observed that miR-375 is upregulated in primary tumor tissues and serum [22,23]. Further, Schaefer et al. reported the combination of six miRNAs including that miR-375 was used; the AUC was significant (0.88) in discriminating normal and tumor tissue [24]. miR-375 is also associated with clinical variables. Including, a high Gleason score, lymph-node-positive status, biochemical recurrence, and metastasis [25–27]. Cheng et al. [28] observed upregulation of miR-375 in serum samples from patients with metastatic, castration-resistant PCa. These results were found in the screening cohort; the serum level of miR-375 was significantly increased in PCa cases as compared with the testing cohort (AUC = 0.77) and a validation cohort. Haldrup et al. [29] confirmed dysregulation of miR-375 using genome-wide miRNA profiling of serum samples and was able to identify 84% of all PCa patients. However, these findings of miR-375 in tumor tissue are not always consistent. Kachakova et al. reported that miR-375 was significantly downregulated in 83.5% of PCa patients compared to benign prostatic hyperplasia (BPH) controls [30]. Although functional studies might define certain miRNAs as onco-miRNAs or tumor-suppressor miRNAs, their expression in prostate tumors might not correlate with these classifications. For instance, normally, miR-375 is upregulated as an onco-miRNA in PCa tumor tissue relative to normal tissue. However, forced expression of miR-375 decreased proliferation and invasion of androgen-independent PC-3 cells [31].

The overexpression of miR-183 in PCa tissues was reported in previous studies [32–34]. Larne et al. proposed a formula that can predict aggressive progression characteristics. This formula, consisting of four miRNAs including miR-183, is associated with tumor grades, PSA levels, metastasis, and survival. More importantly, this signature distinguishes aggressive tumors from non-aggressive PCa with an Area under the ROC Curve (AUC) of 0.90 [35]. Martens-Uzunova et al. found that levels of several miRNAs, including miR-183, significantly differ in lymphocytes and could be used in the evaluation of the progression of PCa [36]. Recently, miR-183 was suggested as one of the oncogenic clusters for PCa after a series of analyses using various data including TCGA [37].

miR-96 was reported as one of the overexpressed miRNAs in malignant prostate tissue compared with normal adjacent prostate tissue [32–34,38–40]. Schaefer et al. reported that miRs-96 showed a significant correlation with the Gleason score. Furthermore, the combination of six miRNAs including miR-96 provided a significant AUC (0.88) in discriminating normal and tumor tissue [24]. Larne et al. developed a formula that can predict poor outcomes, such as grades, PSA level, metastasis, and survival. More importantly, this formula distinguishes aggressive tumors from non-aggressive PCa with an AUC of 0.90 [35]. Martens-Uzunova et al. found miRNA-96 expression was significantly different in lymphocytes from progressed PCa [36]. Recently, miR-96 was suggested as one of the onco-miRNAs after a series of bioinformatic analyses using various data including TCGA [37].

4.2. *miRNAs Associated with Prognosis*

Deregulated miRNA expression has been associated with tumor progression in PCa [41]. Previous studies reported differentially expressed miRNAs associated with PCa progression [21,42–44]. Although those results are not consistent, several miRNAs, such as miR-1, -145, -205, -221, and -375, were suggested as good candidates for the prognosis of prostate cancer [42,44,45]. We identified several miRNAs, miR-1, -127-5p, -139-5p, -145, 296-5p, -302a, -330-5p, -365, -495, -509-3-5p, -511, and -518d-5p, as potential biomarkers for prognosis in this study. Among these miRNAs, some miRNAs were evaluated in previous studies.

miR-1 is known as an oncomiRNA, and is involved in bone metastasis by activating the epidermal growth factor (EGFR) [46]. Previous studies reported that the downregulation of miR-1 in PCa tissues is linked to PCa progression, castration-resistant disease, and metastasis [36,47]. Furthermore, downregulations of miR-1 contribute to the proliferation, migration, and invasion of PCa cells. Therefore, miR-1 was suggested as a candidate prognostic biomarker for PCa in previous studies [22,46,48–52].

miR-139-5p downregulation in prostate tumor tissue has been previously reported [36,53]. Prior findings indicate that miR-139-5p inhibits the proliferation of PCa cells by interfering with the cell cycle [54], functioning as a tumor suppressor in PCa through regulation of SOX5 [55].

miR-145 binds to the 3′UTR of *MYO6* and is regulated inversely, resulting in a decrease in myosin VI; which, is involved in cancer-related cell migration and β-actin in the LNCaP PCa cell line [23]. Ectopic expression of miR-145 in LNCaP cells significantly reduced the proliferation [21,56–58]. miR-145 expressed in endothelial cells of blood vessels but not stromal cells [21]. Several studies reported downregulation of miR-145 in prostate tumor samples [23,24,57–61] and metastatic lymph nodes [36]; especially miR-145, which showed significant downregulation in aggressive PCa [58]. The reduction of miR-145 expression was also correlated with clinical variables, such as the Gleason score, clinical stage, tumor size, and PSA level. Further, miR-145 expression was correlated with risk for biochemical recurrence and shorter disease-free survival [35,50,62,63]. Based on these studies, miR-145 was suggested as a biomarker with a high-level sensitivity and specificity in PCa detection [21].

4.3. miRNA Associated with Racial Disparity

We are interested in investigating the role of miRNAs associated with health disparities in PCa. We used prostate tissue samples obtained from AA and EA patient cohorts. We used microarray analysis and qRT-PCR techniques to confirm our results.

The relative expression of miR-34c was significantly lower in the tumor tissues compared to the benign prostatic hyperplasia (BPH) tissues, and inversely correlated with a high Gleason score [39], PSA level, metastatic status, survival [34,64,65], clinical stage, and status of TMPRSS2-ERG [66]. Low expression of miR-34c was suggested to occur due to DNA methylation, loss of heterozygosity in the 11q23 region, or p53 mutation. Hagman et al. demonstrated that the function of miR-34c in PCa is mediated by targeting MET [67].

Previous studies have shown the tumor suppressor role of miR-30 in various cancers, with this miR-30e being extensively studied and well-characterized [17]. The relative expression of miR-30e was significantly lower in the tumor tissues compared to the normal tissues [23,33]. Recently, a multidimensional function of miR-30e through the regulation of genes involved in various signaling pathways was reported. Ganapathy et al. observed low expression miR-30e in prostate tumors and experimental upregulation led to cell cycle arrest, apoptosis, drug sensitivity of PCa cells, and reduced tumor progression [17].

miR-299-3p, another androgen receptor (AR) targeting miRNA, which showed downregulation in PCa from AA patients, has also been shown to function as a tumor suppressor in a number of cancers including colon cancer and hepatocellular carcinoma [68,69]. Recently, Ganapathy et al. showed loss of expression of miR-299 in prostate tumors, and restored expression of this miRNA improved drug sensitivity and exhibited a tumor suppressor function that is mediated through targeting AR and vascular endothelial growth factor (VEGF)A [18].

miR-135b has been reported to be downregulated in prostate cancer and to play a role in the progression of PCa. Tong et al. developed the 48-miRNA signature, including miR-135b, that predicted biochemical recurrence after prostatectomy [57]. Previous studies reported that downregulation of miR-135b was associated with the status of tumor and tumor metastasis [70]. These data suggested that low expression of miR-135b in the primary tumors may be a risk factor for bone metastatic [71].

Among miRNAs identified in this study, many of them were extensively investigated previously, and we confirmed their results. However, the role of some miRNAs in prostate cancer was not previously reported. This may be partly due to differences in methodology, platforms used, or sample size. These miRNAs observed in this study may help to investigate potential mechanisms in different PCa outcomes between AA and EA men. There are some limitations to this study. First, the small number of PCa samples is a limitation. Therefore, these results need to be validated in larger studies. Furthermore, our results were based on analyses of radical prostatectomy specimens; whereas, a future diagnostic test for PCa should use more clinically relevant non-invasive sample types, such as urine or blood.

5. Conclusions

In summary, miRNA expression studies provide evidence for the role of miRNAs in PCa diagnosis, prognosis, and elimination of health disparities. Despite these promising studies, there is currently a limited number of PCa-related miRNAs used in the clinical setting. Our findings underscore an important opportunity for the implementation of miRNA-based biomarkers, including miR-1, -30e, -34c, -96, -135b, -139, -145, -183, -299-3p, and -375 for diagnosis, prognosis, and elimination of health disparities for men with PCa.

Author Contributions: Conceptualization, R.C., R.O., C.D.O., G.R.-D., J.M., K.Y., J.Y.P.; methodology, R.C., R.O., K.G., J.D., J.Y.P.; software, R.C., R.O., J.Y.P.; validation, R.C.; formal analysis, A.B., H.-Y.L.; investigation, L.W., J.Y.P.; resources, R.C.; data curation, R.C., K.G.; writing—original draft preparation, R.C., R.O., J.Y.P.; writing—review and editing, R.C., R.O., C.D.O., H.-Y.L., J.D., J.M., G.R.-D., L.W., K.Y., K.G., A.B., J.Y.P.; visualization, R.C., J.Y.P.; supervision, J.Y.P.; project administration, R.C.; funding acquisition, R.C. All authors have read and agreed to the published version of the manuscript.

Funding: This research was funded by grants from the Department of Defense Prostate Cancer Research Program (PCRP) (Grant/Award Number: W81XWH-11-1-0563) and National Institutes of Health (Grant/Award Number: R21CA226611) to R.C.

Institutional Review Board Statement: The study was conducted in accordance with the Declaration of Helsinki and approved by the Institutional Review Board (or Ethics Committee) of UCF (SBE-14-10298).

Informed Consent Statement: All patients have written informed consent to be enrolled in the study.

Data Availability Statement: miRNA expression data and clinical data are available upon request.

Acknowledgments: We thank the support of William E. Grizzle who kindly provided us with the prostate tissues from Cooperative Human Tissue Network at the University of Alabama in Birmingham.

Conflicts of Interest: The authors declare no conflict of interest.

References

1. Siegel, R.L.; Miller, K.D.; Fuchs, H.E.; Jemal, A. Cancer Statistics, 2021. *CA Cancer J. Clin.* **2021**, *71*, 7–33. [CrossRef] [PubMed]
2. Siegel, R.L.; Miller, K.D.; Wagle, N.S.; Jemal, A. Cancer statistics, 2023. *CA Cancer J. Clin.* **2023**, *73*, 17–48. [CrossRef] [PubMed]
3. DeSantis, C.E.; Miller, K.D.; Goding Sauer, A.; Jemal, A.; Siegel, R.L. Cancer statistics for African Americans, 2019. *CA Cancer J. Clin.* **2019**, *69*, 211–233. [CrossRef] [PubMed]
4. Byers, T.E.; Wolf, H.J.; Bauer, K.R.; Bolick-Aldrich, S.; Chen, V.W.; Finch, J.L.; Fulton, J.P.; Schymura, M.J.; Shen, T.; Van Heest, S.; et al. The impact of socioeconomic status on survival after cancer in the United States: Findings from the National Program of Cancer Registries Patterns of Care Study. *Cancer* **2008**, *113*, 582–591. [CrossRef]
5. Aladuwaka, S.; Alagan, R.; Singh, R.; Mishra, M. Health Burdens and SES in Alabama: Using Geographic Information System to Examine Prostate Cancer Health Disparity. *Cancers* **2022**, *14*, 4824. [CrossRef]
6. Bartel, D.P. MicroRNAs: Genomics, biogenesis, mechanism, and function. *Cell* **2004**, *116*, 281–297. [CrossRef]
7. Encarnacion-Medina, J.; Ortiz, C.; Vergne, R.; Padilla, L.; Matta, J. MicroRNA Expression Changes in Women with Breast Cancer Stratified by DNA Repair Capacity Levels. *J. Oncol.* **2019**, *2019*, 7820275. [CrossRef] [PubMed]
8. Shi, X.B.; Tepper, C.G.; deVere White, R.W. Cancerous miRNAs and their regulation. *Cell Cycle* **2008**, *7*, 1529–1538. [CrossRef] [PubMed]
9. Asirvatham, A.J.; Magner, W.J.; Tomasi, T.B. miRNA regulation of cytokine genes. *Cytokine* **2009**, *45*, 58–69. [CrossRef] [PubMed]
10. Mello-Grand, M.; Bruno, A.; Sacchetto, L.; Cristoni, S.; Gregnanin, I.; Dematteis, A.; Zitella, A.; Gontero, P.; Peraldo-Neia, C.; Ricotta, R.; et al. Two Novel Ceramide-Like Molecules and miR-5100 Levels as Biomarkers Improve Prediction of Prostate Cancer in Gray-Zone PSA. *Front. Oncol.* **2021**, *11*, 769158. [CrossRef] [PubMed]
11. Giglio, S.; De Nunzio, C.; Cirombella, R.; Stoppacciaro, A.; Faruq, O.; Volinia, S.; Baldassarre, G.; Tubaro, A.; Ishii, H.; Croce, C.M.; et al. A preliminary study of micro-RNAs as minimally invasive biomarkers for the diagnosis of prostate cancer patients. *J. Exp. Clin. Cancer Res.* **2021**, *40*, 79. [CrossRef] [PubMed]
12. Liu, J.; Quan, Z.; Gao, Y.; Wu, X.; Zheng, Y. MicroRNA-199b-3p suppresses malignant proliferation by targeting Phospholipase Cepsilon and correlated with poor prognosis in prostate cancer. *Biochem. Biophys. Res. Commun.* **2021**, *576*, 73–79. [CrossRef]
13. Wang, Y.; Fang, Y.X.; Dong, B.; Du, X.; Wang, J.; Wang, X.; Gao, W.Q.; Xue, W. Discovery of extracellular vesicles derived miR-181a-5p in patient's serum as an indicator for bone-metastatic prostate cancer. *Theranostics* **2021**, *11*, 878–892. [CrossRef] [PubMed]
14. Ronnau, C.G.H.; Fussek, S.; Smit, F.P.; Aalders, T.W.; van Hooij, O.; Pinto, P.M.C.; Burchardt, M.; Schalken, J.A.; Verhaegh, G.W. Upregulation of miR-3195, miR-3687 and miR-4417 is associated with castration-resistant prostate cancer. *World J. Urol.* **2021**, *39*, 3789–3797. [CrossRef] [PubMed]
15. Stoen, M.J.; Andersen, S.; Rakaee, M.; Pedersen, M.I.; Ingebriktsen, L.M.; Bremnes, R.M.; Donnem, T.; Lombardi, A.P.G.; Kilvaer, T.K.; Busund, L.T.; et al. High expression of miR-17-5p in tumor epithelium is a predictor for poor prognosis for prostate cancer patients. *Sci. Rep.* **2021**, *11*, 13864. [CrossRef]
16. Kim, M.Y.; Shin, H.; Moon, H.W.; Park, Y.H.; Park, J.; Lee, J.Y. Urinary exosomal microRNA profiling in intermediate-risk prostate cancer. *Sci. Rep.* **2021**, *11*, 7355. [CrossRef] [PubMed]

17. Ganapathy, K.; Ngo, C.; Andl, T.; Coppola, D.; Park, J.; Chakrabarti, R. Anticancer function of microRNA-30e is mediated by negative regulation of HELLPAR, a noncoding macroRNA, and genes involved in ubiquitination and cell cycle progression in prostate cancer. *Mol. Oncol.* **2022**, *16*, 2936–2958. [CrossRef] [PubMed]
18. Ganapathy, K.; Staklinski, S.; Hasan, M.F.; Ottman, R.; Andl, T.; Berglund, A.E.; Park, J.Y.; Chakrabarti, R. Multifaceted Function of MicroRNA-299-3p Fosters an Antitumor Environment Through Modulation of Androgen Receptor and VEGFA Signaling Pathways in Prostate Cancer. *Sci. Rep.* **2020**, *10*, 5167. [CrossRef] [PubMed]
19. Cooperberg, M.R.; Hilton, J.F.; Carroll, P.R. The CAPRA-S score: A straightforward tool for improved prediction of outcomes after radical prostatectomy. *Cancer* **2011**, *117*, 5039–5046. [CrossRef]
20. Ostling, P.; Leivonen, S.K.; Aakula, A.; Kohonen, P.; Makela, R.; Hagman, Z.; Edsjo, A.; Kangaspeska, S.; Edgren, H.; Nicorici, D.; et al. Systematic analysis of microRNAs targeting the androgen receptor in prostate cancer cells. *Cancer Res.* **2011**, *71*, 1956–1967. [CrossRef]
21. Wach, S.; Nolte, E.; Szczyrba, J.; Stohr, R.; Hartmann, A.; Orntoft, T.; Dyrskjot, L.; Eltze, E.; Wieland, W.; Keck, B.; et al. MicroRNA profiles of prostate carcinoma detected by multiplatform microRNA screening. *Int. J. Cancer* **2012**, *130*, 611–621. [CrossRef] [PubMed]
22. Hudson, R.S.; Yi, M.; Esposito, D.; Watkins, S.K.; Hurwitz, A.A.; Yfantis, H.G.; Lee, D.H.; Borin, J.F.; Naslund, M.J.; Alexander, R.B.; et al. MicroRNA-1 is a candidate tumor suppressor and prognostic marker in human prostate cancer. *Nucleic Acids Res.* **2012**, *40*, 3689–3703. [CrossRef]
23. Szczyrba, J.; Loprich, E.; Wach, S.; Jung, V.; Unteregger, G.; Barth, S.; Grobholz, R.; Wieland, W.; Stohr, R.; Hartmann, A.; et al. The microRNA profile of prostate carcinoma obtained by deep sequencing. *Mol. Cancer Res.* **2010**, *8*, 529–538. [CrossRef] [PubMed]
24. Schaefer, A.; Jung, M.; Mollenkopf, H.J.; Wagner, I.; Stephan, C.; Jentzmik, F.; Miller, K.; Lein, M.; Kristiansen, G.; Jung, K. Diagnostic and prognostic implications of microRNA profiling in prostate carcinoma. *Int. J. Cancer* **2010**, *126*, 1166–1176. [CrossRef]
25. Selth, L.A.; Townley, S.; Gillis, J.L.; Ochnik, A.M.; Murti, K.; Macfarlane, R.J.; Chi, K.N.; Marshall, V.R.; Tilley, W.D.; Butler, L.M. Discovery of circulating microRNAs associated with human prostate cancer using a mouse model of disease. *Int. J. Cancer* **2012**, *131*, 652–661. [CrossRef]
26. Brase, J.C.; Johannes, M.; Schlomm, T.; Falth, M.; Haese, A.; Steuber, T.; Beissbarth, T.; Kuner, R.; Sultmann, H. Circulating miRNAs are correlated with tumor progression in prostate cancer. *Int. J. Cancer* **2011**, *128*, 608–616. [CrossRef]
27. Nguyen, H.L.; Yang, X.; Omiecinski, C.J. Expression of a novel mRNA transcript for human microsomal epoxide hydrolase (EPHX1) is regulated by short open reading frames within its 5′-untranslated region. *RNA* **2013**, *19*, 752–766. [CrossRef]
28. Cheng, H.H.; Mitchell, P.S.; Kroh, E.M.; Dowell, A.E.; Chery, L.; Siddiqui, J.; Nelson, P.S.; Vessella, R.L.; Knudsen, B.S.; Chinnaiyan, A.M.; et al. Circulating microRNA profiling identifies a subset of metastatic prostate cancer patients with evidence of cancer-associated hypoxia. *PLoS ONE* **2013**, *8*, e69239. [CrossRef]
29. Haldrup, C.; Kosaka, N.; Ochiya, T.; Borre, M.; Hoyer, S.; Orntoft, T.F.; Sorensen, K.D. Profiling of circulating microRNAs for prostate cancer biomarker discovery. *Drug Deliv. Transl. Res.* **2014**, *4*, 19–30. [CrossRef] [PubMed]
30. Kachakova, D.; Mitkova, A.; Popov, E.; Popov, I.; Vlahova, A.; Dikov, T.; Christova, S.; Mitev, V.; Slavov, C.; Kaneva, R. Combinations of serum prostate-specific antigen and plasma expression levels of let-7c, miR-30c, miR-141, and miR-375 as potential better diagnostic biomarkers for prostate cancer. *DNA Cell Biol.* **2015**, *34*, 189–200. [CrossRef]
31. Costa-Pinheiro, P.; Ramalho-Carvalho, J.; Vieira, F.Q.; Torres-Ferreira, J.; Oliveira, J.; Goncalves, C.S.; Costa, B.M.; Henrique, R.; Jeronimo, C. MicroRNA-375 plays a dual role in prostate carcinogenesis. *Clin. Epigenetics* **2015**, *7*, 42. [CrossRef] [PubMed]
32. Mihelich, B.L.; Khramtsova, E.A.; Arva, N.; Vaishnav, A.; Johnson, D.N.; Giangreco, A.A.; Martens-Uzunova, E.; Bagasra, O.; Kajdacsy-Balla, A.; Nonn, L. miR-183-96-182 cluster is overexpressed in prostate tissue and regulates zinc homeostasis in prostate cells. *J. Biol. Chem.* **2011**, *286*, 44503–44511. [CrossRef]
33. Kristensen, H.; Thomsen, A.R.; Haldrup, C.; Dyrskjot, L.; Hoyer, S.; Borre, M.; Mouritzen, P.; Orntoft, T.F.; Sorensen, K.D. Novel diagnostic and prognostic classifiers for prostate cancer identified by genome-wide microRNA profiling. *Oncotarget* **2016**, *7*, 30760–30771. [CrossRef]
34. Tsuchiyama, K.; Ito, H.; Taga, M.; Naganuma, S.; Oshinoya, Y.; Nagano, K.; Yokoyama, O.; Itoh, H. Expression of microRNAs associated with Gleason grading system in prostate cancer: miR-182-5p is a useful marker for high grade prostate cancer. *Prostate* **2013**, *73*, 827–834. [CrossRef]
35. Larne, O.; Martens-Uzunova, E.; Hagman, Z.; Edsjo, A.; Lippolis, G.; den Berg, M.S.; Bjartell, A.; Jenster, G.; Ceder, Y. miQ—A novel microRNA based diagnostic and prognostic tool for prostate cancer. *Int. J. Cancer* **2013**, *132*, 2867–2875. [CrossRef] [PubMed]
36. Martens-Uzunova, E.S.; Jalava, S.E.; Dits, N.F.; van Leenders, G.J.; Moller, S.; Trapman, J.; Bangma, C.H.; Litman, T.; Visakorpi, T.; Jenster, G. Diagnostic and prognostic signatures from the small non-coding RNA transcriptome in prostate cancer. *Oncogene* **2012**, *31*, 978–991. [CrossRef] [PubMed]
37. Schitcu, V.H.; Raduly, L.; Nutu, A.; Zanoaga, O.; Ciocan, C.; Munteanu, V.C.; Cojocneanu, R.; Petrut, B.; Coman, I.; Braicu, C.; et al. MicroRNA Dysregulation in Prostate Cancer. *Pharm. Pers. Med.* **2022**, *15*, 177–193. [CrossRef] [PubMed]
38. Mishra, S.; Lin, C.L.; Huang, T.H.; Bouamar, H.; Sun, L.Z. MicroRNA-21 inhibits p57Kip2 expression in prostate cancer. *Mol. Cancer* **2014**, *13*, 212. [CrossRef] [PubMed]
39. Walter, B.A.; Valera, V.A.; Pinto, P.A.; Merino, M.J. Comprehensive microRNA Profiling of Prostate Cancer. *J. Cancer* **2013**, *4*, 350–357. [CrossRef] [PubMed]

40. Nguyen, H.C.; Xie, W.; Yang, M.; Hsieh, C.L.; Drouin, S.; Lee, G.S.; Kantoff, P.W. Expression differences of circulating microRNAs in metastatic castration resistant prostate cancer and low-risk, localized prostate cancer. *Prostate* **2013**, *73*, 346–354. [CrossRef]
41. Lee, R.C.; Feinbaum, R.L.; Ambros, V. The *C. elegans* heterochronic gene lin-4 encodes small RNAs with antisense complementarity to lin-14. *Cell* **1993**, *75*, 843–854. [CrossRef] [PubMed]
42. Pang, Y.; Young, C.Y.; Yuan, H. MicroRNAs and prostate cancer. *Acta Biochim. Biophys. Sin.* **2010**, *42*, 363–369. [CrossRef] [PubMed]
43. Bentwich, I. Prediction and validation of microRNAs and their targets. *FEBS Lett.* **2005**, *579*, 5904–5910. [CrossRef] [PubMed]
44. Wahid, F.; Shehzad, A.; Khan, T.; Kim, Y.Y. MicroRNAs: Synthesis, mechanism, function, and recent clinical trials. *Biochim. Biophys. Acta* **2010**, *1803*, 1231–1243. [CrossRef]
45. Rigoutsos, I. New tricks for animal microRNAS: Targeting of amino acid coding regions at conserved and nonconserved sites. *Cancer Res.* **2009**, *69*, 3245–3248. [CrossRef] [PubMed]
46. Chang, Y.S.; Chen, W.Y.; Yin, J.J.; Sheppard-Tillman, H.; Huang, J.; Liu, Y.N. EGF Receptor Promotes Prostate Cancer Bone Metastasis by Downregulating miR-1 and Activating TWIST1. *Cancer Res.* **2015**, *75*, 3077–3086. [CrossRef] [PubMed]
47. Ambs, S.; Prueitt, R.L.; Yi, M.; Hudson, R.S.; Howe, T.M.; Petrocca, F.; Wallace, T.A.; Liu, C.G.; Volinia, S.; Calin, G.A.; et al. Genomic profiling of microRNA and messenger RNA reveals deregulated microRNA expression in prostate cancer. *Cancer Res.* **2008**, *68*, 6162–6170. [CrossRef] [PubMed]
48. Kojima, S.; Chiyomaru, T.; Kawakami, K.; Yoshino, H.; Enokida, H.; Nohata, N.; Fuse, M.; Ichikawa, T.; Naya, Y.; Nakagawa, M.; et al. Tumour suppressors miR-1 and miR-133a target the oncogenic function of purine nucleoside phosphorylase (PNP) in prostate cancer. *Br. J. Cancer* **2012**, *106*, 405–413. [CrossRef]
49. Liu, Y.N.; Yin, J.J.; Abou-Kheir, W.; Hynes, P.G.; Casey, O.M.; Fang, L.; Yi, M.; Stephens, R.M.; Seng, V.; Sheppard-Tillman, H.; et al. MiR-1 and miR-200 inhibit EMT via Slug-dependent and tumorigenesis via Slug-independent mechanisms. *Oncogene* **2013**, *32*, 296–306. [CrossRef]
50. Karatas, O.F.; Guzel, E.; Suer, I.; Ekici, I.D.; Caskurlu, T.; Creighton, C.J.; Ittmann, M.; Ozen, M. miR-1 and miR-133b are differentially expressed in patients with recurrent prostate cancer. *PLoS ONE* **2014**, *9*, e98675. [CrossRef]
51. Stope, M.B.; Stender, C.; Schubert, T.; Peters, S.; Weiss, M.; Ziegler, P.; Zimmermann, U.; Walther, R.; Burchardt, M. Heat-shock protein HSPB1 attenuates microRNA miR-1 expression thereby restoring oncogenic pathways in prostate cancer cells. *Anticancer Res.* **2014**, *34*, 3475–3480. [PubMed]
52. Liu, Y.N.; Yin, J.; Barrett, B.; Sheppard-Tillman, H.; Li, D.; Casey, O.M.; Fang, L.; Hynes, P.G.; Ameri, A.H.; Kelly, K. Loss of Androgen-Regulated MicroRNA 1 Activates SRC and Promotes Prostate Cancer Bone Metastasis. *Mol. Cell. Biol.* **2015**, *35*, 1940–1951. [CrossRef] [PubMed]
53. Song, C.J.; Chen, H.; Chen, L.Z.; Ru, G.M.; Guo, J.J.; Ding, Q.N. The potential of microRNAs as human prostate cancer biomarkers: A meta-analysis of related studies. *J. Cell. Biochem.* **2018**, *119*, 2763–2786. [CrossRef] [PubMed]
54. Sun, Q.; Weng, D.; Li, K.; Li, S.; Bai, X.; Fang, C.; Luo, D.; Wu, P.; Chen, G.; Wei, J. MicroRNA-139-5P inhibits human prostate cancer cell proliferation by targeting Notch1. *Oncol. Lett.* **2018**, *16*, 793–800. [CrossRef] [PubMed]
55. Yang, B.; Zhang, W.; Sun, D.; Wei, X.; Ding, Y.; Ma, Y.; Wang, Z. Downregulation of miR-139-5p promotes prostate cancer progression through regulation of SOX5. *Biomed. Pharmacother.* **2019**, *109*, 2128–2135. [CrossRef] [PubMed]
56. Fuse, M.; Nohata, N.; Kojima, S.; Sakamoto, S.; Chiyomaru, T.; Kawakami, K.; Enokida, H.; Nakagawa, M.; Naya, Y.; Ichikawa, T.; et al. Restoration of miR-145 expression suppresses cell proliferation, migration and invasion in prostate cancer by targeting FSCN1. *Int. J. Oncol.* **2011**, *38*, 1093–1101. [CrossRef] [PubMed]
57. Tong, A.W.; Fulgham, P.; Jay, C.; Chen, P.; Khalil, I.; Liu, S.; Senzer, N.; Eklund, A.C.; Han, J.; Nemunaitis, J. MicroRNA profile analysis of human prostate cancers. *Cancer Gene Ther.* **2009**, *16*, 206–216. [CrossRef]
58. Wang, L.; Tang, H.; Thayanithy, V.; Subramanian, S.; Oberg, A.L.; Cunningham, J.M.; Cerhan, J.R.; Steer, C.J.; Thibodeau, S.N. Gene networks and microRNAs implicated in aggressive prostate cancer. *Cancer Res.* **2009**, *69*, 9490–9497. [CrossRef]
59. Ozen, M.; Creighton, C.J.; Ozdemir, M.; Ittmann, M. Widespread deregulation of microRNA expression in human prostate cancer. *Oncogene* **2008**, *27*, 1788–1793. [CrossRef] [PubMed]
60. Shen, J.; Hruby, G.W.; McKiernan, J.M.; Gurvich, I.; Lipsky, M.J.; Benson, M.C.; Santella, R.M. Dysregulation of circulating microRNAs and prediction of aggressive prostate cancer. *Prostate* **2012**, *72*, 1469–1477. [CrossRef] [PubMed]
61. Porkka, K.P.; Pfeiffer, M.J.; Waltering, K.K.; Vessella, R.L.; Tammela, T.L.; Visakorpi, T. MicroRNA expression profiling in prostate cancer. *Cancer Res.* **2007**, *67*, 6130–6135. [CrossRef] [PubMed]
62. Avgeris, M.; Stravodimos, K.; Fragoulis, E.G.; Scorilas, A. The loss of the tumour-suppressor miR-145 results in the shorter disease-free survival of prostate cancer patients. *Br. J. Cancer* **2013**, *108*, 2573–2581. [CrossRef] [PubMed]
63. Leite, K.R.; Tomiyama, A.; Reis, S.T.; Sousa-Canavez, J.M.; Sanudo, A.; Camara-Lopes, L.H.; Srougi, M. MicroRNA expression profiles in the progression of prostate cancer—From high-grade prostate intraepithelial neoplasia to metastasis. *Urol. Oncol.* **2013**, *31*, 796–801. [CrossRef] [PubMed]
64. Hagman, Z.; Larne, O.; Edsjo, A.; Bjartell, A.; Ehrnstrom, R.A.; Ulmert, D.; Lilja, H.; Ceder, Y. miR-34c is downregulated in prostate cancer and exerts tumor suppressive functions. *Int. J. Cancer* **2010**, *127*, 2768–2776. [CrossRef]
65. Hao, Y.; Zhao, Y.; Zhao, X.; He, C.; Pang, X.; Wu, T.C.; Califano, J.A.; Gu, X. Improvement of prostate cancer detection by integrating the PSA test with miRNA expression profiling. *Cancer Investig.* **2011**, *29*, 318–324. [CrossRef]

66. Casanova-Salas, I.; Rubio-Briones, J.; Calatrava, A.; Mancarella, C.; Masia, E.; Casanova, J.; Fernandez-Serra, A.; Rubio, L.; Ramirez-Backhaus, M.; Arminan, A.; et al. Identification of miR-187 and miR-182 as Biomarkers of Early Diagnosis and Prognosis in Patients with Prostate Cancer Treated with Radical Prostatectomy. *J. Urol.* **2014**, *192*, 252–259. [CrossRef] [PubMed]
67. Hagman, Z.; Haflidadottir, B.S.; Ansari, M.; Persson, M.; Bjartell, A.; Edsjo, A.; Ceder, Y. The tumour suppressor miR-34c targets MET in prostate cancer cells. *Br. J. Cancer* **2013**, *109*, 1271–1278. [CrossRef] [PubMed]
68. Wang, J.Y.; Jiang, J.B.; Li, Y.; Wang, Y.L.; Dai, Y. MicroRNA-299-3p suppresses proliferation and invasion by targeting VEGFA in human colon carcinoma. *Biomed. Pharmacother.* **2017**, *93*, 1047–1054. [CrossRef]
69. Dang, S.; Zhou, J.; Wang, Z.; Wang, K.; Dai, S.; He, S. MiR-299-3p functions as a tumor suppressor via targeting Sirtuin 5 in hepatocellular carcinoma. *Biomed. Pharmacother.* **2018**, *106*, 966–975. [CrossRef] [PubMed]
70. Wang, N.; Tao, L.; Zhong, H.; Zhao, S.; Yu, Y.; Yu, B.; Chen, X.; Gao, J.; Wang, R. miR-135b inhibits tumour metastasis in prostate cancer by targeting STAT6. *Oncol. Lett.* **2016**, *11*, 543–550. [CrossRef]
71. Olivan, M.; Garcia, M.; Suarez, L.; Guiu, M.; Gros, L.; Mendez, O.; Rigau, M.; Reventos, J.; Segura, M.F.; de Torres, I.; et al. Loss of microRNA-135b Enhances Bone Metastasis in Prostate Cancer and Predicts Aggressiveness in Human Prostate Samples. *Cancers* **2021**, *13*, 6202. [CrossRef] [PubMed]

cancers

MDPI

Article

Leukocytic Infiltration of Intraductal Carcinoma of the Prostate: An Exploratory Study

Mame-Kany Diop [1,2], Oscar Eduardo Molina [3], Mirela Birlea [1], Hélène LaRue [3], Hélène Hovington [3], Bernard Têtu [3,4], Louis Lacombe [3,5], Alain Bergeron [3,5], Yves Fradet [3,5] and Dominique Trudel [1,2,6,*]

1 Centre de Recherche du Centre Hospitalier de l'Université de Montréal (axe Cancer) and Institut du Cancer de Montréal, 900 Saint-Denis, Montréal, QC H2X 0A9, Canada; mame-kany.diop.chum@ssss.gouv.qc.ca (M.-K.D.); mirela.birlea.chum@ssss.gouv.qc.ca (M.B.)
2 Department of Pathology and Cellular Biology, Université de Montréal, 2900 Boulevard Édouard-Montpetit, Montréal, QC H3T 1J4, Canada
3 Centre de Recherche du CHU de Québec-Université Laval (axe Oncologie), Hôpital L'Hôtel-Dieu de Québec, 9 McMahon, Québec, QC G1R 3S3, Canada; oscar-eduardo.molina.1@ulaval.ca (O.E.M.); h_larue@videotron.ca (H.L.); helene.hovington@crchudequebec.ulaval.ca (H.H.); bernard.tetu.1@ulaval.ca (B.T.); louis.lacombe@crchudequebec.ulaval.ca (L.L.); alain.bergeron@crchudequebec.ulaval.ca (A.B.); yves.fradet@crchudequebec.ulaval.ca (Y.F.)
4 Department of Pathology, CHU de Québec-Université Laval, 11 Côte du Palais, Québec, QC G1R 2J6, Canada
5 Department of Surgery, Université Laval, 2325 rue de l'Université, Québec, QC G1V 0A6, Canada
6 Department of Pathology, Centre Hospitalier de l'Université de Montréal, 1051 Sanguinet, Montréal, QC H2X 0C1, Canada
* Correspondence: dominique.trudel.med@ssss.gouv.qc.ca; Tel.: +1-514-890-8000

Simple Summary: Men with a particular type of prostate cancer, called intraductal carcinoma of the prostate (IDC-P), are more likely to die from their cancer than men without IDC-P. No researchers have yet compared the immune infiltrate of IDC-P to the immune infiltrate of prostate cancer. In this study, we quantified immune cells specifically in IDC-P and compared the cell densities in IDC-P to those in the adjacent cancer, tumor margins and benign tissues. We found that the immune infiltrate of IDC-P was generally reduced compared to the surrounding tissues, especially regarding antigen-presenting cells. Following validation in larger cohorts, the characterization of the immune microenvironment of IDC-P could allow a better understanding of the immune response to lethal prostate cancer and enable the development of new therapies.

Abstract: Intraductal carcinoma of the prostate (IDC-P) is an aggressive histological subtype of prostate cancer (PCa) detected in approximately 20% of radical prostatectomy (RP) specimens. As IDC-P has been associated with PCa-related death and poor responses to standard treatment, the purpose of this study was to explore the immune infiltrate of IDC-P. Hematoxylin- and eosin-stained slides from 96 patients with locally advanced PCa who underwent RP were reviewed to identify IDC-P. Immunohistochemical staining of CD3, CD8, CD45RO, FoxP3, CD68, CD163, CD209 and CD83 was performed. For each slide, the number of positive cells per mm^2 in the benign tissues, tumor margins, cancer and IDC-P was calculated. Consequently, IDC-P was found in a total of 33 patients (34%). Overall, the immune infiltrate was similar in the IDC-P-positive and the IDC-P-negative patients. However, FoxP3$^+$ regulatory T cells ($p < 0.001$), CD68$^+$ and CD163$^+$ macrophages ($p < 0.001$ for both) and CD209$^+$ and CD83$^+$ dendritic cells ($p = 0.002$ and $p = 0.013$, respectively) were less abundant in the IDC-P tissues compared to the adjacent PCa. Moreover, the patients were classified as having immunologically "cold" or "hot" IDC-P, according to the immune-cell densities averaged in the total IDC-P or in the immune hotspots. The CD68/CD163/CD209-immune hotspots predicted metastatic dissemination ($p = 0.014$) and PCa-related death ($p = 0.009$) in a Kaplan–Meier survival analysis. Further studies on larger cohorts are necessary to evaluate the clinical utility of assessing the immune infiltrate of IDC-P with regards to patient prognosis and the use of immunotherapy for lethal PCa.

Citation: Diop, M.-K.; Molina, O.E.; Birlea, M.; LaRue, H.; Hovington, H.; Têtu, B.; Lacombe, L.; Bergeron, A.; Fradet, Y.; Trudel, D. Leukocytic Infiltration of Intraductal Carcinoma of the Prostate: An Exploratory Study. *Cancers* **2023**, *15*, 2217. https://doi.org/10.3390/cancers15082217

Academic Editor: Kouji Izumi

Received: 23 February 2023
Revised: 3 April 2023
Accepted: 7 April 2023
Published: 9 April 2023

Keywords: prostate cancer; intraductal carcinoma of the prostate; radical prostatectomy; T-lymphocytes; antigen-presenting cells

1. Introduction

Despite the tremendous advances made in cancer immunotherapy in the last decade [1–3], the efficacy of immunological approaches remains modest for advanced prostate cancer (PCa) [4–6]. Sipuleucel-T, an autologous cellular-immunotherapy vaccine based on antigen-presenting cells (APC), was approved by the Food and Drug Administration (FDA) in 2010 for the treatment of advanced PCa; Sipuleucel-T offers a slight 4-month overall survival benefit compared to placebo in men with metastatic castration-resistant PCa (mCRPC) [7]. More recently, a checkpoint inhibitor, pembrolizumab, was approved by the FDA for cancers with high microsatellite instability or mismatch-repair deficiency, regardless of the tumor origin [8]. However, barely 3% of men with advanced PCa have such alterations [9]. Other immunotherapy drugs are yet to be approved.

Although ongoing clinical trials are exploring immunotherapy-based combinatorial strategies for advanced PCa, it is crucial to better understand the immune response associated with PCa to better identify men who could benefit from these approaches. Most studies evaluating the immune infiltrate of PCa focused on T lymphocytes and found that a higher expression of tumor-infiltrating lymphocytes (TILs) is associated with worse PCa prognosis [10–15].

Intraductal carcinoma of the prostate (IDC-P) is an aggressive histologic entity of PCa associated with poor prognosis [16]. It is characterized by the proliferation of malignant prostatic epithelial cells in pre-existing prostatic ducts [17]. Current evidence suggests that most IDC-P arises from the retrograde invasion of conventional prostatic adenocarcinoma into prostatic ducts [18–20]. In a systemic review of 38 PCa cohorts, Porter et al. found that the prevalence of IDC-P increased from 2.1% in low-risk PCa patients to 36.7% in high-risk PCa patients, even reaching 56.0% in patients with metastatic disease [21]. Accordingly, men with IDC-P tend to have more advanced PCa, as shown by their higher pathologic (p) T stages and higher Gleason scores [22–24]. Furthermore, IDC-P still independently predicts biochemical recurrence (BCR) and the development of metastasis and CRPC [18,21,25,26]; furthermore, it has been linked to poor responses to treatment and worse PCa-specific and overall survival [27–34]. There is currently no consensus on the clinical management of IDC-P [35–37].

Because of its association with lethal PCa and its resistance to current therapies, we believe that the immune infiltrate of IDC-P is distinct from that in surrounding tissues, and that its evaluation will allow a better understanding of the microenvironment of advanced PCa. Here, we show that the immune infiltrate of IDC-P is different from that found in the adjacent invasive carcinoma. In addition, we found that the immune infiltrate in IDC-P can be categorized as "cold", "intermediate" or "hot", depending on the immune-cell densities averaged in the total IDC-P or in IDC-P-immune hotspots. We found that the patients with "hot" CD68-, CD163- and CD209-immune hotspots experienced shorter metastasis-free and PCa-specific survival.

2. Materials and Methods

2.1. Patients and Ethics

Radical prostatectomy (RP) specimens from 96 men with locally advanced hormone-naïve PCa who underwent surgery between 1996 and 1998 at the CHU de Québec-Université Laval were included in this study. Locally advanced PCa was defined as either pT3- or pT4-stage PCa or pT2-stage PCa with positive margins. Each participant signed an informed consent form to participate at the local cancer biobank (URO-1 biobank), allowing the use of their tissues and clinical and pathological data for cancer research. This study was conducted following approval by the CHU de Québec-Université Laval Research

Ethics Committee (research project 2012-1059) and the CHUM Research Ethics Committee (research project MP-02-2018-7450).

2.2. Selection of the Representative Blocks and Identification of IDC-P

Hematoxylin and eosin (H&E) slides were reviewed to select one representative formalin-fixed paraffin-embedded (FFPE) tissue block per patient. The corresponding H&E slide had to be representative of the grade group (GG) assigned at diagnosis, containing between 30% and 70% of cancer and as small a number of calcifications as possible; furthermore, the selected block had to allow at least eight additional tissue sections.

The presence of IDC-P was assessed on the selected H&E slides by one trained observer (M.-K.D.) and a pathologist with expertise in IDC-P (D.T.). Intraductal carcinoma of the prostate was identified when cancer cells invaded the lumen of obvious pre-existing ducts to form dense-to-solid cribriform patterns or loose patterns, provided that either marked pleomorphism, frequent mitotic activity, comedonecrosis or abnormally large nuclei were present, as defined by Guo and Epstein [18].

2.3. Immunohistochemistry

Consecutive 5-µm-thick sections of the selected FFPE block were cut, dried overnight at 37 °C and deparaffinized. Heat-induced antigen retrieval was performed using a PT Link (Dako, Burlington, ON, Canada) at 92 °C for 20 min in citrate buffer, pH 6.1 (EnVision™ FLEX, K8004, Dako), for CD3, CD45RO, CD68 and CD209 stainings or Tris/EDTA, pH 9 (EnVision™ FLEX, K8005, Dako), for CD8, FoxP3, CD163 and CD83 stainings. Slides were then incubated for 10 min in 3% hydrogen peroxide. Using the IDetect Super Stain Horseradish Peroxidase (HRP) polymer kit (ID Labs, London, ON, Canada), slides were first incubated for 10 min with Super Block blocking buffer and then with primary antibodies at room temperature (Table 1). With washes between each step, slides were then incubated for 30 min with HRP-polymer-conjugated antibodies and for 5 min with 3,3′-diaminobenzidine (DAB) tetrahydrochloride solution. Lastly, slides were counterstained with hematoxylin, dehydrated and mounted with MM 24 low-viscosity mounting medium (Leica Microsystems, Hurham, NC, USA).

Table 1. Primary antibodies used in this study.

Antibody	Clone	Company	Dilution	Incubation Time
Anti-CD3	SP7	Abcam, Toronto, ON, Canada	1/500	Overnight
Anti-CD8	4B11	Novocastra, Newcastle upon Tyne, England	1/600	Overnight
Anti-CD45RO	UCHL-1	Abcam, Toronto, ON, Canada	1/6000	Overnight
Anti-FoxP3	236A/E7	Abcam, Toronto, ON, Canada	1/600	Overnight
Anti-CD68	KP1	Abcam, Toronto, ON, Canada	1/800	2 h
Anti-CD163	2G12	Abcam, Toronto, ON, Canada	1/2000	1 h
Anti-CD209	120612	R&D Systems, Minneapolis, MN, USA	1/80	Overnight
Anti-CD83	1H4B	Novocastra, Newcastle-upon-Tyne, UK	1/200	Overnight

2.4. Quantification of Immunohistochemistry Staining

The immunohistochemistry (IHC) slides were scanned using a Nanozoomer whole-slide scanner (Hamamatsu, Bridgewater, NJ, USA).

For each slide, 10 high-power fields at 200× magnification (0.460 mm^2), or less when less tissue was available, were randomly selected in isolated benign areas (containing ducts), tumor margins (areas on the periphery of the tumor) and within the cancer. The number of positive cells in each area was then calculated using one of the two following methods: manual use of the NDP.view2 software (Hamamatsu Photonics) by two trained observers (O.E.M. and H.L.); or manually by one trained observer (O.E.M) and in a semi-automatic fashion through the Calopix software (TRIBVN Healthcare, Châtillon, France). Ten percent of the slides were reviewed by an experienced pathologist (B.T.).

Positive cells in IDC-P were quantified using the NDP.view2 software (Hamamatsu Photonics). On slides containing IDC-P, each individual IDC-P lesion was encircled using the freehand-region tool in NDP.view2, and positive cells were manually counted by a trained observer (M.-K.D.) to obtain the number of positive cells/mm^2 for each IDC-P lesion and the mean number of positive cells/mm^2 in the total IDC-P of the slide. Immune hotspots were defined as the highest number of positive cells/mm^2 in IDC-P lesions with an area greater than the median area of all IDC-P lesions on the slide. Slides were reviewed by an experienced pathologist (D.T.).

The observers were blinded to the clinical outcomes of the patients.

2.5. Clinical-Data Collection and Endpoints

Age, pre-operative prostate-specific antigen (PSA) serum concentrations, pT stage, modified Gleason grading system/GG grading [17,38] and margin status were collected from patient files. Clinical follow-up data were collected from the day of RP. Biochemical recurrence was defined as two consecutive PSA test results over 0.3 ng/mL after RP, one PSA test result over 0.3 ng/mL after post-operative treatment or any increase in serum PSA that required post-operative treatment by a urologist. Castration-resistant prostate cancer was defined as disease progression, including rise in serum PSA and development of metastases, despite castrate levels of serum testosterone [39]. Definitive androgen deprivation therapy (ADT) was defined as any hormonotherapy that was given to a patient as primary treatment (not neoadjuvant or adjuvant) after suspected or confirmed disease progression.

2.6. Statistical Analyses

Data analyses were conducted using IBM SPSS Statistics for Windows, version 28.0 (Armonk, NY, USA: IBM Corp.), according to the REMARK guidelines [40]. Descriptive statistical analysis for quantitative variables used mean, median, standard deviation, standard error, inter-quartile range (IQR) and, for qualitative variables, percentage. Univariate analyses were performed using the independent-samples *t*-test, Mann–Whitney *U* test, Welch's *t*-test, Pearson's chi-square test, Fisher's exact test and the paired-samples sign test. To evaluate the correlation between cell densities, we performed Pearson correlations [41]. The Benjamini–Hochberg procedure was used to control for multiple comparisons with a 10% false-discovery rate. Time to BCR, metastasis, CRPC, definitive ADT, PCa-specific death and overall survival were measured from the date of RP until the date of the event or last follow-up date; these events were evaluated using the Kaplan–Meier method and log-rank test. Statistical significance was established for two-sided p-values < 0.05.

Bar charts were generated in Excel (Microsoft Corporation, version 18.2301.1131.0). Survival curves were created in IBM SPSS Statistics. Other charts were built using R (R Core Team, 2022, Vienna, Austria) and RStudio (RStudio Team, 2022, Boston, MA, USA). The ggplot2 [42] and ggbreak [43] packages were used to generate jitter plots and parallel coordinates charts, while the plot function was used to generate correlation matrix and the heatmap.2 function of the gplots package [44] was used for heatmap and hierarchical clustering.

3. Results

3.1. Clinicopathological Characteristics of Patients

The clinicopathological characteristics of the 96 patients included in this study are presented in Table 2. A total of 33 patients (34%) had IDC-P on their selected block. The patients in the IDC-P-negative group and in the IDC-P-positive group had similar median follow-ups of 15.8 years and 14.3 years ($p = 0.105$), respectively. As expected, the presence of IDC-P was associated with higher pT stages ($p < 0.001$) and GGs ($p = 0.001$). Indeed, the pT3b and pT4 stages were found in 58% (19/33) of the patients in the IDC-P-positive group compared to 21% (13/63) of the patients in the IDC-P-negative group. Furthermore, high grades (GGs 4 and 5) were diagnosed in 36% (12/33) of the patients from the IDC-P-positive group compared to 10% (6/63) of the patients from the IDC-P-negative group. Accordingly, the men with IDC-P had higher rates of lymph-node involvement (42% vs. 21%, $p = 0.032$). Moreover, IDC-P was associated with the development of BCR (73% vs. 35%, $p < 0.001$), CRPC (36% vs. 8%, $p < 0.001$) and metastases (39% vs. 6%, $p < 0.001$). In addition, IDC-P was associated with higher rates of PCa-specific death (33% vs. 5%, $p < 0.001$) and overall death (73% vs. 41%, $p = 0.005$). No statistically significant differences were found in the rates of positive margins ($p = 1.000$) and lymphovascular invasion ($p = 0.332$) between the two groups.

Table 2. Clinicopathological characteristics of patients according to the presence or absence of intraductal carcinoma of the prostate (IDC-P) on representative slides.

Characteristics	Total Cohort	IDC-P Status		*p*-Value
		Negative	Positive	
	n = 96 (%)	*n* = 63 (%)	*n* = 33 (%)	
Mean age at diagnosis (SD)	63.5 (5)	62.8 (5)	64.9 (5)	0.064 [a]
Mean pre-operative PSA (SD)	13.4 (14)	13.6 (16)	12.9 (10)	0.889 [b]
Stage pT, *n* (%)				**<0.001** [b]
pT2	32 (33)	26 (41)	6 (18)	
pT3a	32 (33)	24 (38)	8 (24)	
pT3b	30 (31)	13 (21)	17 (52)	
pT4	2 (2)	0	2 (6)	
Grade group, *n* (%)				**0.001** [c]
1	45 (47)	37 (59)	8 (24)	
2	24 (25)	14 (22)	10 (30)	
3	9 (9)	6 (10)	3 (9)	
4	10 (10)	3 (5)	7 (21)	
5	8 (8)	3 (5)	5 (15)	
Lymph-node involvement, *n* (%)	27 (28)	13 (21)	14 (42)	**0.032** [d]
Lymphovascular invasion, *n* (%)	25 (26)	14 (22)	11 (33)	0.332 [d]
Positive margins, *n* (%)	75 (78)	49 (78)	26 (79)	1.000 [d]
Biochemical recurrence, *n* (%)	46 (48)	22 (35)	24 (73)	**<0.001** [d]
Castration-resistant PCa, *n* (%)	17 (18)	5 (8)	12 (36)	**<0.001** [d]
Metastasis, *n* (%)	17 (18)	4 (6)	13 (39)	**<0.001** [d]
PCa-related death, *n* (%)	14 (15)	3 (5)	11 (33)	**<0.001** [e]
Overall death, *n* (%)	50 (52)	26 (41)	24 (73)	**0.005** [d]
Median follow-up in years (IQR)	15.5 (10–19)	15.8 (10–19)	14.3 (8–18)	0.105 [b]

IDC-P: intraductal carcinoma of the prostate; SD: standard deviation; PSA: prostate-specific antigen; PCa: prostate cancer; IQR: inter-quartile range. Bold entities indicate statistically significant *p*-values. [a] Independent-samples *t*-test, [b] Mann–Whitney *U* test; [c] Welch's *t*-test; [d] Pearson's chi-square; [e] Fisher's exact test.

3.2. Quantification of $CD3^+$, $CD8^+$, $CD45RO^+$, $FoxP3^+$, $CD68^+$, $CD163^+$, $CD209^+$ and $CD83^+$ Cells in Benign Tissues, Margins, Cancer and IDC-P

The immune cells were detected through the immunohistochemical staining of CD3 (T lymphocytes), CD8 (cytotoxic T lymphocytes), CD45RO (memory T cells), FoxP3 (regulatory T cells), CD68 (macrophages), CD163 (M2-type macrophages), CD209 (immature dendritic cells) and CD83 (mature dendritic cells) (Figure 1). The FoxP3 expression was localized in the nuclei of the T cells, whereas CD3, CD8, CD45RO, CD209, CD83, CD68 and CD163 expression was localized in the cell membrane. These eight markers were quantified in isolated benign tissues, cancer margins and within the whole cancer area (regions with invasive carcinoma selected randomly and independently of the presence of IDC-P).

The average cell densities (mean number of positive cells per mm^2) ranged from 3 to 836 for CD3, 4 to 163 for CD8, 1 to 238 for CD45RO, 0 to 45 for FoxP3, 1 to 335 for CD68, 0 to 280 for CD163, 0 to 59 for CD209 and 0 to 40 for CD83 (Figure 2). The cell densities tended to be higher in the margins compared to the benign and cancer compartments, except for the $CD68^+$ macrophages, which tended to be more abundant in the cancer compartment and the $CD83^+$ dendritic cells in benign tissues ($p > 0.05$). Furthermore, no significant differences were seen in the mean ranks of the immune cells between the IDC-P-negative and the IDC-P-positive samples in the same compartment, excluding the FoxP3$^+$ cells, which were more abundant in the margins of the IDC-P-positive samples (mean ranks: 55.0 vs. 41.0, U = 608, p = 0.016) (Figure 2).

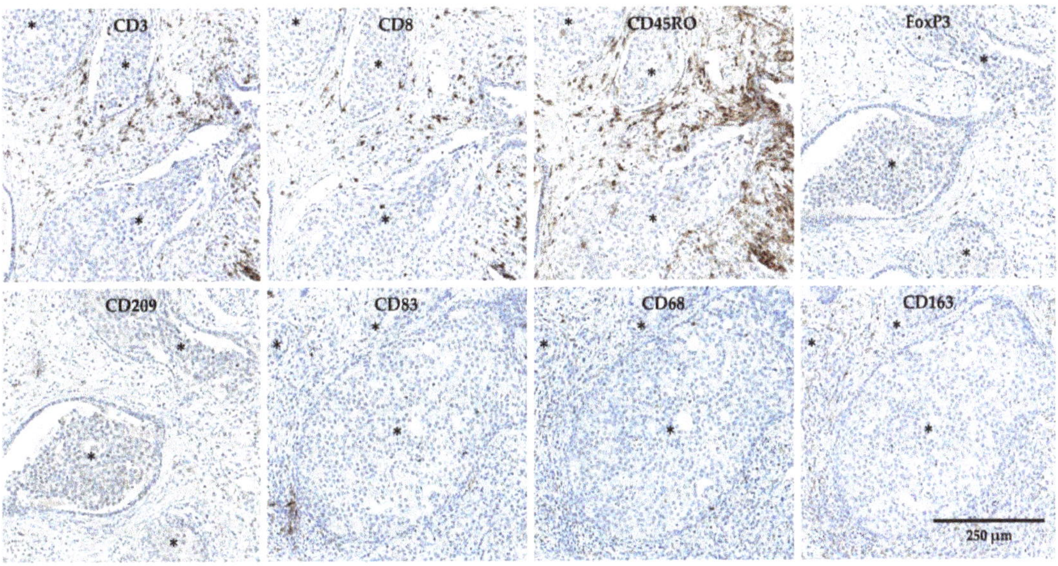

Figure 1. Example of immunohistochemical staining for CD3, CD8, CD45RO, FoxP3, CD209, CD83, CD68 and CD163 in cancer, including intraductal carcinoma of the prostate (IDC-P, asterisks), of the same tissue block. Scale bar: 250 µm.

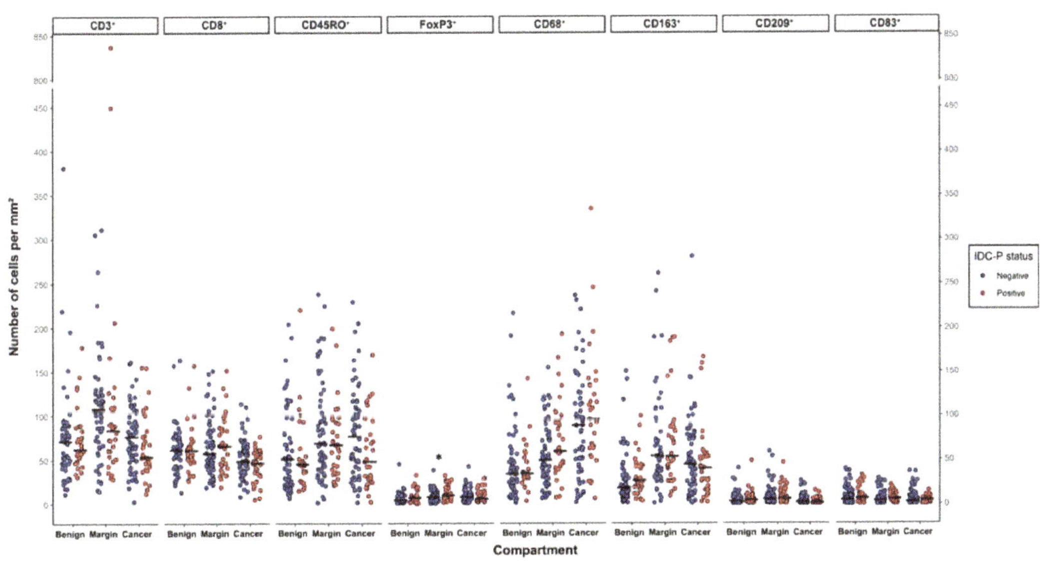

Figure 2. Leucocyte densities depending on IDC-P status. Dots represent individual patients. Horizontal bars represent medians. For each compartment, mean ranks according to IDC-P status were compared using the Mann–Whitney U test. * p = 0.016.

Next, to further evaluate the inflammation associated with IDC-P, we specifically assessed the immune infiltrate within the IDC-P areas (Figure 1). The mean area of IDC-P per slide was 6.5 mm^2 and the median was 3.2 mm^2, with a minimum area of 0.1 mm^2 and a maximum area of 25.6 mm^2. The immune infiltrate of IDC-P varied broadly between samples for CD3, CD8, CD45RO and CD68, with median (range) counts of 48 (6–244)/mm^2, 39 (5–174)/mm^2, 38 (8–150)/mm^2 and 44 (12–211)/mm^2, respectively. Only a small portion of macrophages in the IDC-P seemed to express CD163, with a median count of 4 (0–51)/mm^2. By contrast, FoxP3$^+$, CD209$^+$ and CD83$^+$ cells were scarce in the IDC-P, ranging from 0 to 15 cells/mm^2, 0 to 4 cells/mm^2 and 0 to 4 cells/mm^2, respectively.

When we compared the cell densities in the IDC-P to the other compartments, we found significant differences. Paired-samples sign tests were conducted to assess the variations in the mean number of immune cells within the same slide and the results are presented in Figure 3. Regardless of the compartment, benign, margins or cancer, CD163$^+$ macrophages ($p < 0.001$ for all three compartments) and CD209$^+$ ($p < 0.001$ for benign and margins and $p = 0.002$ for cancer) or CD83$^+$ ($p < 0.001$ for benign and margins and $p = 0.013$ for cancer) dendritic cells were typically less abundant in the IDC-P (Figure 3). Furthermore, CD68$^+$ macrophages ($p = 0.036$ for margins and $p < 0.001$ for cancer) and FoxP3$^+$ regulatory T lymphocytes ($p < 0.001$ for both) were typically less abundant in the IDC-P compared to margins and cancer (Figure 3b,c). Notably, except for the CD68$^+$ macrophages, which were generally more abundant in the cancer than in the tumor margins, leucocytes were typically more abundant in the tumor margins than in the cancer (Figure 3b,c and Supplementary Figures S1 and S2).

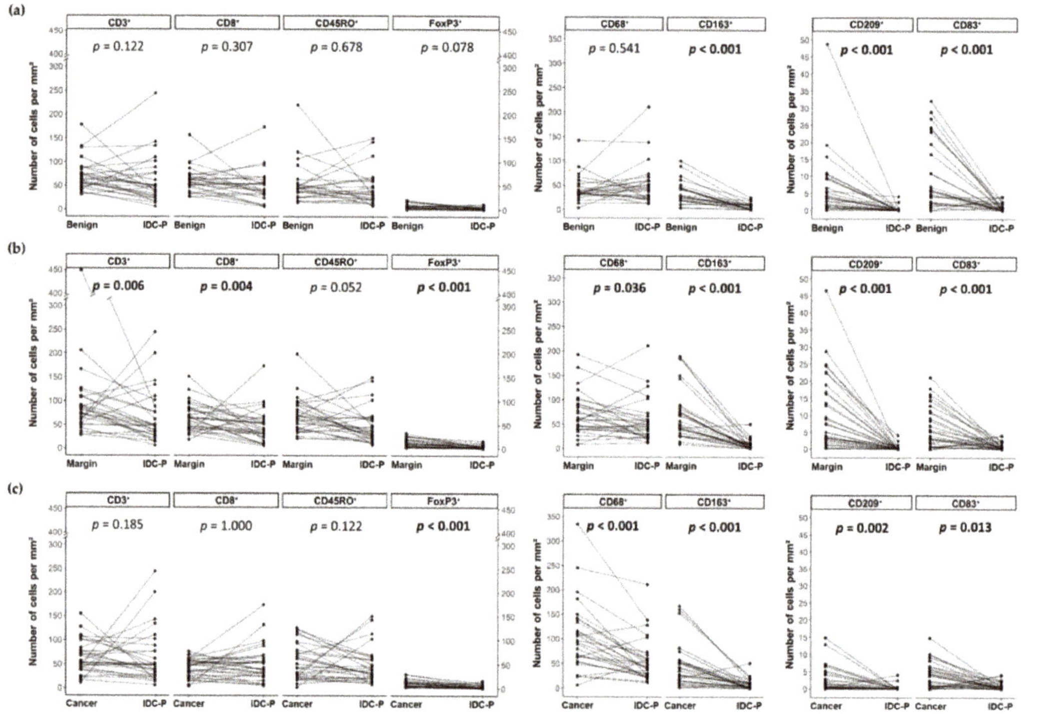

Figure 3. Parallel coordinate plots showing the changes in cell density for each IDC-P-positive patient between the IDC-P compartment and benign tissues (**a**), margins (**b**) and cancer (**c**). Paired-samples sign tests were performed. Bold entities indicate statistically significant *p*-values. IDC-P: intraductal carcinoma of the prostate.

Interestingly, no significant differences were found between the variations in the mean number of T lymphocytes ($CD3^+$, $CD8^+$, $CD45RO^+$ and $FoxP3^+$) and $CD68^+$ macrophages in the IDC-P compared to the benign tissues (Figure 3a). Indeed, as shown in Figure 3, the decrease in the densities of the T cells in the IDC-P was more balanced, with a considerable number of patients having more positive cells in IDC-P tissues compared to benign tissues. Furthermore, most of the patients had more $CD3^+$ (p = 0.006) and $CD8^+$ (p = 0.004) T cells and tended to have more $CD45RO^+$ T cells (p = 0.052) in the margins compared to IDC-P (Figure 3b), while the $CD3^+$, $CD8^+$ and $CD45RO^+$ cell densities were less often decreased in IDC-P tissues compared to cancer or benign tissues (Figure 3a,c), resulting in a non-significant difference between the two compartments. Notably, we observed $CD45RO^+$ cell clusters surrounding the IDC-P tissues in 56% (15/27) of the cases and the number of $CD45RO^+$ cells/mm^2 in the IDC-P increased with the presence of surrounding $CD45RO^+$ cell clusters (mean $CD45RO^+$/mm^2 ± SD: 63 ± 45 vs. 32 ± 19, p = 0.025).

Parallel coordinate plots showing the changes in cell density for each IDC-P-positive patient in the general cancer or in the margins compared to the other compartments are available in the Supplementary Materials (Supplementary Figures S1 and S2).

3.3. Correlation between Immune-Cell Densities in IDC-P

Unsurprisingly, we found a strong correlation between the $CD3^+$-T-lymphocyte densities and those of the $CD8^+$ cytotoxic T lymphocytes (r = 0.90, p < 0.001), $CD45RO^+$ memory T lymphocytes (r = 0.87, p < 0.001) and $FoxP3^+$ regulatory T lymphocytes (r = 0.72, p < 0.001) in the IDC-P tissues (Figure 4a). The $CD8^+$ and $CD45RO^+$ T-cell densities were also strongly correlated in the IDC-P tissues (r = 0.80, p < 0.001). The $CD163^+$-M2-type-macrophage densities were not significantly correlated with the $CD68^+$ cells (r = 0.27, p = 0.196; Figure 4b), nor were the $CD209^+$ and $CD83^+$ dendritic cells (r = 0.13, p = 0.514; Figure 4c). Interestingly, the T-lymphocyte densities in the IDC-P tissues were moderately correlated with the $CD163^+$-M2-macrophage densities (r = 0.59, p = 0.002; Figure 4b) and, albeit to a lesser extent, with those of the $CD83^+$ mature dendritic cells (r = 0.48, p = 0.013) (Figure 4c) and $CD68^+$ macrophages (r = 0.41, p = 0.047; Figure 4b), but not with those of the $CD209^+$ immature dendritic cells (r = 0.02, p = 0.938; Figure 4c).

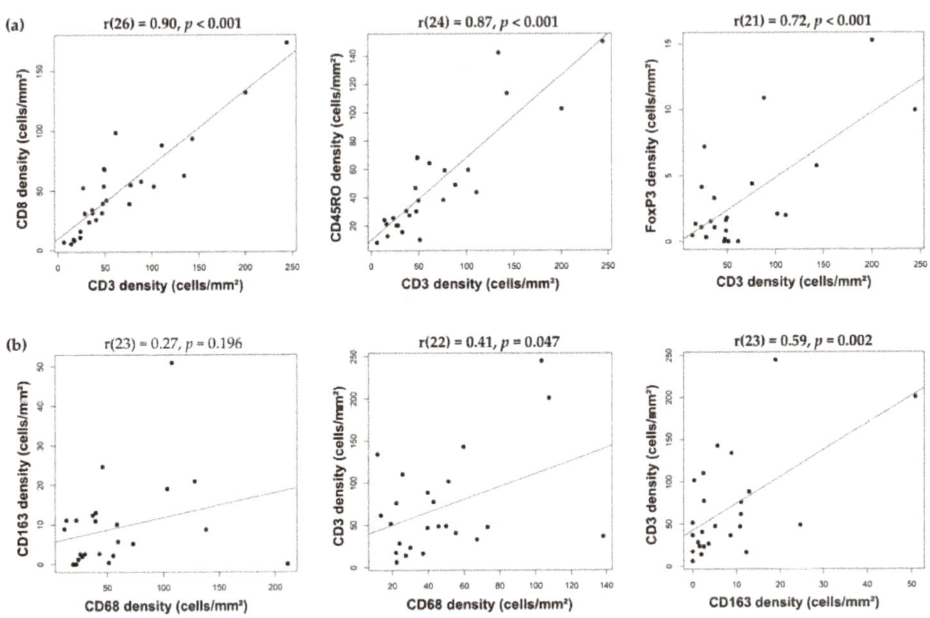

Figure 4. *Cont.*

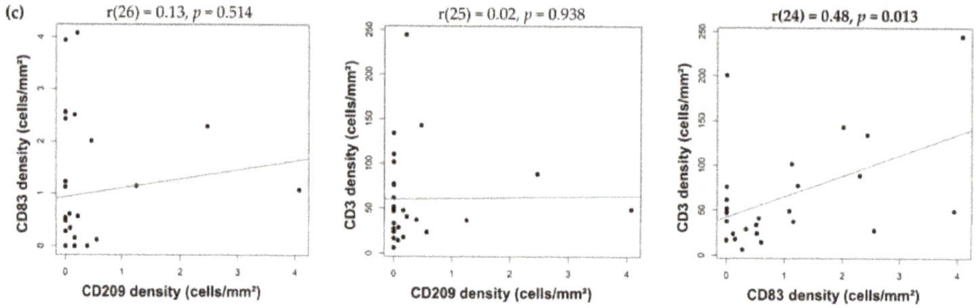

Figure 4. Linear regression and Pearson correlation for cell densities between the different cell types in IDC-P. Correlation between T cells and T cell subtypes (**a**), macrophages and T cells (**b**) and dendritic cells and T cells (**c**). Dots represent individual patients. Bold entities indicate statistically significant correlation.

3.4. Clusterization of IDC-P-Positive Patients According to Immune-Cell Densities

The mean numbers of positive cells per mm^2 according to the patients' outcomes after five and 10 years of follow-up are presented in Figure 5. No significant differences were seen in the mean ranks of the leukocytes in the IDC-P tissues between patients with different outcomes, except for CD68$^+$ cells, which were more abundant in the men who died of their PCa (mean ranks: 18.0 vs. 10.2, $U = 21$, adjusted $p = 0.047$) and the men who died regardless of cause (mean ranks: 17.8 vs. 12.7, $U = 40$, adjusted $p = 0.047$) (Figure 5b).

We further explored the immune infiltrate of IDC-P by examining the immune signatures of each patient according to the average immune-cell densities in the total IDC-P. Three patients were excluded due to the absence of more than three IHC slides. The mean numbers of positive immune cells per mm^2 in the IDC-P tissues were standardized using z-score normalization to generate a heatmap representing the unsupervised hierarchical clustering of both the rows and the columns. Two main groups were identified according to the expression of the eight immune-cell markers: men with a low expression of immune markers, hereafter referred to as "cold" IDC-P; and men with a higher expression of immune markers, hereafter referred to as "hot/intermediate" IDC-P (Figure 6a).

The median follow-up of the 30 patients with IDC-P was 164 months (IQR: 89–209). We generated Kaplan–Meier curves to explore the association between the expression of the immune markers and the clinical outcomes, according to the two groups: "cold" or "hot/intermediate" IDC-P (Figure 6b). Although, in this small cohort, statistical significance was not reached, there was a trend toward better prognoses for patients with immunologically "cold" IDC-P. Only 19% of the men with "hot/intermediate" IDC-P were BCR-free after 10 years of follow-up compared to twice as many men with "cold" IDC-P. The need for definitive ADT, which is an indication of recurrence, was also lower in the "cold" IDC-P group (10-year definitive ADT-free survival rates: 70% for the "cold" group vs. 43% for the "hot/intermediate" group). At ten years of follow-up, 32% of the patients with "cold" IDC-P developed CRPC, 25% developed metastasis and 25% died of their PCa compared to 35%, 41% and 31% of the patients with "hot/intermediate" IDC-P, respectively. Finally, under one third of the men with "cold" IDC-P died within 10 years of follow-up, compared to nearly half of the patients with "hot/intermediate" IDC-P.

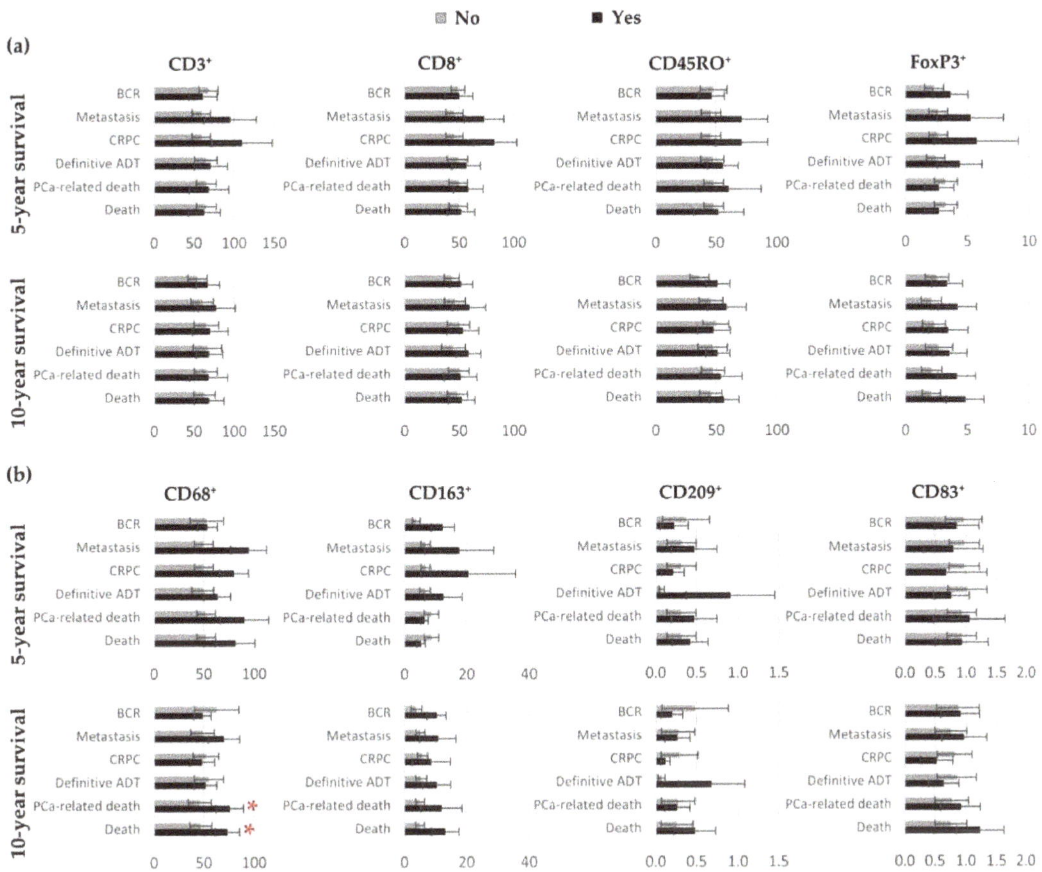

Figure 5. Bar charts representing the mean number of positive T cells (**a**) and antigen-presenting cells (**b**) in the total IDC-P according to patients' outcomes five and ten years post-surgery. Error bars represent standard errors. For each cell marker, mean ranks according to survival status were compared using the Mann–Whitney *U* test and Benjamini–Hochberg corrections were applied to control for multiple comparisons. * Statistically significant *p*-values. ADT: androgen-deprivation therapy; BCR: biochemical recurrence; CRPC: castration-resistant prostate cancer; IDC-P: intraductal carcinoma of the prostate; PCa: prostate cancer.

We then examined the association between the cell densities in the IDC-P-immune hotspots and prognosis. The dependence of the mean numbers of cells per mm^2 on the outcomes after five and 10 years of follow-up are illustrated in Figure 7. No significant differences were seen in the T-cells densities between the groups (Figure 7a). However, higher densities were seen in the hotspots in the patients who died of their cancer or of other causes within five years for $CD68^+$ macrophages (mean ranks: 24.3 vs. 12.7, $U = 5$, adjusted $p = 0.035$ and mean ranks: 23.8 vs. 13.0, $U = 11$, adjusted $p = 0.035$, respectively) or within 10 years for $CD163^+$ macrophages (mean ranks: 18.7 vs. 9.9, $U = 16$, adjusted $p = 0.012$ and mean ranks: 20.6 vs. 10.6, $U = 27$, adjusted $p = 0.006$, respectively) (Figure 7b). Greater $CD163^+$-cell densities were also associated with the development of metastasis during the first 10 years of follow-up (mean ranks: 17.3 vs.10.1, $U = 26$, adjusted $p = 0.035$) (Figure 7b). Furthermore, higher $CD209^+$-cell densities predicted the need for definitive ADT within five (mean ranks: 21.9 vs. 12.4, $U = 29$, adjusted $p = 0.005$) and 10 years (mean ranks: 18.4 vs. 11.0, $U = 40$, adjusted $p = 0.031$) (Figure 7b).

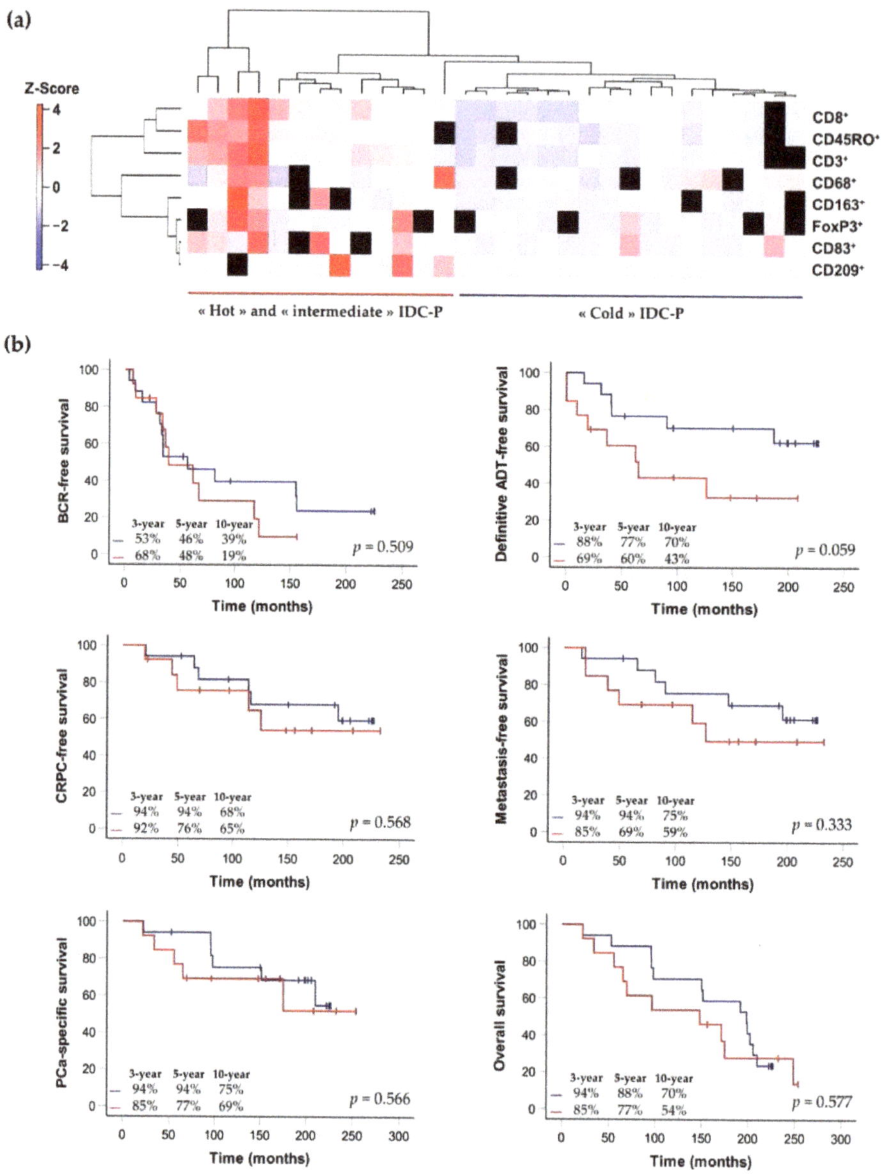

Figure 6. Hierarchical clustering of the eight immune-cell markers according to average cell densities in the total IDC-P (**a**) and Kaplan–Meier curves exploring survival rates of patients with immunologically "cold" IDC-P (blue) and patients with immunologically "hot/intermediate" IDC-P (red) (**b**). (**a**) On the left side: cell-density scale from dark blue (low) to dark red (high). Each row corresponds to a patient and missing slides/quantification data are represented by black squares. The IDC-P-positive patients with more than three missing quantification data were excluded, bringing the total number of patients to 30. (**b**) The *p*-values were calculated using the log-rank test. Three-, five- and ten-year survival rates are indicated in the bottom left of each graph. ADT: androgen-deprivation therapy; BCR: biochemical recurrence; CRPC: castration-resistant prostate cancer; IDC-P: intraductal carcinoma of the prostate; PCa: prostate cancer.

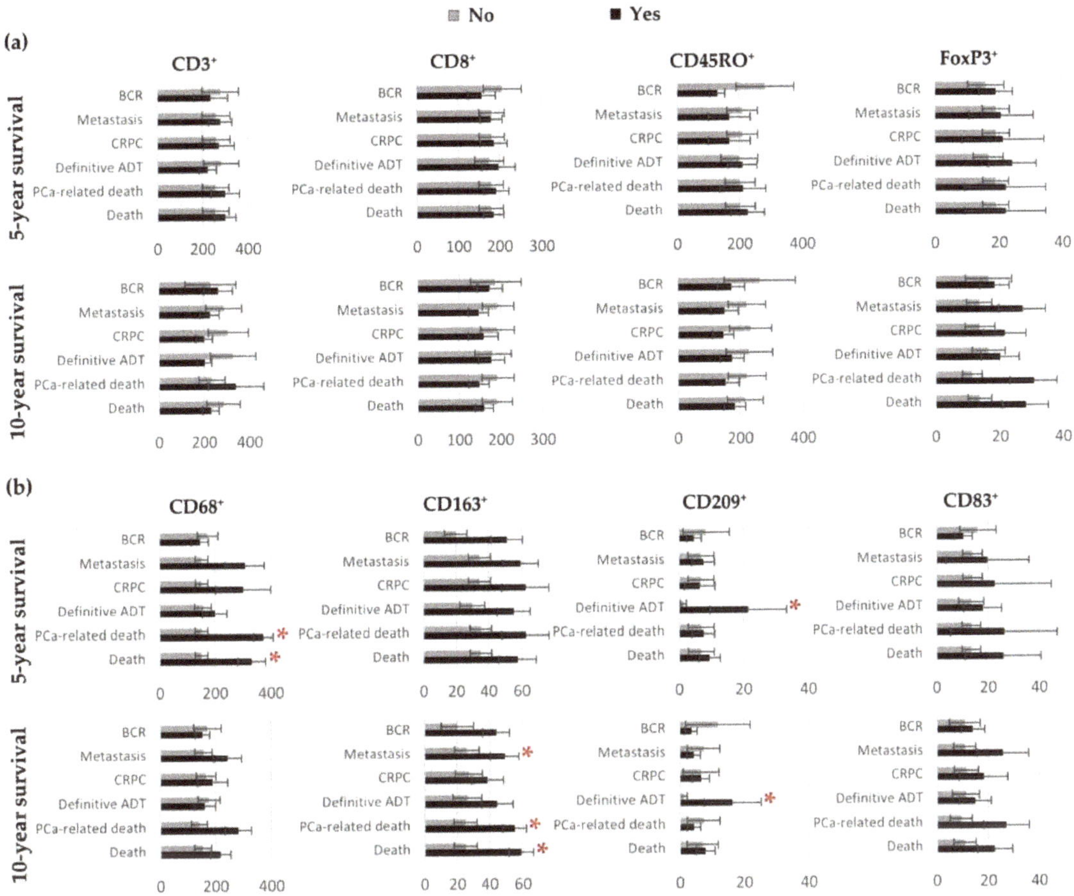

Figure 7. Bar charts representing the mean number of positive T cells (**a**) and antigen-presenting cells (**b**) in IDC-P-immune hotspots according to patients' outcomes five- and ten-years post-surgery. Error bars represent standard errors. For each cell marker, mean ranks according to survival status were compared using the Mann–Whitney *U* test and Benjamini–Hochberg corrections were applied to control for multiple comparisons. * Statistically significant *p*-values. ADT: androgen-deprivation therapy; BCR: biochemical recurrence; CRPC: castration-resistant prostate cancer; IDC-P: intraductal carcinoma of the prostate; PCa: prostate cancer.

The immune signatures of the patients were generated using the cell densities of the three markers significantly associated with prognosis in the IDC-P-immune hotspots CD68, CD163 and CD209. One additional patient was excluded due to the absence of more than one IHC slide. Again, the cell densities in the IDC-P tissues were standardized using z-score normalization to generate a heatmap representing unsupervised hierarchical clustering. Two main groups were identified according to the expression of the three immune-cell markers in the hotspots: men with a low or intermediate expression of immune markers, constituting the "cold/intermediate" group; and men with a higher expression of immune markers, constituting the "hot" group, largely due to the presence of macrophages (Figure 8a).

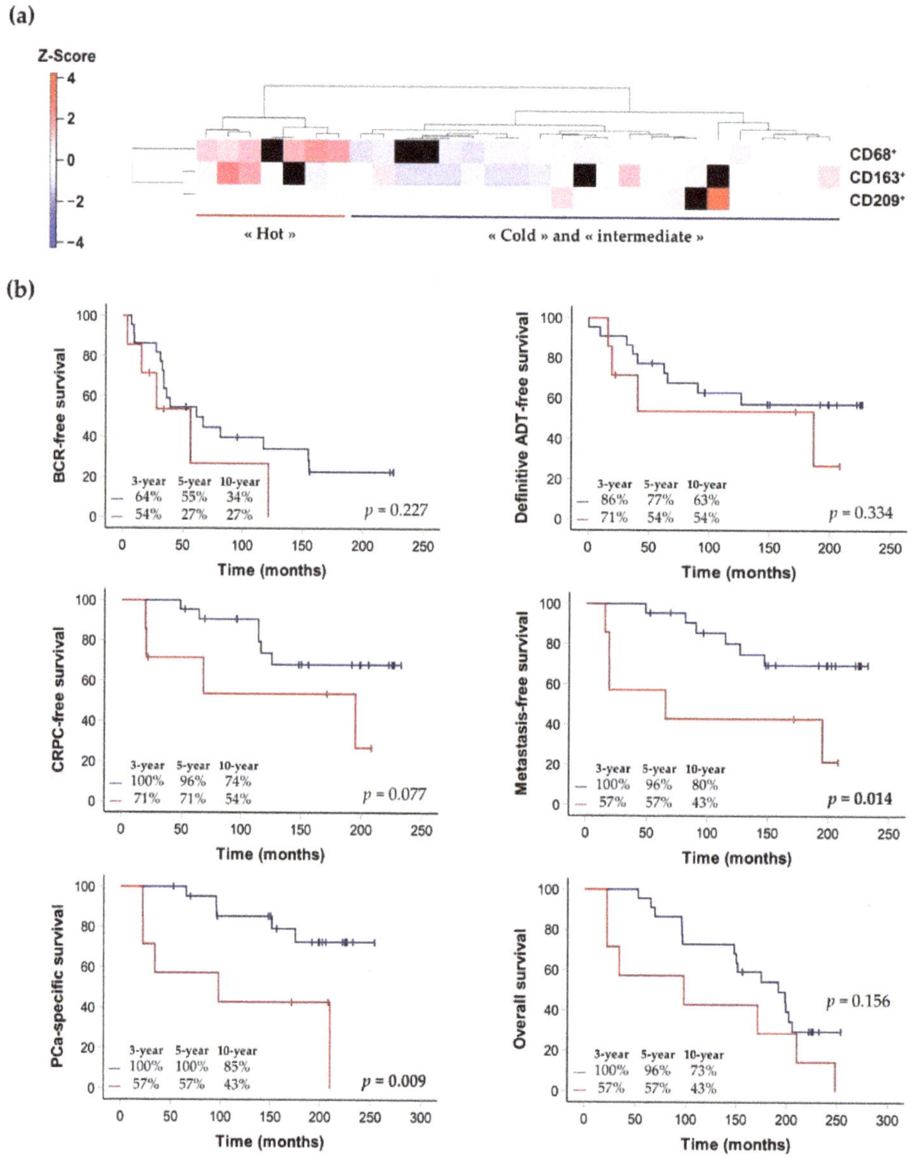

Figure 8. Hierarchical clustering of the three selected immune-cell markers according to cell densities in hotspots (**a**) and Kaplan–Meier curves exploring survival rates of patients with immunologically "cold/intermediate" IDC-P (blue) and patients with immunologically "hot" IDC-P (red), depending on the density in hotspots (**b**). (**a**) On the left side: cell-density scale from dark blue (low) to dark red (high). Each row corresponds to a patient and missing slides/quantification data are represented by black squares. One IDC-P-positive patient with two missing quantification data was excluded, bringing the total number of patients to 29. (**b**) The p-values were calculated using the log-rank test. Three-, five- and ten-year survival rates are indicated in the bottom left of each graph. ADT: androgen-deprivation therapy; BCR: biochemical recurrence; CRPC: castration-resistant prostate cancer; IDC-P: intraductal carcinoma of the prostate; PCa: prostate cancer.

We also generated Kaplan–Meier curves to explore the association between the expression of CD68, CD163 and CD209 and the clinical outcomes, according to the two groups: "cold/intermediate" or "hot" IDC-P hotspots (Figure 8b). The median follow-up of the 29 patients was 172 months (IQR: 96–209). Higher expressions of immune APC still tended to be associated with worse prognoses. Despite our small number of patients, we found that the median time to metastasis (number of events = 11) and PCa-related death (number of events = 10) was significantly shorter in the patients with "hot" APC hotspots (65 months, 95% confidence interval (CI): 0–184 vs. median survival not yet reached in patients in the "cold/intermediate" group, with $p = 0.014$ for metastasis; and 98 months, 95% CI: 0–262 vs. median survival not yet reached in patients in the "cold/intermediate" group, with $p = 0.009$ for PCa-specific death) (Figure 8b).

When clinico-pathological characteristics of patients with immunologically "cold", "intermediate" or "hot" IDC-P were compared, extraprostatic extension was the only characteristic that was found to be more frequent in the "cold" total-IDC-P group than in the "hot/intermediate" total-IDC-P group (88% vs. 54%, $p = 0.049$; Table 3).

Table 3. Association of clinical and pathological variables with immunologically "cold", "intermediate" or "hot" IDC-P.

Characteristics	Total IDC-P			CD68/CD163/CD209 Hotspots		
	Cold $n = 17$	Hot and Intermediate $n = 13$	*p*-Value	Cold and Intermediate $n = 22$	Hot $n = 7$	*p*-Value
Mean age at diagnosis (SD)	64.6 (5)	65.5 (6)	0.650 [a]	65.9 (5)	61.7 (7)	0.149 [a]
Mean pre-operative PSA (SD)	11.4 (9)	13.5 (10)	0.476 [a]	13.4 (10)	8.7 (4)	0.524 [a]
Stage pT *, *n* (%)			1.000 [a]			0.162 [a]
pT2	2 (12)	3 (23)		4 (8)	1 (14)	
pT3a	6 (35)	2 (15)		8 (36)	0 (0)	
pT3b-pT4	9 (53)	8 (62)		10 (46)	6 (86)	
Grade group *, *n* (%)			0.575 [a]			0.182 [a]
1–2	10 (59)	6 (46)		14 (64)	2 (29)	
3	1 (6)	1 (8)		1 (5)	1 (14)	
4–5	6 (35)	6 (46)		7 (32)	4 (57)	
Lymph-node involvement, *n* (%)	6 (35)	7 (54)	0.460 [b]	8 (36)	4 (57)	0.403 [c]
Lymphovascular invasion, *n* (%)	5 (29)	5 (39)	0.694 [c]	6 (27)	3 (50)	0.352 [c]
Positive margins, *n* (%)	13 (77)	12 (92)	0.355 [c]	17 (77)	7 (100)	0.296 [c]
Extraprostatic extension, *n* (%)	15 (88)	7 (54)	**0.049** [c]	17 (77)	4 (57)	0.357 [c]
Seminal vesicle invasion, *n* (%)	10 (59)	8 (62)	1.000 [b]	11 (50)	6 (86)	0.187 [c]
Median follow-up in years (IQR)	16.5 (8–18)	12.4 (5–16)	0.263 [a]	15.3 (8–19)	8.2 (2–17)	0.149 [a]

IDC-P: intraductal carcinoma of the prostate; SD: standard deviation; PSA: prostate-specific antigen; PCa: prostate cancer; IQR: inter-quartile range. * pT3b–pT4 stages and grade groups 1–2 and 4–5 were combined because of the small number of patients. Bold entities indicate statistically significant *p*-values. [a] Mann–Whitney *U* test; [b] Pearson's chi-square test; [c] Fisher's exact test.

Notably, four men were in both the "hot/intermediate" IDC-P group, according to the cell densities in the total IDC-P ($n = 13$) and in the "hot" IDC-P group, according to the hotspots ($n = 7$). In addition, three out of the seven men (43%) in the latter group had comedonecrosis in at least one of their slides (CD68: one slide, comedonecrosis in 3/196 affected ducts; CD163: one slide, comedonecrosis in 2/78 affected ducts, CD209: two slides, comedonecrosis in 1/190 and 1/111 affected ducts) and only CD68$^+$ cells were found in the necrotic region of one slide.

4. Discussion

Intraductal carcinoma of the prostate is linked to metastasis and lethality in PCa [16]. In this exploratory study, we are the first to explore the immune infiltrate of IDC-P, an aggressive histologic subtype of PCa characterized by the growth of cancer cells within the prostatic ducts. We found that the immune microenvironment of IDC-P is distinct from that of the adjacent invasive carcinoma. Specifically, $CD163^+$ M2-type macrophages and $CD68^+$ macrophages, $FoxP3^+$ T cells and $CD209^+$ and $CD83^+$ dendritic cells are often less abundant in IDC-P than in the adjacent invasive PCa. Furthermore, the IDC-P patients were separated into groups, according to the immune-cell densities in the total IDC-P or in the IDC-P-immune hotspots. Regardless of category, patients with "colder" IDC-P tend to have better survival rates than patients with more leucocytes in IDC-P. Moreover, we found an association between the development of metastasis and PCa-specific death in men with higher expressions of CD68, CD163 and CD209 in IDC-P-immune hotspots.

Until now, TILs in PCa were assessed in areas containing conventional invasive carcinoma, or without addressing the presence of IDC-P. However, IDC-P alone has been associated with shorter disease-specific survival in men with localized PCa and men with high-risk PCa [16], making it an attractive lesion in which to study the immune response associated with lethal PCa. We found that the immune infiltrates of IDC-P were mainly reduced compared to randomly selected regions in the benign tissues, the tumor margins and, most importantly, in the adjacent invasive cancers. An explanation for this could be related to the association of IDC-P with hypoxia [45]. Indeed, hypoxic environments are believed to be highly immunosuppressive [46]. Furthermore, in our study, the immunosuppressive environment in IDC-P was even more pronounced in association with APC (dendritic cells and macrophages). These findings suggest that the immune environment of IDC-P is different from those in the adjacent carcinoma and other surrounding tissues, and might be better suitable for the study of the tumor microenvironment in the context of aggressive PCa.

Most studies assessing tumor-infiltrating immune cells in PCa and clinical outcomes suggested that the high expression of TILs is associated with poor prognosis. The first studies on this topic date back to the 1990s, when Vesalainen et al. [47] and then Irani et al. [48] visually semi-quantified TILs in H&E-stained PCa tissues. The first group ($n = 325$) found that a low expression of TILs was associated with the development of distant metastasis (univariate analysis: $p = 0.016$) and with lethal disease in patients without metastasis at diagnosis (multivariate hazard ratio (HR): 0.67, CI: 0.47–0.95, $p = 0.012$) and patients with organ-confined disease and without metastasis at diagnosis (multivariate HR: 0.44, 95% CI: 0.23–0.84, $p = 0.041$) [47]. The second group ($n = 161$) found that a high expression of stromal TILs was associated with an increased risk of post-RP BCR (multivariate relative risk (RR): 2.35, 95% CI: 1.08–5.08, $p = 0.03$) [48].

From the 2000s onwards, the quantification of leucocytes on IHC-stained PCa tissues was performed, with most studies focusing on T lymphocytes. Ness et al. [10] found that a high expression of $CD8^+$ in the epithelial compartment and in the total tumor was an independent predictor of shorter BCR-free survival in tissue microarrays (TMAs) from 535 RP specimens (multivariate HR: 1.45, CI 95%: 1.03–2.03, $p = 0.032$ and multivariate HR: 1.57, CI 95%: 1.13–2.17, $p = 0.007$, respectively). However, in their cohort of 11 RP and 68 transurethral-resection-tissue specimens, McArdle et al. [11] noted that an increased density of $CD4^+$ cells, but not of $CD8^+$ cells, was independently associated with poorer disease-specific survival (multivariate HR: 2.29, 95% CI: 1.25–4.22, $p = 0.008$). Using a digital approach, Richardsen et al. [12] observed that men with metastatic PCa ($n = 32$) had a higher expression of $CD3^+$ T cells in the epithelial ($p = 0.007$) and stromal ($p < 0.0001$) compartments than men with non-metastatic disease ($n = 27$). Kärjä et al. [13] added B lymphocytes in their study and found that high expressions of $CD4^+$, $CD8^+$ and $CD20^+$ were independent predictors of shorter BCR-free survival in TMAs from 188 RP specimens (multivariate HR: 0.18, 95% CI: 0.07–0.44, $p = 0.012$). Furthermore, Flammiger et al. [49] found that very low or very high expressions of $CD3^+$ cells were associated with shorter BCR-free survival compared to the intermediate expression of $CD3^+$ cells in a large cohort of TMAs collected from 2144 RP specimens (univariate analysis: $p = 0.0188$), while $CD20^+$-cell density was not associated with prognosis. The same researchers [50] then suggested that a high expression of $FoxP3^+$ T cells was associated with reduced BCR-free survival in a univariate analysis ($p = 0.0151$), but this result was not upheld by their multivariate analysis (n = 1463). Similarly, Davidsson et al. [15] observed in their TMA cohort that a high expression of regulatory T lymphocytes increased the odds of dying of PCa by 12% (multivariate odds ratio: 1.12; 95% CI: 1.02–1.23), but that this was not the case with helper or cytotoxic T cells (n = 663). More recently, Kaur et al. [14] used an automated quantification method to assess $CD3^+$, $CD8^+$ and $FoxP3^+$ lymphocytes in a TMA cohort comprising 312 PCa patients, including 212 (68%) African-American patients. With BCR and the development of metastasis as endpoints, only high densities of $FoxP3^+$ cells (top tertile) remained significantly associated with an increased risk of metastasis according to the researchers' multivariate analysis (HR: 12.89, 95% CI: 1.59–104.40, p = 0.02).

Very few studies examined APC in PCa tissues. In the aforementioned study by Richardsen et al. [12], higher percentages of $CD68^+$ cells were seen in the epithelial and stromal primary-tumor compartments of non-metastatic cancers compared to metastatic cancers (48% vs. 28%, p = 0.029 in the epithelial compartment; 54% vs. 14%, p = 0.008 in the stromal compartment, respectively) (n = 59). Moreover, Comito et al. [51] focused on $CD68^+$ and $CD163^+$ macrophages in hotspots identified in RP specimens from 93 patients with clinically localized PCa. They found that M1 macrophages were more abundant in organ-confined diseases upon final evaluation compared to cancers that presented with extraprostatic extension ($\approx$18 cells/mm^2 vs. 5 cells/mm^2). In contrast, M2 macrophages were associated with extraprostatic extension (multivariate RR: 0.30, 95% CI: 0.09–0.89, p = 0.03). Patients with a prevalence of M2 macrophages also tended to have shorter BCR-free survival than patients with a prevalence of M1 macrophages, but statistical significance was not reached. In addition, Calagua et al. [52] found a correlation between $CD8^+$ T cells and APC niches (R^2 = 0.57, p = 0.0001) through multiplex immunofluorescence, suggesting an important role of APC in T-cell response (n = 20).

In our study, we found a correlation between T cells and APC in IDC-P, particularly with M2 macrophages (r = 0.59, p = 0.002) and mature dendritic cells (r = 0.48, p = 0.013). In contrast, no correlation was found between T cells and immature dendritic cells. Despite the immunosuppressive microenvironment of IDC-P, we separated our IDC-P patients into groups according to their immune-cell densities: patients with immunologically "cold" IDC-P and patients with immunologically "hot" IDC-P. Probably due to the small number of patients with IDC-P and, hence, the limited statistical power of our study, we did not find any significant differences in survival between the men with globally "cold" IDC-P and the men with globally "hot/intermediate" IDC-P. However, when we examined the immune hotspots in IDC-P, we found that the $CD68^+$ and $CD163^+$ macrophages and $CD209^+$ immature dendritic cells were associated with poor prognosis. Immune hotspots have been studied in breast cancer, among others, in which they were found to be associated with better prognosis in estrogen-receptor-negative tumors [53], but were also associated with poorer prognosis in estrogen-receptor-positive tumors [54]. In our cohort, CD68/CD163/CD209-immune hotspots predicted progression to metastatic disease and cancer-specific survival. Altogether, and in accordance with most PCa studies, our results tend to show that increased IDC-P infiltration is associated with poorer prognosis.

The reasons why higher immune-cell densities are associated with worse prognoses in PCa are still not understood. They could be related to the tumors themselves, as well as the tumor microenvironment. Some studies sought explanations by examining alterations in gene expression. Amongst these studies, Kaur et al. [14] showed that higher T-lymphocyte densities were associated with ERG expression (median: 309 vs. 188 $CD3^+$ T cells/mm^2; p = 0.0004) and PTEN loss (median: 317 vs. 192 $CD3^+$ T cells/mm^2; p = 0.001). Similarly, Calagua et al. [52] found that the deletion of *BRCA* and/or *RB1* was more frequent in their subset of 11 immunogenic patients than in the localized PCa data obtained from the TCGA Firehose legacy (*BRCA2* deletion: p = 0.053, *RB1* deletion: p = 0.017, co-deletion of *BRCA2/RB1*: p = 0.053, focal co-deletion of *BRCA2/RB1*: p = 0.039; n = 489). Both ERG expression and PTEN loss [55,56], as well as the co-loss of BRCA2/RB1, have been associated with aggressive forms of PCa [57]. Interestingly, a few limited studies linked $BRCA^{mut}$ to IDC-P [16].

Our study has limitations that warrant discussion. The main limitation is the small number of patients with IDC-P in our cohort (n = 33). However, IDC-P is often focal, with more than 75% of specimens with IDC-P harboring IDC-P in less than 5% of the full tumor volume [58]. Furthermore, the evaluation of the inflammatory infiltrate of adjacent invasive carcinoma, tumor margins and benign glands requires spatial localization, which cannot be provided by biopsies and TMAs. These limitations in sample availability could explain why the immune infiltrate of IDC-P have not yet been described. Our findings must still be replicated in larger independent cohorts, but our work was essential to begin to unravel the signification of the immune infiltrate in IDC-P. Larger cohorts will also allow to separately evaluate men with immunologically "intermediate" IDC-P and the performance of multivariate analyses. Moreover, we only examined one representative block per patient, meaning that the patients in the IDC-P-negative group could have had IDC-P in other tissue blocks. However, despite this, IDC-P was still associated with poor prognoses and adverse pathological features in our cohort [16]. Furthermore, we performed single-color IHC to characterize the immune cells in PCa instead of multiplex immunofluorescence, which would have permitted us to assess the colocalization of the markers and quantify all the markers on the same slides, in addition to allow for the confirmation of the presence of basal cells around IDC-P. In addition, we examined T lymphocytes and macrophages, but other key immune cells [59], such as B lymphocytes, natural killer cells, classical neutrophiles and monocytes and myeloid-derived suppressor cells [60] should be included in further research. Futures studies will incorporate these leucocytes in addition to other key actors in the immune response. However, our study highlights the importance of evaluating IDC-P in the study of the immune environment of PCa.

5. Conclusions

In conclusion, we found that the immune infiltrate of IDC-P is different from that in the adjacent invasive carcinoma, while the overall immune infiltration is not affected by the IDC-P status. Antigen-presenting cells are particularly less abundant in IDC-P compared to cancer in general. Moreover, IDC-P can be classified as immunologically "cold" or "hot", depending on the immune-cell densities. In this study, these groups were associated with different clinical outcomes, and CD68/CD163/CD209-immune hotspots predicted progression to metastatic disease and cancer-specific survival. Our study highlights the need to better characterize the immune microenvironment of IDC-P and evaluate its involvement in the poor prognoses of men with IDC-P.

Supplementary Materials: The following supporting information can be downloaded at: https://www.mdpi.com/article/10.3390/cancers15082217/s1. Figure S1: Parallel coordinate plots showing the changes in immune-cell density between the cancer compartments and benign tissues (a), margins (b) and IDC-P (c) in patients with IDC-P; Figure S2: Parallel coordinate plots showing the changes in immune-cell density between the margin and benign tissues (a), cancer regions (b) and IDC-P (c) in patients with IDC-P.

Author Contributions: Conceptualization, M.-K.D. and D.T.; methodology, M.-K.D. and D.T.; formal analysis, M.-K.D.; investigation, M.-K.D., O.E.M., M.B., H.L., B.T. and D.T.; resources, H.H., A.B. and Y.F.; writing—original draft preparation, M.-K.D. and D.T.; writing—review and editing, M.-K.D., O.E.M., H.L., B.T., L.L., A.B. and D.T.; visualization, D.T. and M.-K.D.; supervision, D.T., A.B. and Y.F.; funding acquisition, H.L., B.T., L.L., A.B., Y.F. and D.T. All authors have read and agreed to the published version of the manuscript.

Funding: This research was funded by Prostate Cancer Canada with funds from the Movember Foundation, grant number 2012-927, the Canadian Institutes of Health Research—Institute of Cancer Research (CIHR-ICR) and the Cancer Research Society (CRS), grant number CRP-154487, startup funds from the Institut du cancer de Montréal and by internal funds from the Laboratoire d'Uro-Oncologie Expérimentale. M.-K.D. received salary support from the Université de Montréal and the Institut du cancer de Montréal. D.T. receives salary support from the Fonds de recherche du Québec-Santé (FRQS) (Clinical Research Scholar, Junior 2). The CRCHUM and CRCHUQc-UL receive support from the FRQS.

Institutional Review Board Statement: The study was conducted in accordance with the Declaration of Helsinki and approved by the Ethics Committee of the CHU de Québec-Université Laval (protocol code: 2012-1059; date of approval: 10 September 2012) and the Ethics Committee of the CHUM (protocol code: MP-02-2018-7450, date of approval: 28 September 2017).

Informed Consent Statement: Informed consent was obtained from all subjects involved in the study.

Data Availability Statement: The data presented in this study are available on request from the corresponding author. The data are not publicly available due to ethical restrictions.

Acknowledgments: URO-1 Biobank at CHU de Québec-Université Laval is affiliated with the Réseau de Recherche sur le cancer of the FRQS and registered to the Canadian Tumor Repository Network (CTRNet). We thank the patients for agreeing to donate their prostate specimens and data for research and all staff members who participated in the biobanking of biological samples and data.

Conflicts of Interest: The authors declare no conflict of interest. The funders had no role in the design of the study; in the collection, analyses, or interpretation of data; in the writing of the manuscript; or in the decision to publish the results.

References

1. Havel, J.J.; Chowell, D.; Chan, T.A. The evolving landscape of biomarkers for checkpoint inhibitor immunotherapy. *Nat. Rev. Cancer* **2019**, *19*, 133–150. [CrossRef] [PubMed]
2. Zhang, Y.; Zhang, Z. The history and advances in cancer immunotherapy: Understanding the characteristics of tumor-infiltrating immune cells and their therapeutic implications. *Cell. Mol. Immunol.* **2020**, *17*, 807–821. [CrossRef] [PubMed]
3. Kruger, S.; Ilmer, M.; Kobold, S.; Cadilha, B.L.; Endres, S.; Ormanns, S.; Schuebbe, G.; Renz, B.W.; D'Haese, J.G.; Schloesser, H.; et al. Advances in cancer immunotherapy 2019—Latest trends. *J. Exp. Clin. Cancer Res.* **2019**, *38*, 268. [CrossRef] [PubMed]
4. Gulley, J.L.; Borre, M.; Vogelzang, N.J.; Ng, S.; Agarwal, N.; Parker, C.C.; Pook, D.W.; Rathenborg, P.; Flaig, T.W.; Carles, J.; et al. Phase III Trial of PROSTVAC in Asymptomatic or Minimally Symptomatic Metastatic Castration-Resistant Prostate Cancer. *J. Clin. Oncol.* **2019**, *37*, 1051–1061. [CrossRef]
5. Narayan, V.; Barber-Rotenberg, J.S.; Jung, I.Y.; Lacey, S.F.; Rech, A.J.; Davis, M.M.; Hwang, W.T.; Lal, P.; Carpenter, E.L.; Maude, S.L.; et al. PSMA-targeting TGFβ-insensitive armored CAR T cells in metastatic castration-resistant prostate cancer: A phase 1 trial. *Nat. Med.* **2022**, *28*, 724–734. [CrossRef]
6. Antonarakis, E.S.; Piulats, J.M.; Gross-Goupil, M.; Goh, J.; Ojamaa, K.; Hoimes, C.J.; Vaishampayan, U.; Berger, R.; Sezer, A.; Alanko, T.; et al. Pembrolizumab for Treatment-Refractory Metastatic Castration-Resistant Prostate Cancer: Multicohort, Open-Label Phase II KEYNOTE-199 Study. *J. Clin. Oncol.* **2020**, *38*, 395–405. [CrossRef]
7. Kantoff, P.W.; Higano, C.S.; Shore, N.D.; Berger, E.R.; Small, E.J.; Penson, D.F.; Redfern, C.H.; Ferrari, A.C.; Dreicer, R.; Sims, R.B.; et al. Sipuleucel-T immunotherapy for castration-resistant prostate cancer. *N. Engl. J. Med.* **2010**, *363*, 411–422. [CrossRef]
8. Le, D.T.; Uram, J.N.; Wang, H.; Bartlett, B.R.; Kemberling, H.; Eyring, A.D.; Skora, A.D.; Luber, B.S.; Azad, N.S.; Laheru, D.; et al. PD-1 Blockade in Tumors with Mismatch-Repair Deficiency. *N. Engl. J. Med.* **2015**, *372*, 2509–2520. [CrossRef]
9. Abida, W.; Cheng, M.L.; Armenia, J.; Middha, S.; Autio, K.A.; Vargas, H.A.; Rathkopf, D.; Morris, M.J.; Danila, D.C.; Slovin, S.F.; et al. Analysis of the Prevalence of Microsatellite Instability in Prostate Cancer and Response to Immune Checkpoint Blockade. *JAMA Oncol.* **2019**, *5*, 471–478. [CrossRef]
10. Ness, N.; Andersen, S.; Valkov, A.; Nordby, Y.; Donnem, T.; Al-Saad, S.; Busund, L.T.; Bremnes, R.M.; Richardsen, E. Infiltration of CD8+ lymphocytes is an independent prognostic factor of biochemical failure-free survival in prostate cancer. *Prostate* **2014**, *74*, 1452–1461. [CrossRef]
11. McArdle, P.A.; Canna, K.; McMillan, D.C.; McNicol, A.M.; Campbell, R.; Underwood, M.A. The relationship between T-lymphocyte subset infiltration and survival in patients with prostate cancer. *Br. J. Cancer* **2004**, *91*, 541–543. [CrossRef]
12. Richardsen, E.; Uglehus, R.D.; Due, J.; Busch, C.; Busund, L.T. The prognostic impact of M-CSF, CSF-1 receptor, CD68 and CD3 in prostatic carcinoma. *Histopathology* **2008**, *53*, 30–38. [CrossRef]
13. Kärjä, V.; Aaltomaa, S.; Lipponen, P.; Isotalo, T.; Talja, M.; Mokka, R. Tumour-infiltrating lymphocytes: A prognostic factor of PSA-free survival in patients with local prostate carcinoma treated by radical prostatectomy. *Anticancer. Res.* **2005**, *25*, 4435–4438.
14. Kaur, H.B.; Guedes, L.B.; Lu, J.; Maldonado, L.; Reitz, L.; Barber, J.R.; De Marzo, A.M.; Tosoian, J.J.; Tomlins, S.A.; Schaeffer, E.M.; et al. Association of tumor-infiltrating T-cell density with molecular subtype, racial ancestry and clinical outcomes in prostate cancer. *Mod. Pathol.* **2018**, *31*, 1539–1552. [CrossRef]
15. Davidsson, S.; Ohlson, A.L.; Andersson, S.O.; Fall, K.; Meisner, A.; Fiorentino, M.; Andrén, O.; Rider, J.R. CD4 helper T cells, CD8 cytotoxic T cells, and FOXP3(+) regulatory T cells with respect to lethal prostate cancer. *Mod. Pathol.* **2013**, *26*, 448–455. [CrossRef]
16. Pantazopoulos, H.; Diop, M.K.; Grosset, A.A.; Rouleau-Gagné, F.; Al-Saleh, A.; Boblea, T.; Trudel, D. Intraductal Carcinoma of the Prostate as a Cause of Prostate Cancer Metastasis: A Molecular Portrait. *Cancers* **2022**, *14*, 820. [CrossRef]
17. Humphrey, P.A.; Moch, H.; Cubilla, A.L.; Ulbright, T.M.; Reuter, V.E. The 2016 WHO Classification of Tumours of the Urinary System and Male Genital Organs-Part B: Prostate and Bladder Tumours. *Eur. Urol.* **2016**, *70*, 106–119. [CrossRef]

18. Guo, C.C.; Epstein, J.I. Intraductal carcinoma of the prostate on needle biopsy: Histologic features and clinical significance. *Mod. Pathol.* **2006**, *19*, 1528–1535. [CrossRef]
19. Haffner, M.C.; Weier, C.; Xu, M.M.; Vaghasia, A.; Gürel, B.; Gümüşkaya, B.; Esopi, D.M.; Fedor, H.; Tan, H.-L.; Kulac, I.; et al. Molecular evidence that invasive adenocarcinoma can mimic prostatic intraepithelial neoplasia (PIN) and intraductal carcinoma through retrograde glandular colonization. *J. Pathol.* **2016**, *238*, 31–41. [CrossRef]
20. Miyai, K.; Divatia, M.K.; Shen, S.S.; Miles, B.J.; Ayala, A.G.; Ro, J.Y. Heterogeneous clinicopathological features of intraductal carcinoma of the prostate: A comparison between "precursor-like" and "regular type" lesions. *Int. J. Clin. Exp. Pathol.* **2014**, *7*, 2518–2526.
21. Porter, L.H.; Lawrence, M.G.; Ilic, D.; Clouston, D.; Bolton, D.M.; Frydenberg, M.; Murphy, D.G.; Pezaro, C.; Risbridger, G.P.; Taylor, R.A. Systematic Review Links the Prevalence of Intraductal Carcinoma of the Prostate to Prostate Cancer Risk Categories. *Eur. Urol.* **2017**, *72*, 492–495. [CrossRef] [PubMed]
22. McNeal, J.E.; Yemoto, C.E.M. Spread of Adenocarcinoma Within Prostatic Ducts and Acini: Morphologic and Clinical Correlations. *Am. J. Surg. Pathol.* **1996**, *20*, 802–814. [CrossRef] [PubMed]
23. Wilcox, G.; Soh, S.; Chakraborty, S.; Scardino, P.T.; Wheeler, T.M. Patterns of high-grade prostatic intraepithelial neoplasia associated with clinically aggressive prostate cancer. *Hum. Pathol.* **1998**, *29*, 1119–1123. [CrossRef] [PubMed]
24. Cohen, R.J.; Chan, W.C.; Edgar, S.G.; Robinson, E.; Dodd, N.; Hoscek, S.; Mundy, I.P. Prediction of pathological stage and clinical outcome in prostate cancer: An improved pre-operative model incorporating biopsy-determined intraductal carcinoma. *Br. J. Urol.* **1998**, *81*, 413–418. [CrossRef]
25. Zhao, T.; Liao, B.; Yao, J.; Liu, J.; Huang, R.; Shen, P.; Peng, Z.; Gui, H.; Chen, X.; Zhang, P.; et al. Is there any prognostic impact of intraductal carcinoma of prostate in initial diagnosed aggressively metastatic prostate cancer? *Prostate* **2015**, *75*, 225–232. [CrossRef]
26. Kato, M.; Kimura, K.; Hirakawa, A.; Kobayashi, Y.; Ishida, R.; Kamihira, O.; Majima, T.; Funahashi, Y.; Sassa, N.; Matsukawa, Y.; et al. Prognostic parameter for high risk prostate cancer patients at initial presentation. *Prostate* **2018**, *78*, 11–16. [CrossRef]
27. Zhao, J.; Liu, J.; Sun, G.; Zhang, M.; Chen, J.; Shen, P.; Liu, Z.; Liao, B.; Zhang, X.; Gong, J.; et al. The Prognostic Value of the Proportion and Architectural Patterns of Intraductal Carcinoma of the Prostate in Patients with De Novo Metastatic Prostate Cancer. *J. Urol.* **2019**, *201*, 759–768. [CrossRef]
28. Kato, M.; Tsuzuki, T.; Kimura, K.; Hirakawa, A.; Kinoshita, F.; Sassa, N.; Ishida, R.; Fukatsu, A.; Kimura, T.; Funahashi, Y.; et al. The presence of intraductal carcinoma of the prostate in needle biopsy is a significant prognostic factor for prostate cancer patients with distant metastasis at initial presentation. *Mod. Pathol.* **2016**, *29*, 166–173. [CrossRef]
29. Zhao, J.; Sun, G.; Liao, B.; Zhang, X.; Armstrong, C.M.; Yin, X.; Liu, J.; Chen, J.; Yang, Y.; Zhao, P.; et al. Novel nomograms for castration-resistant prostate cancer and survival outcome in patients with de novo bone metastatic prostate cancer. *BJU Int.* **2018**, *122*, 994–1002. [CrossRef]
30. Zhao, J.; Shen, P.; Sun, G.; Chen, N.; Liu, J.; Tang, X.; Huang, R.; Cai, D.; Gong, J.; Zhang, X.; et al. The prognostic implication of intraductal carcinoma of the prostate in metastatic castration-resistant prostate cancer and its potential predictive value in those treated with docetaxel or abiraterone as first-line therapy. *Oncotarget* **2017**, *8*, 55374–55383. [CrossRef]
31. Dinerman, B.F.; Khani, F.; Golan, R.; Bernstein, A.N.; Cosiano, M.F.; Margolis, D.J.; Hu, J.C. Population-based study of the incidence and survival for intraductal carcinoma of the prostate. *Urol. Oncol.* **2017**, *35*, 673.e9–673.e14. [CrossRef]
32. Saeter, T.; Vlatkovic, L.; Waaler, G.; Servoll, E.; Nesland, J.M.; Axcrona, K.; Axcrona, U. Intraductal Carcinoma of the Prostate on Diagnostic Needle Biopsy Predicts Prostate Cancer Mortality: A Population-Based Study. *Prostate* **2017**, *77*, 859–865. [CrossRef]
33. Tom, M.C.; Nguyen, J.K.; Lucianò, R.; Mian, O.Y.; Stephans, K.L.; Ciezki, J.P.; Smile, T.D.; Wei, W.; McKenney, J.K.; Magi-Galluzzi, C.; et al. Impact of Cribriform Pattern and Intraductal Carcinoma on Gleason 7 Prostate Cancer Treated with External Beam Radiotherapy. *J. Urol.* **2019**, *202*, 710–716. [CrossRef]
34. Kimura, K.; Tsuzuki, T.; Kato, M.; Saito, A.M.; Sassa, N.; Ishida, R.; Hirabayashi, H.; Yoshino, Y.; Hattori, R.; Gotoh, M. Prognostic value of intraductal carcinoma of the prostate in radical prostatectomy specimens. *Prostate* **2014**, *74*, 680–687. [CrossRef]
35. van Leenders, G.; van der Kwast, T.H.; Iczkowski, K.A. The 2019 International Society of Urological Pathology Consensus Conference on Prostate Cancer Grading. *Eur. Urol.* **2021**, *79*, 707–709. [CrossRef]
36. Epstein, J.I.; Amin, M.B.; Fine, S.W.; Algaba, F.; Aron, M.; Baydar, D.E.; Beltran, A.L.; Brimo, F.; Cheville, J.C.; Colecchia, M.; et al. The 2019 Genitourinary Pathology Society (GUPS) White Paper on Contemporary Grading of Prostate Cancer. *Arch. Pathol. Lab. Med.* **2021**, *145*, 461–493. [CrossRef]
37. Varma, M. Intraductal Carcinoma of the Prostate: A Guide for the Practicing Pathologist. *Adv. Anat. Pathol.* **2021**, *28*, 276–287. [CrossRef]
38. Amin, M.B.; Edge, S.; Greene, F.; Byrd, D.R.; Brookland, R.K.; Washington, M.K.; Gershenwald, J.E.; Compton, C.C.; Hess, K.R.; Sullivan, D.C.; et al. *AJCC Cancer Staging Manual*, 8th ed.; Springer International Publishing: Cham, Switzerland, 2017; p. 1032.
39. Scher, H.I.; Halabi, S.; Tannock, I.; Morris, M.; Sternberg, C.N.; Carducci, M.A.; Eisenberger, M.A.; Higano, C.; Bubley, G.J.; Dreicer, R.; et al. Design and end points of clinical trials for patients with progressive prostate cancer and castrate levels of testosterone: Recommendations of the Prostate Cancer Clinical Trials Working Group. *J. Clin. Oncol.* **2008**, *26*, 1148–1159. [CrossRef]
40. Altman, D.G.; McShane, L.M.; Sauerbrei, W.; Taube, S.E. Reporting Recommendations for Tumor Marker Prognostic Studies (REMARK): Explanation and elaboration. *PLoS Med.* **2012**, *9*, e1001216. [CrossRef]

41. Schober, P.; Boer, C.; Schwarte, L.A. Correlation Coefficients: Appropriate Use and Interpretation. *Anesth. Analg.* **2018**, *126*, 1763–1768. [CrossRef]
42. Wickham, H. *ggplot2: Elegant Graphics for Data Analysis*, 2nd ed.; Springer: New York, NY, USA, 2016; p. 276.
43. Xu, S.; Chen, M.; Feng, T.; Zhan, L.; Zhou, L.; Yu, G. Use ggbreak to Effectively Utilize Plotting Space to Deal With Large Datasets and Outliers. *Front. Genet.* **2021**, *12*, 774846. [CrossRef] [PubMed]
44. Warnes, G.; Bolker, B.; Bonebakker, L.; Gentleman, R.; Huber, W.; Liaw, A.; Lumley, T.; Maechler, M.; Magnusson, A.; Moeller, S.; et al. *gplots: Various R Programming Tools for Plotting Data*; R Package Version 3.1.3; CRAN: Wien, Austria, 2022.
45. Chua, M.L.K.; Lo, W.; Pintilie, M.; Murgic, J.; Lalonde, E.; Bhandari, V.; Mahamud, O.; Gopalan, A.; Kweldam, C.F.; van Leenders, G.; et al. A Prostate Cancer "Nimbosus": Genomic Instability and SChLAP1 Dysregulation Underpin Aggression of Intraductal and Cribriform Subpathologies. *Eur. Urol.* **2017**, *72*, 665–674. [CrossRef] [PubMed]
46. Motz, G.T.; Santoro, S.P.; Wang, L.P.; Garrabrant, T.; Lastra, R.R.; Hagemann, I.S.; Lal, P.; Feldman, M.D.; Benencia, F.; Coukos, G. Tumor endothelium FasL establishes a selective immune barrier promoting tolerance in tumors. *Nat. Med.* **2014**, *20*, 607–615. [CrossRef] [PubMed]
47. Vesalainen, S.; Lipponen, P.; Talja, M.; Syrjänen, K. Histological grade, perineural infiltration, tumour-infiltrating lymphocytes and apoptosis as determinants of long-term prognosis in prostatic adenocarcinoma. *Eur. J. Cancer* **1994**, *30*, 1797–1803. [CrossRef] [PubMed]
48. Irani, J.; Goujon, J.M.; Ragni, E.; Peyrat, L.; Hubert, J.; Saint, F.; Mottet, N. High-grade inflammation in prostate cancer as a prognostic factor for biochemical recurrence after radical prostatectomy. Pathologist Multi Center Study Group. *Urology* **1999**, *54*, 467–472. [CrossRef]
49. Flammiger, A.; Bayer, F.; Cirugeda-Kühnert, A.; Huland, H.; Tennstedt, P.; Simon, R.; Minner, S.; Bokemeyer, C.; Sauter, G.; Schlomm, T.; et al. Intratumoral T but not B lymphocytes are related to clinical outcome in prostate cancer. *Apmis* **2012**, *120*, 901–908. [CrossRef]
50. Flammiger, A.; Weisbach, L.; Huland, H.; Tennstedt, P.; Simon, R.; Minner, S.; Bokemeyer, C.; Sauter, G.; Schlomm, T.; Trepel, M. High tissue density of FOXP3+ T cells is associated with clinical outcome in prostate cancer. *Eur. J. Cancer* **2013**, *49*, 1273–1279. [CrossRef]
51. Comito, G.; Giannoni, E.; Segura, C.P.; Barcellos-de-Souza, P.; Raspollini, M.R.; Baroni, G.; Lanciotti, M.; Serni, S.; Chiarugi, P. Cancer-associated fibroblasts and M2-polarized macrophages synergize during prostate carcinoma progression. *Oncogene* **2014**, *33*, 2423–2431. [CrossRef]
52. Calagua, C.; Ficial, M.; Jansen, C.S.; Hirz, T.; Del Balzo, L.; Wilkinson, S.; Lake, R.; Ku, A.T.; Voznesensky, O.; Sykes, D.B.; et al. A Subset of Localized Prostate Cancer Displays an Immunogenic Phenotype Associated with Losses of Key Tumor Suppressor Genes. *Clin. Cancer Res.* **2021**, *27*, 4836–4847. [CrossRef]
53. Nawaz, S.; Heindl, A.; Koelble, K.; Yuan, Y. Beyond immune density: Critical role of spatial heterogeneity in estrogen receptor-negative breast cancer. *Mod. Pathol.* **2015**, *28*, 766–777. [CrossRef]
54. Heindl, A.; Sestak, I.; Naidoo, K.; Cuzick, J.; Dowsett, M.; Yuan, Y. Relevance of Spatial Heterogeneity of Immune Infiltration for Predicting Risk of Recurrence After Endocrine Therapy of ER+ Breast Cancer. *J. Natl. Cancer Inst.* **2018**, *110*, 166–175. [CrossRef]
55. Leinonen, K.A.; Saramäki, O.R.; Furusato, B.; Kimura, T.; Takahashi, H.; Egawa, S.; Suzuki, H.; Keiger, K.; Ho Hahm, S.; Isaacs, W.B.; et al. Loss of PTEN is associated with aggressive behavior in ERG-positive prostate cancer. *Cancer Epidemiol. Biomarkers Prev.* **2013**, *22*, 2333–2344. [CrossRef]
56. Robinson, D.; Van Allen, E.M.; Wu, Y.M.; Schultz, N.; Lonigro, R.J.; Mosquera, J.M.; Montgomery, B.; Taplin, M.E.; Pritchard, C.C.; Attard, G.; et al. Integrative clinical genomics of advanced prostate cancer. *Cell* **2015**, *161*, 1215–1228. [CrossRef]
57. Chakraborty, G.; Armenia, J.; Mazzu, Y.Z.; Nandakumar, S.; Stopsack, K.H.; Atiq, M.O.; Komura, K.; Jehane, L.; Hirani, R.; Chadalavada, K.; et al. Significance of BRCA2 and RB1 Co-loss in Aggressive Prostate Cancer Progression. *Clin. Cancer Res.* **2020**, *26*, 2047–2064. [CrossRef]
58. Trudel, D.; Downes, M.R.; Sykes, J.; Kron, K.J.; Trachtenberg, J.; van der Kwast, T.H. Prognostic impact of intraductal carcinoma and large cribriform carcinoma architecture after prostatectomy in a contemporary cohort. *Eur. J. Cancer* **2014**, *50*, 1610–1616. [CrossRef]
59. Kwon, J.T.W.; Bryant, R.J.; Parkes, E.E. The tumor microenvironment and immune responses in prostate cancer patients. *Endocr. Relat. Cancer* **2021**, *28*, T95–T107. [CrossRef]
60. Veglia, F.; Sanseviero, E.; Gabrilovich, D.I. Myeloid-derived suppressor cells in the era of increasing myeloid cell diversity. *Nat. Rev. Immunol.* **2021**, *21*, 485–498. [CrossRef]

cancers

Article

Comparison of Four Validated Nomograms (Memorial Sloan Kettering Cancer Center, Briganti 2012, 2017, and 2019) Predicting Lymph Node Invasion in Patients with High-Risk Prostate Cancer Candidates for Radical Prostatectomy and Extended Pelvic Lymph Node Dissection: Clinical Experience and Review of the Literature

Giovanni Battista Di Pierro [1,*], Stefano Salciccia [1], Marco Frisenda [1], Antonio Tufano [1], Alessandro Sciarra [1], Emiliano Scarrone [1], Francesco Del Giudice [1], Vincenzo Asero [1], Giulio Bevilacqua [1], Martina Moriconi [1], Antonio Carbone [2], Antonio Pastore [2], Stefano Signore [3], Pierluigi Bove [4], Flavio Forte [5], Paolo Emiliozzi [6], Andrea Tubaro [7], Cosimo De Nunzio [7] and Vittorio Canale [1]

1 Department "Materno Infantile e Scienze Urologiche", Policlinico Umberto I, Sapienza University of Rome, 00161 Rome, Italy
2 Department of Urology, ICOT Latina, University Sapienza, 04100 Latina, Italy
3 Sant'Eugenio Hospital, 00144 Rome, Italy
4 San Carlo di Nancy Hospital, 00165 Rome, Italy
5 Vannini Hospital, 00177 Rome, Italy
6 San Camillo Hospital, 00152 Rome, Italy
7 Department of Urology, Ospedale Sant'Andrea, University Sapienza, 00189 Rome, Italy
* Correspondence: giovannibattista.dipierro@uniroma1.it; +39-0649977000

Citation: Di Pierro, G.B.; Salciccia, S.; Frisenda, M.; Tufano, A.; Sciarra, A.; Scarrone, E.; Del Giudice, F.; Asero, V.; Bevilacqua, G.; Moriconi, M.; et al. Comparison of Four Validated Nomograms (Memorial Sloan Kettering Cancer Center, Briganti 2012, 2017, and 2019) Predicting Lymph Node Invasion in Patients with High-Risk Prostate Cancer Candidates for Radical Prostatectomy and Extended Pelvic Lymph Node Dissection: Clinical Experience and Review of the Literature. *Cancers* **2023**, *15*, 1683. https://doi.org/10.3390/cancers15061683

Academic Editor: Kouji Izumi

Received: 30 January 2023
Revised: 2 March 2023
Accepted: 8 March 2023
Published: 9 March 2023

Simple Summary: The indication for ePLND at the time of RP is based on a risk assessment of LNI through validated nomograms such as the MSKCC; Briganti 2012; Briganti 2017 and Briganti 2019. However, in daily practice, a relevant percentage of cases, including those with the high-risk disease, show no LNI at the final histopathological assay pathology (pN0) after ePLND. Furthermore, currently available evidence does not demonstrate the superiority of one nomogram over the others, and there is still lacking data to support the routine use of one predictive model over another, even in more aggressive diseases. Therefore, we evaluated the accuracy of the most used nomograms (MSKCC, Briganti 2012, Briganti 2017, and Briganti 2019) for predicting LNI and compared them in our sub-cohort of high-risk PC patients treated with ePLND. We found that the predictive performance of the four nomograms as well as their ability to avoid unnecessary ePLND, are virtually the same, even in high-risk PC patients.

Abstract: Background: The indication for extended pelvic lymph node dissection (ePLND) at the time of radical prostatectomy (RP) is based on nomograms predicting the risk of lymph node invasion (LNI). However, limited data are available on the comparison of these predictive models in high-risk prostate cancer (PC) patients. Therefore, we compared the accuracy of the most used nomograms (MSKCC, Briganti 2012, 2017, and 2019) in the setting of high-risk PC patients submitted to ePLND. Methods: 150 patients with high-risk PC disease treated from 2019 to 2022 were included. Before RP + ePLND, we assessed the MSKCC, Briganti 2012, 2017, and 2019 nomograms for each patient, and we compared the prediction of LNI with the final histopathological analysis of the ePLND using pathologic results as a reference. Results: LNI was found in 39 patients (26%), and 71.3% were cT2. The percentage of patients with estimated LNI risk above the cut-off was significantly higher in pN+ cases than in pN0 for all Briganti nomograms. The percentage of patients at risk of LNI, according to Briganti Nomogram (2012, 2017, and 2019), was significantly higher in pN+ cases than in pN0 ($p < 0.04$), while MSKCC prediction didn't vary significantly between pN0 and pN+ groups ($p = 0.2$). All nomograms showed high sensitivity (Se > 0.90), low specificity (Sp < 0.20), and similar AUC (range: 0.526–0.573) in predicting pN+. Particularly, 74% of cases patients with MSKCC estimated risk > 7% showed pN0 compared to 71% with Briganti 2012 > 5%, 69% with Briganti 2017 > 7%, and 70% with Briganti 2019 > 7%. Conclusions: Despite the high-risk disease, in our patients treated with ePLND emerges a still high number of pN0 cases and a similar low specificity of nomograms in predicting LNI.

Keywords: prostatic neoplasm; extended pelvic lymph node dissection; nomograms; radical prostatectomy

1. Introduction

Prostate cancer (PC) is the most common urological cancer in men. In patients with non-metastatic disease eligible for radical prostatectomy (RP), current European Urological Association (EAU) guidelines recommend performing an extended pelvic lymph node dissection (ePLND) according to the risk for lymph node invasion (LNI) estimated by validated nomograms [1–4]. Overall, although current evidence shows no improved survival when associating an ePLND to RP [5] and no significant differences in terms of oncological outcomes between limited PLND and ePLND [6], the prognostic and staging role of ePLND is undiscussed [2,6]. Indeed, despite recent efforts to devlop new imaging techniques for nodal staging, they do not represent reliable tool to predict LNI due to (the) lack of sensitivity, and ePLND still remains the gold standard for the detection of lymph node invasion [2,5–10].

Since the performance of ePLND is associated with increased morbidity and higher costs [5], in everyday clinical practice, the indication for ePLND is usually assessed by available nomograms such as the Briganti 2012, Briganti 2017, Briganti 2019 or the MSKCC nomograms [2–4,7,8]. Recently, the Briganti 2019 nomogram has also incorporated the multiparametric magnetic resonance imaging (mpMRI) findings and mpMRI-targeted biopsy as parameters to be considered, with a threshold of 7% which would result in missing 1.5% of patients with LNI [7].

To date, in the literature, there are several studies investigating the accuracy of nomograms [8,11–21]. However, few studies have directly compared the accuracy of MSKCC, Briganti 2012, 2017, and 2019 nomograms. In addition, limited data are available on the comparison of these predictive models in a selected population with only high-risk prostate cancer (PC).

The aim of the present study is to compare the accuracy of the most used nomograms (MSKCC, Briganti 2012, 2017, and 2019) predicting LNI, specifically in patients with high-risk PC candidates to ePLND at the time of RP.

2. Materials and Methods

From 2019 to 2022, all patients with high-risk PC treated with RP and ePLND at our departments were retrospectively examined and included in the analysis. High-risk PC was defined according to both the EAU and D'Amico classification. All diagnostic and therapeutic procedures reflected our routine clinical practice in a department at a high volume for the management of PC disease. Inclusion criteria were: diagnosis of high-risk PC; no distant metastases at clinical staging; RP as chosen primary treatment decision after discussion of treatment options. Exclusion criteria were previous or current androgen deprivation therapy, chemotherapies, pelvic radiation therapy, or treatments with other agents that could influence prostate tumor growth and diffusion.

2.1. Nomogram Evaluation

Briganti 2012 [3], Briganti 2017 [4], Briganti 2019 [7], and MSKCC [8] nomograms were evaluated using preoperative clinical and pathological features in order to establish the probability of LNI. As previously described, the MSKCC nomogram is based on preoperative PSA, clinical stage, primary and secondary biopsy Gleason pattern as well as negative and positive biopsy cores; the Briganti 2012 nomogram is based on pretreatment preoperative PSA, clinical stage, primary and secondary biopsy Gleason score and percentage of positive cores; the Briganti 2017 based on includes preoperative PSA; clinical stage, biopsy Gleason grade, percentage of positive cores with the highest and with the lowest grade disease; the Briganti 2019 is based on pretreatment preoperative PSA, clinical stage, grade group at MR-targeted biopsy, the maximum diameter of the index lesion at mpMR, and the percentage of cores with clinically significant PC at systematic biopsy.

2.2. *Surgical Procedure and Pathologic Evaluation*

All the Procedures were performed using a standard robot-assisted (RARP) or pure laparoscopic (LRP) radical prostatectomy approach. Anatomical ePLND was performed in a standardized manner as previously described and included the removal of the nodes overlying the external iliac artery and vein, the nodes within the obturator fossa, and the nodes medial and lateral nodes to the internal iliac artery [22].

All histological specimens of prostatic biopsy and RP were analyzed by our uropathologists, with a long experience in the PC field. In all cases, they reported the Gleason score and grade groups according to the World Health Organization (WHO)/ISUP guidelines at biopsy and at surgery, pathologic staging using TNM classification, surgical margin (SM) status, and perineural invasion (PNI) were routinely defined in all cases. Lymph node involvement was defined as the presence of positive pelvic lymph nodes for PC at the histopathological assay. The outcome of our study was lymph node involvement, defined as the presence of positive pelvic lymph nodes for PC at final pathology. The number of lymph nodes removed at surgery and the percentage of positive LNs for PC in pN+ cases were reported.

2.3. *Statistical Analysis*

Data analyses were performed using STATA version 17.0 (Stata Corp., College Station, TX, USA).

Descriptive statistical methods such as number and percentage of cases, mean $\pm$ SD, median, and range were used. For the comparison of quantitative data, a Mann–Whitney test was used, whereas for qualitative data, a Fisher's Exact test and chi-square test were used. Pearson correlation analysis was also performed. We assessed the accuracy of the available nomograms MSKCC, Briganti 2012, Briganti 2017, and Briganti 2019 to predict LNI defined at final pathology. Regression coefficients were used to calculate the risk of LN positivity according to each model, and the discrimination accuracy of these models was quantified using the area under the receiver operating characteristic (ROC) curve (AUC). Sensitivity, specificity, positive predictive value (PPV), and negative predictive value (NPV) of the different clinical variables in predicting pathologic LN status were evaluated. Statistical significance was fixed at $p < 0.05$.

3. Results

Overall, 150 patients with high-risk PC submitted to RP with ePLND were included in the present analysis. The baseline characteristics of the included population are described in Table 1. PIRADS 4 was the most frequently observed (47.5%) at mpRMI pattern; 84% of them were cN0, and 71.3% were cT2.

At final pathology, LNI was found in 39 patients (26.1%), and the mean $\pm$ SD percentage of positive LNs was 16.1 $\pm$ 12.9 (Table 1).

The percentage of patients with an estimated risk for N+ at nomograms above the recommended cut-off threshold was significantly higher in pN+ cases than in pN0 for all Briganti nomograms ($p < 0.04$) but not for MSKCC nomogram ($p = 0.2$). The site of positive LNs at final pathology analysis was not described in most cases and was simply classified as left or right.

Table 1. Baseline characteristics of the whole population.

Number of cases	150
Age (years)	64.7 ± 5.35; 66: (49–71)
BMI	25.4 ± 3.3; 26: (20.9–37.8)
Preoperative total PSA (ng/mL)	17.0 ± 12.3; 14.0: (2.4–66.0)
PSAD	0.28 ± 0.19; 0.20: (0.03–0.48)
Prostate volume (cc)	47.1 ± 20.1; 39.5: (20.0–89.0)
mMR PIRADS score total cases	
PIRADS 2	3 (2.0%)
PIRADS 3	14 (9.5%)
PIRADS 4	71 (47.5%)
PIRADS 5	62 (41.0%)
Prostate Tumor size (mm) at mMR	13.5 ± 5.1; 12.5: (5.4–31.1)
Clinical T staging	
T1c	15 (10.1%)
T2	107 (71.3%)
T3a	16 (10.6%)
T3b	12 (8.0%)
Clinical N staging	
N0	126 (84.0%)
N1	24 (16.0%)
Biopsy outcomes	
% Positive samples PC	63.7 ± 27.1; 59.8: (9.0–100.0)
% Positive clinically significant PC	56.7 ± 30.5; 52.0: (10.0–100.0)
Max % PC tissue per core	60.1 ± 28.2; 51.0: (8.0–100.0)
ISUP grading at biopsy	
1	5 (3.3%)
2	13 (8.7%)
3	47 (31.7%)
4	58 (38.0%)
5	27 (18.3%)
Nomograms results (% estimated risk for N+)	
MSKCC	33.5 ± 19.7; 31.0: (5.0–84.0)
Briganti 2012	26.1 ± 19.7; 19.6: (6.0–85.0)
Briganti 2017	43.3 ± 25.4; 41.0: (5.0–95.0)
Briganti 2019	24.9 ± 20.0; 19.0: (5.0–84.0)
Percentage of patients with estimated risk for N+ at nomogram over the cut-off	
MSKCC (>7%)	93.8 %
Briganti 2012 (>5%)	94.0 %
Briganti 2017 (>7%)	90.1 %
Briganti 2019 (>7%)	85.7 %
Number of suspected lymph nodes at imaging	2.8 ± 1.9; 3: (1–6)
Surgical technique at radical prostatectomy	
- Pure Laparoscopic	44 (29.0%)
- Robot assisted	106 (71.0%)
Pathological stage (T)	
pT2	39 (26.2%)
pT3a	68 (45.1%)
pT3b	42 (28.0%)
pT4	1 (0.7%)
Pathological stage (N)	
N0	111 (73.9%)
N+	39 (26.1%)

Table 1. *Cont.*

Number of lymph nodes removed at surgery	
- Total cases	24.1 ± 9.01; 21: (12–46)
- N+ cases	24.3 ± 9.1; 22: (13–45)
- N0 cases	23.9 ± 8.9; 23: (11–44)
Percentage of positive lymph nodes	16.1 ± 12.9; 12.0: (5.1-67.3)
ISUP grading at surgery	
1	3 (2.3%)
2	9 (6.1%)
3	49 (32.3%)
4	60 (40.1%)
5	29 (19.2%)
Surgical margin at surgery (R)	
- Negative	108 (72.0%)
- positive	42 (28.0%)
PNI at surgery	
positive	78 (52.0%)
negative	72 (48.0%)
Cribriform/IDC at surgery	
- positive	28 (18.7%)
- negative	122 (81.3%)
Postoperative total PSA (ng/mL)	0.32 ± 1.45; 0.02: (0.01–5.0)
Biochemical progression	28 (17.3%)
Time to biochemical progression (months)	7.1 ± 10.6; 3.0 (2–25)

Mean ± SD, median, (range). Number of cases (%).

When considering nomograms results as continuous variables, mean ± SD estimated risk for pN+ showed some differences among MSKCC (33.5 ± 19.7), Briganti 2012 (26.1 ± 19.7), Briganti 2017 (43.3 ± 25.4) and Briganti 2019 (24.9 ± 20.0) nomograms (Table 1).

3.1. Comparative Analysis between pN0 and pN+ Cases

A comparative analysis between pN0 and pN+ cases is reported in Table 2.

The mean ± SD number of LNs removed was similar between pN0 (23.8 ± 8.4) and pN+ (25.0 ± 8.1) cases ($p = 0.2$). Only preoperative PSA and the maximal percentage of PC tissue per core at biopsy were significantly higher in pN+ (mean value 17.6 ± 15.1 ng/mL and 71.3 ± 24.1, respectively) when compared to pN0 cases (mean value 10.9 ± 10.0 ng/mL and 56.5 ± 27.6, respectively) cases (all $p < 0.01$).

Considering nomograms results as a continuous variable, none of the four preoperative nomograms (although mean values were always higher in pN+ than in the pN0 group) showed percentages of estimated risk for pN+ significantly different between pN0 and pN+ cases (all $p > 0.05$) (Table 2).

Pearson correlation analysis showed no statistically significant correlation between the pN result and each of the four nomograms examined as continuous variables ($p > 0.1$), whereas a statistically significant correlation was found with preoperative PSA (r = 0.2155; $p = 0.008$).

Different pathologic parameters at RP, such as pT stage, ISUP grading, and surgical margins but not the number of nodes surgically removed (r = 0.0793, $p = 0.334$), significantly correlated with pN status (Table 3).

Table 2. Comparative analysis based on pN results.

Pathological Lymph Node Status	pN0	pN1	*p* Value
Number cases	111	39	-
Age (years)	65.0 ± 7.1; 67.0: (48–73)	65.5 ± 7.2; 66.0: (50–72)	0.40
BMI	26.3 ± 3.1; 26.9: (22–35)	26.8 ± 3.4; 26.1: (23–37.7)	0.30
Preoperative total PSA (ng/mL)	10.9 ± 10.0; 8.7: (1.6–66.0)	17.6 ± 15.1; 12.0 (3.7–65.2)	0.01
PSAD	0.20 ± 0.7; 0.15: (0.05–0.60)	0.39 ± 0.06; 0.40: (0.35–0.5)	0.06
Prostate volume (cc)	45.6 ± 21.0; 38.0: (23.0–89.0)	48.7 ± 13.5; 49.0: (40.0–65.0)	0.30
mMR PIRADS score			
PIRADS 2	3 (2.0%)	0 (0%)	0.30
PIRADS 3	17 (11.2%)	5 (3.5%)	
PIRADS 4	72 (48.3%)	94 (62.6%)	
PIRADS 5	58 (38.5%)	51 (33.9%)	
Prostate Tumor size (mm) at mMR	14.0 ± 6.2; 12.4:(5.3–31.0)	13.9 ± 6.4; 13.0: (6.9–28.0)	0.50
Clinical T staging			
T1c	17 (11.5%)	0 (0%)	0.004
T2	116 (77.4%)	129 (86.1%)	
T3a	10 (6.6%)	13 (8.5%)	
T3b	7 (4.5%)	8 (5.4%)	
Clinical N staging			
N0	141 (94.3%)	118 (78.9%)	0.002
N1	9 (5.7%)	32 (21.1%)	
Biopsy outcomes:			
% Positive samples PC	59.8 ± 25.8; 58.0: (9.0–100)	62.4 ± 29.8; 62.0: (11.4–100)	0.20
% Positive clinically significant PC	54.2 ± 29.5; 50.3: (8.0–100)	52.1 ± 31.5; 49.5: (11.0–100)	0.30
Max % PC tissue per core	56.5 ± 27.6; 50.0: (6.0–100)	71.3 ± 24.1; 67.6: (32.1–100)	0.001
ISUP grading at biopsy			
1	5 (3.1%)	4 (2.5%)	0.50
2	18 (12.2%)	20 (13.6%)	
3	47 (31.6%)	47 (31.4%)	
4	57 (37.8%)	55 (36.5%)	
5	23 (15.3%)	24 (16.0%)	
Nomograms results (% estimated risk for N+)			
MSKCC	32.1 ± 18.9; 29.0: (4–81)	37.1 ± 18.2; 34.8: (7–75)	0.08
Briganti 2012	25.2 ± 19.7; 18.0: (4–80)	28.1 ± 18.5; 21.1: (7–84)	0.20
Briganti 2017	42.0 ± 26.6; 39.1: (4–94)	47.8 ± 24.3; 45.9: (7–90)	0.09
Briganti 2019	23.5 ± 19.8; 16.9: (4–82)	28.2 ± 21.3; 22.0: (4–78)	0.10
Percentage of patients with estimated risk for N+ at nomogram over the cut-off			
MSKCC (>7%)	92.8%	98.0%	0.20
Briganti 2012 (>5%)	91.2%	100%	0.03
Briganti 2017 (>7%)	86.4%	97.5%	0.04
Briganti 2019 (>7%)	80.7%	97.1%	0.03
Number of suspected lymph nodes at imaging	1.3±0.48; 1.0 (1–2)	2.9±1.6; 3.0 (1–5)	0.03
Surgical technique at radical prostatectomy			
- Pure Laparoscopic	23 (15.2%)	21 (13.8%)	0.70
- Robot-assisted	51 (33.8%)	55 (36.2%)	

Table 2. *Cont.*

Pathological Lymph Node Status	pN0	pN1	*p* Value
Pathological stage (T)			
pT2	62 (41.2%)	12 (7.8%)	0.02
pT3a	63 (42.3%)	77 (51.1%)	
pT3b	25 (16.5%)	60 (40.2%)	
pT4	0 (0%)	1 (0.9%)	
Number of Lymph nodes removed at surgery	23.8 ± 8.4; 23.0: (12–46)	25.0 ± 8.1; 24.0: (13–45)	0.20
ISUP grading at surgery			
1	5 (3.2%)	0 (0%)	0.04
2	30 (20.2%)	25 (17.0%)	
3	52 (34.5%)	47 (31.1%)	
4	34 (23.0%)	22 (14.3%)	
5	29 (19.1%)	56 (37.6%)	
Surgical margin at surgery (R)			
- Negative	113 (75.5%)	90 (60.3%)	0.01
- Positive	37 (24.5%)	60 (39.7%)	
PNI at surgery			
- negative	69 (45.9%)	57 (37.8%)	0.06
- positive	81 (54.1%)	93 (62.2%)	
Cribriform/IDC at surgery			
- negative	126 (84.3%)	40 (26.8%)	0.02
- positive	23 (15.7%)	110 (73.2%)	
Postoperative total PSA (ng/mL)	0.14 ± 0.4; 0.02: (0.01–2.8)	0.82 ± 2.9; 0.02: (0.01–4.8)	0.03
Biochemical progression (number of cases and %)	24 (15.8%)	39 (26.1%)	0.05
Time to biochemical progression	10.1 ± 12.8; 7.8: (3–22)	3.2 ± 1.4; 3.1: (3–7)	0.02

Mean ± SD, median, (range). Number of cases (%).

Table 3. Pearson correlation coefficient among pathological N stage (pN) and the other clinical and pathological variables.

Correlation	Coefficient	*p* Value
pN-age	−0.0353	0.670
pN-BMI	0.0524	0.524
pN-prostate volume	0.1577	0.545
pN-risk class	0.0511	0.534
pN-preoperative PSA	0.2155	0.008
pN-PSAD	0.4878	0.055
pN-PIRADS score	0.1275	0.215
pN-prostate tumor volume at imaging	0.0064	0.950
pN-percentage positive core at biopsy	0.0358	0.663
pN-MSKCC nomogram	0.119	0.149
pN-Briganti 2012 nomogram	0.0762	0.390
pN-Briganti 2017 nomogram	0.1188	0.192
pN-Briganti 2019 nomogram	0.1175	0.251
pN-number of suspected N at imaging	0.3313	<0.001

Table 3. *Cont.*

Correlation	Coefficient	p Value
pN-surgical technique	0.1979	0.0152
pN-pT stage	0.3148	<0.001
pN-ISUP grading at surgery	0.1622	0.049
pN-number of lymph nodes removed at surgery	0.0793	0.334
pN-surgical margins	0.2887	0.00034
pN-PNI	0.1249	0.127
pN-cribriform/IDC	0.143	0.08
pN-postoperative PSA	0.2068	0.013

3.2. Sensitivity, Specificity, PPV, NPV, and AUC Results in Predicting pN Status

The performance of the four nomograms in predicting pN status at final pathology is reported in Table 4.

Table 4. Sensitivity, specificity, Positive predictive value (PPV), Negative predictive value (NPV), and AUC of different variables in predicting pN+ status at surgery.

	Sensitivity (CI 95%)	Specificity (CI 95%)	PPV (CI 95%)	NPV (CI 95%)	AUC (CI 95%)
MSKCC nomogram > 7%	0.973 (0.845–1.000)	0.078 (0.043–0.147)	0.248 (0.181–0.340)	0.905 (0.851–0.938)	0.526 (0.489–0.562)
Briganti 2012 nomogram > 5%	0.991 (0.889–1.000)	0.093 (0.049–0.171)	0.285 (0.220–0.351)	0.957 (0.911–0.991)	0.548 (0.518–0.578)
Briganti 2017 nomogram > 7%	0.973 (0.840–1.000)	0.140 (0.090–0.230)	0.352 (0.251–0.487)	0.919 (0.851–0.959)	0.555 (0.509–0.601)
Briganti 2019 Nomogram > 7%	0.959 (0.789–1.000)	0.183 (0.124–0.291)	0.301 (0.212–0.408)	0.931 (0.855–0.972)	0.573 (0.513–0.633)

In our population, nomograms showed similar high sensitivity (0.973, 0.991, 0.973, and 0.959, respectively, for MSKCC, Briganti 2012, Briganti 2017, and Briganti 2019) and low specificity (0.078, 0.093, 0.140 and 0.183 respectively for MSKCC, Briganti 2012, Briganti 2017 and Briganti 2019) at the recommended threshold of estimated risk (of >5% or >7%). AUC values were similar, with 0.526, 0.548, 0.555, and 0.573 for the four nomograms, respectively (Figure 1).

74% of cases with MSKCC estimated risk > 7% showed no LNI (pN0) at final pathology compared to 71% of cases with Briganti 2012 > 5%, 69% with Briganti 2017 > 7% and, 70% with Briganti 2019 > 7% (Figure 2). When the MSKCC nomogram was performed, 74% of patients with more than 7% risk of LNI showed no LNI at histopathological node assay.

3.3. Regression Analysis: Predictors for pN+ Result at Final Pathology

A logistic regression analysis was carried out to identify predictors of positive PLN involvement at final pathology (pN+) (Table 5).

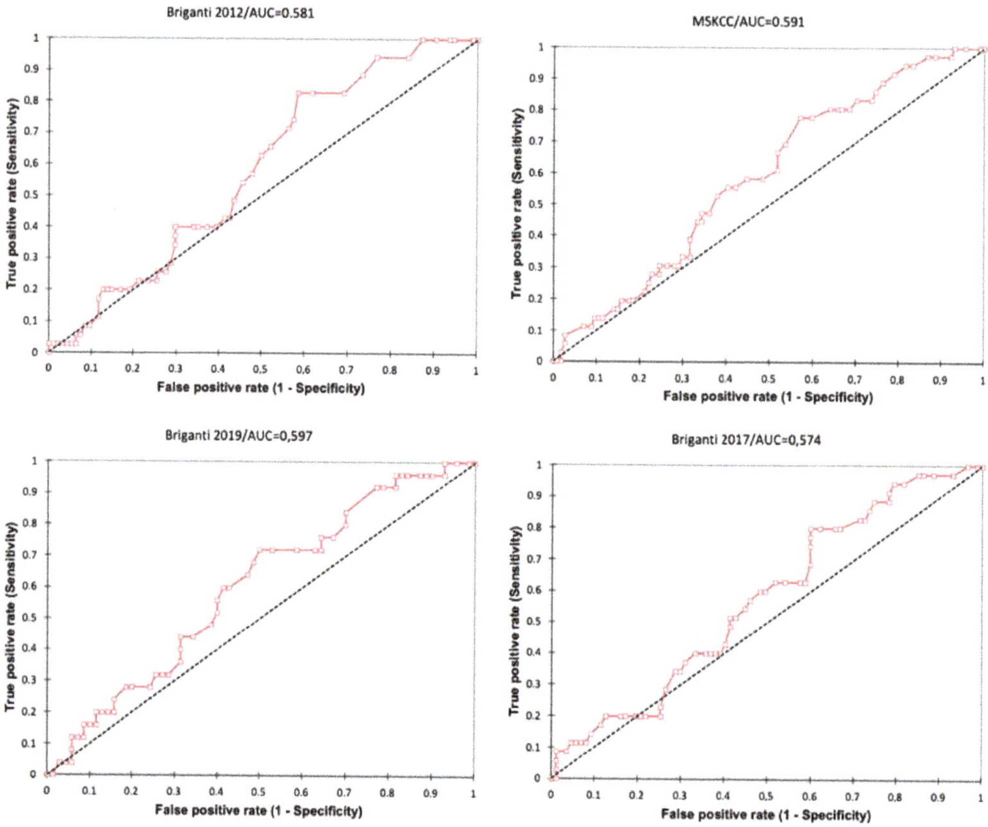

Cut-off	AUC	SE	95% CI	
Briganti 2019_>7%	0.573	0.031	0.513	0.633
Briganti 2017_>7%	0.555	0.023	0.509	0.601
Briganti 2012_>5%	0.548	0.015	0.518	0.578
MSKCC_>7%	0.526	0.019	0.489	0.562

Figure 1. Receiver operating characteristic (ROC) curve and relative Area Under the Curve (AUC) in predicting LNI (pN+) of the currently available MSKCC, Briganti 2012, Briganti 2017, and Briganti 2019 nomograms.

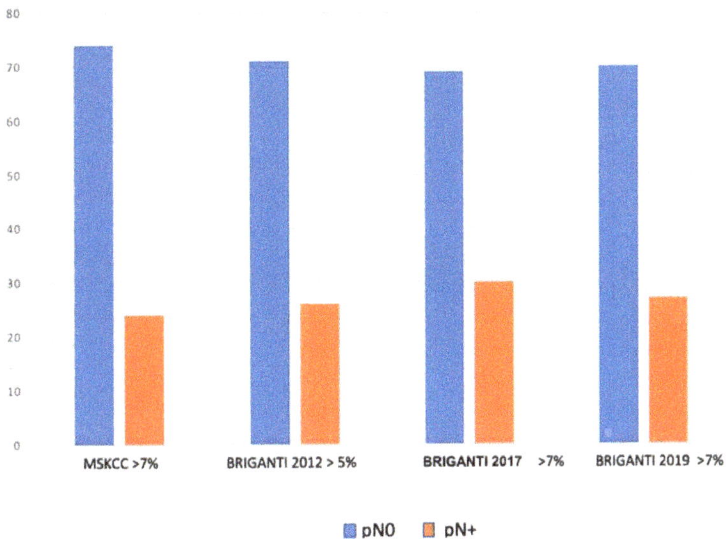

Figure 2. Bar-chart showing pN0 and pN+ cases distribution according to the MSKCC (at estimated risk > 7%), Briganti 2012 (at estimated risk > 5%), Briganti 2017 (at the estimated risk > 7%), Briganti 2019 (at estimated risk > 7%) nomograms.

Table 5. Logistic regression analysis to identify predictors for positive lymph node (pN+).

		Univariable				Multivariable			
		OR	95% CI_lower	95% CI_upper	*p*-Value	OR	95% CI_lower	95% CI_upper	*p*-Value
Preoperative PSA		Ref	–	–	–				
	>10	1.771	0.818	3.807	0.141				
MSKCC		Ref	–	–	–				
	>7%	3.000	0.371	23.561	0.401				
Briganti 2012		Ref	–	–	–				
	>5%	7.752	0.359	159.823	0.210				
Briganti 2017		Ref	–	–	–				
	>7%	5.610	0.611	42.812	0.213				
Briganti 2019		Ref	–	–	–				
	>7%	5.565	0.786	45.235	0.135				
Pathologic stage	pT2	Ref	–	–	–	Ref	–	–	–
	pT3a	6.724	1.932	24.485	0.003	6.52	1.825	24.001	0.005
	pT3b	14.129	3.651	54.231	0.001	11.211	2.621	42.308	0.002
ISUP at surgery	1	Ref	–	–	–				
	2	3.845	0.161	96.270	0.502				
	3	4.215	0.1812	98.528	0.413				
	4	2.759	0.111	71.521	0.499				
	5	7.775	0.357	186.632	0.310				

Odds Ratio (OR), 95% Confidential Interval (CI).

At the univariable analysis, the risk of pN+ significantly increased according to the pT stage, 6.7 times in pT3a ($p = 0.003$) and 14.1 times in pT3b cases ($p = 0.001$).

According to the various nomograms, the risk of pN+ increased 3.0 times for an MSKCC estimated risk > 7%, 7.7 times for a Briganti 2012 estimated risk > 5%, 5.6 times for a Briganti 2017 estimated risk > 7% and 5.5 times for a Briganti 2019 estimated risk > 7%, without statical significance (all $p > 0.1$).

At the multivariable analysis, the pT stage maintained an independent predictive value in terms of risk for pN+ ($p < 0.05$).

4. Discussion

According to EAU guidelines [2], the indication for ePLND at the time of RP is based on risk assessment by validated nomograms such as the MSKCC, Briganti 2012, Briganti 2017, and Briganti 2019 [3,4,7,8]. Using a cut-off of 5% or 7% in terms of estimated risk for pN+ results in missing a very low percentage of cases with LNI [3,4,7,8]. On the other hand, in daily practice, a relevant percentage of cases show no LNI at the final histopathological assay (pN0) after ePLND [2–21]. In fact, it has been demonstrated that when the choice of whether to perform ePLND relies on well-established preoperative nomograms, most patients, including those with high-risk diseases, have no LNI at final pathology [2–21].

To date, various comparisons among nomograms in different patient cohorts have been published (Table 6).

Table 6. Studies investigating the accuracy of most frequently used nomograms to predict the probability of lymph node metastases before radical prostatectomy.

Study	Sensitivity	Specificity	PPV	NPV	Accuracy AUC (CI 95% Range)
Hinev et al. 2014 [11]	N.R.	N.R.	N.R.	N.R.	**Briganti 2012:** 87.5 **MSKCC:** 77
Bandini et al. 2017 [12]	**Briganti 2012:** 90.0 **MSKCC:** 89.9	**Briganti 2012:** 46.1 **MSKCC:** 46.4	N.R.	**Briganti 2012:** 98.7 **MSKCC:** 98.7	**Briganti 2012:** 79.8 **MSKCC:** 79.9
Hueting et al. 2018 [13]	N.R.	N.R.	N.R.	N.R.	**Briganti 2012:** 76 (73–79) **MSKCC:** 75 (72–78)
Gandaglia et al. 2020 [18]	N.R.	N.R.	N.R.	N.R.	**Briganti 2019:** 79 **Briganti 2017:** 75 **Briganti 2012:** 65 **MSKCC:** 74
Diamand et al. 2020 [14]	N.R.	N.R.	N.R.	N.R.	**Briganti 2019:** 80 (75–86) **Briganti 2012:** 80 (74–87)
Milonas et al. 2020 [8]	**MSKCC:** 88.9	**MSKCC:** 45.2	**MSKCC:** N.R.	**MSKCC:** 96.8	**MSKCC:** 79 (73.8–84.2)

Table 6. *Cont.*

Study	Sensitivity	Specificity	PPV	NPV	Accuracy AUC (CI 95% Range)
Oderda et al. 2020 [15]	N.R.	N.R.	N.R.	N.R.	**Briganti 2019:** 76 (70–81) **Briganti 2017:** 80 (75–86) **Briganti 2012:** 83 (81–84) **MSKCC:** 83 (81–84)
Fukagawa et al. 2021 [19]	**Briganti 2019:** 94.7	**Briganti 2019:** 32.0	N.R.	**Briganti 2019:** 98.8	**Briganti 2019:** 71 **Briganti 2017:** 72 **Briganti 2012:** 74 **MSKCC:** 73
Meijer et al. 2021 [16]	N.R.	N.R.	N.R.	N.R.	**Briganti 2019:** 82 (76–87) **Briganti 2017:** 76 (70–82) **MSKCC:** 77 (72–83)
Frego et al. 2022 [20]	N.R.	N.R.	N.R.	N.R.	**Briganti 2019:** 82 **Briganti 2012:** 84

PPV = positive predicted value; NPV = negative predicted value; AUC = area under the curve; N.R. = not reported.

M. Bandini et al. [12] compared four different nomograms: Cagiannos, Godoy, the 2012 Briganti, and the online MSKCC nomograms. Despite several comprehensive analytical steps, they did not prove the superiority of one nomogram over another. Furthermore, all nomograms achieved the same accuracy for predicting LNI, and their ability to avoid unnecessary PLND was similar.

Hueting et al. [13] performed an external validation of 16 predictive models in 1001 Dutch patients with PCa, excluding the Briganti 2017 and 2019 nomograms. LNI was identified in 276 patients (28%). They showed that the Briganti 2012 (AUC 0.76) and MSKCC nomograms (AUC 0.75) were the most accurate, with similar miscalibration with a tendency to underestimation. No direct comparison between nomograms, however, was performed.

Again, Oderda et al. [15] performed a multi-institutional external validation of several nomograms for the prediction of LNI. Overall, 1158 patients (9.6%) had LNI, with a mean of 17.7 and 3.2 resected and positive nodes, respectively. No significant differences in AUCs were observed between the MSKCC (0.83), Briganti 2012 (0.83), Partin 2016 (0.78), Yale (0.80), Briganti 2017 (0.80), and Briganti 2019 (0.76) models.

However, these results do not match with Hinev et al. [11] findings which surprisingly showed that the 2012 Briganti nomogram is far superior to the MSKCC nomogram, reporting a calculated AUC of 0.875 vs. 0.77. More recently, Diamand et al. [14] found the same AUC of 0.8 for both Briganti 2012 and 2019 but with a better net benefit for the 2019 model.

Similarly, in a recent external validation of the Briganti 2019 nomogram, this tool was characterized by higher AUC compared to the Briganti 2012 and 2017 nomograms and the Memorial Sloan Kettering Cancer Center risk calculator (79% vs. 75% vs. 65% vs. 74%) and demonstrated the highest net benefit on decision curve analyses [18].

The results of this study [18] suggest that adding valid imaging, such as mpMRI, can improve the predictive power of these tools.

However, available evidence does not demonstrate the superiority of one nomogram over the others. No data exist to support the routine use of one predictive model over another, even in more aggressive diseases.

Based on these considerations, we aimed to evaluate the accuracy of the most used nomograms for predicting LNI and to compare them in our sub-cohort of high-risk PC patients treated with ePLND.

Overall, we found that the predictive performance of the MSKCC, Briganti 2012, 2017, and 2019 nomograms about LNI are virtually the same. Indeed, despite higher PCa aggressiveness in the present cohort, our findings are in line with those in other series reporting on the general population: the AUC values were similar (0.526, 0.548, 0.555, and 0.573 for the MSKCC, Briganti 2012, Briganti 2017, and Briganti 2019 models, respectively) and the four nomograms showed similar high sensitivity (0.973, 0.991, 0.973, and 0.959 for MSKCC, Briganti 2012, Briganti 2017, and Briganti 2019, respectively) and very low specificity (0.078, 0.093, 0.140, and 0.183 for MSKCC, Briganti 2012, Briganti 2017, and Briganti 2019, respectively).

Theoretically, in the present sub-cohort of patients, the role of ePLND should be undiscussed, and, therefore, preoperative nomograms should play a limited role in deciding whether to perform ePLND. Specifically, when analyzing patients' characteristics, we observed that most of them showed unfavorable tumor features: 74% of cases showed >pT2 disease and high ISUP grade (59% of patients with grade > 3) at final pathology. Nonetheless, it is relevant to underline that 74% of cases with MSKCC estimated risk > 7% showed no LNI (pN0) at final pathology compared to 71% of cases with Briganti 2012 > 5%, 69% with Briganti 2017 > 7% and 70% with Briganti 2019 > 7%. These findings demonstrate that these models tend to overestimate the LNI risk, also in patients diagnosed with high-risk disease. In other words, their ability to avoid unnecessary ePLND is similar; also, in this surgical setting, where we should expect greater accuracy. In addition, our results further corroborate that mpMRI may not be capable of detecting small pelvic lymph node metastases and MRI data on the index lesion are not enough for accurate LNI prediction: mpMRI is highly operator-dependent, and its misinterpretation could account for the performance of the Briganti 2019 nomogram as compared to older nomograms [23]. Therefore, this study confirms that, in a real-life setting, mpMRI and MRI-targeted biopsy may provide a limited additional value in improving the accuracy of clinical predictors of LNI. Indeed, it is well-established that the sensitivity and specificity of mpMRI in the direct detection of metastatic nodes, based on morphological characteristics, are not sufficient [24]. Moreover, in a previous experience, we observed that even a defined standardization of lymph node involvement, such as node rads, did not show superior results to the current nomograms, clearly suggesting the limits of MRI in the lymph node staging (25). Therefore, the question of whether we really need to perform so many ePLNDs remains unanswered. The answer will probably come from future refinements and the widespread adoption of PSMA-PET, which has proven to be superior to conventional imaging for high-risk PCa patients with pelvic nodal metastases [25–29]. It is likely that, in the future, ePLND will be guided directly by PSMA-PET or nomograms integrating PSMA PET/CT data. In fact, as recently demonstrated by Meijer et al., the addition of PSMA-PET to the previously developed nomograms showed substantially improved predictive performances, which suggests that PSMA-PET is a likely future candidate for a modern predictive nomogram [16]. Moreover, in a recent comparative study between ^{68} Ga-PSMA PET/CT and mpMRI in the diagnosis of lymph node metastases, Franklin A et al. observed that preoperative ^{68} Ga-PSMA/PET CT was more sensitive in identifying histological pelvic LNM than 3-T mpMRI. Moreover, they observed that men with a negative ^{68} Ga-PSMA PET/CT have a lower risk of LNI than predicted with MSKCC and Briganti nomograms [27].

Our study is not devoid of limitations: (I) this is a retrospective analysis; (II) some data, such as localization of positive LNs, were not available; (III) multiple surgeons performed ePLND, multiple pathologists reported on the histopathology in the RP and ePLND specimens, and scans were reported by multiple radiologists. Nonetheless, all patients were diagnosed and treated at high-volume tertiary referral centers by experienced surgeons and dedicated expert radiologists and uro-pathologists.

5. Conclusions

Although we considered only high-risk PC cases candidate for ePLND, a high percentage of them continues to show no LNI at final histopathology. In addition, we confirm the similar predictive value in terms of LNI estimation among the four most frequently used validated nomograms, with similar high sensitivity but low specificity.

Author Contributions: Study conception and design: G.B.D.P., A.S., S.S. (Stefano Salciccia), V.C. and A.T. (Antonio Tufano); Patient enrolment and management: M.F., A.T. (Antonio Tufano), E.S., F.D.G., G.B., S.S. (Stefano Signore), V.A., M.M. and P.B.; Collection of clinical data: F.F., P.E., V.C., M.F., V.A., M.M. and S.S. (Stefano Signore); Statistical analysis, biostatistics, and computational analysis: Interpretation of results: G.B.D.P., A.S., S.S. (Stefano Salciccia), A.P., C.D.N. and A.T. (Andrea Tubaro); Writing, review, and/or revision of the manuscript: G.B.D.P., A.S., S.S. (Stefano Salciccia), A.C. and A.T (Andrea Tubaro). All authors have read and agreed to the published version of the manuscript.

Funding: This research received no external funding.

Institutional Review Board Statement: The study was conducted in accordance with the Declaration of Helsinki, and approved by the Ethics Committee of the Policlinico Umberto I Hospital (Rome, Italy).

Informed Consent Statement: Informed consent was obtained from all subjects involved in the study.

Data Availability Statement: The data presented in this study are available on reasonable request from the corresponding author.

Conflicts of Interest: The authors declare no conflict of interest related to the present study.

Abbreviations

PC = prostate cancer; RP= radical prostatectomy; LNI = lymph node invasion; LNs = lymph nodes; SM = surgical margins; ePLND = extended pelvic lymph node dissection; mpMRI = multiparametric magnetic resonance imaging; RARP = robot-assisted radical prostatectomy (RARP); LRP = laparoscopic radical prostatectomy; ROC = receiver operating characteristic; AUC = area under the curve; PPV = positive predictive value; NPV = negative predictive value.

References

1. Gupta, P.; Mohammad, T.; Dahiya, R.; Roy, S.; Noman, O.M.A.; Alajmi, M.F.; Hussain, A.; Hassan, M.I. Evaluation of binding and inhibition mechanism of dietary phytochemicals with sphingosine kinase 1: Towards targeted anticancer therapy. *Sci. Rep.* **2019**, *9*, 18727. [CrossRef] [PubMed]
2. Mottet, N.; van den Bergh, R.C.N. Prostate Cancer: European Association of Urology (EAU) Guidelines 2022. Available online: https://uroweb.org/guideline/prostate-cancer/ (accessed on 2 March 2023).
3. Briganti, A.; Larcher, A.; Abdollah, F.; Capitanio, U.; Gallina, A.; Suardi, N.; Bianchi, M.; Sun, M.; Freschi, M.; Salonia, A.; et al. Updated nomogram predicting lymph node invasion in patients with prostate cancer undergoing extended pelvic lymph node dissection: The essential importance of percentage of positive cores. *Eur. Urol.* **2012**, *61*, 480–487. [CrossRef] [PubMed]
4. Gandaglia, G.; Fossati, N.; Zaffuto, E.; Bandini, M.; Dell'Oglio, P.; Bravi, C.A.; Fallara, G.; Pellegrino, F.; Nocera, L.; Karakiewicz, P.I.; et al. Development and Internal Validation of a Novel Model to Identify the Candidates for Extended Pelvic Lymph Node Dissection in Prostate Cancer. *Eur. Urol.* **2017**, *72*, 632–640. [CrossRef] [PubMed]
5. Fossati, N.; Willemse, P.M.; Van den Broeck, T.; van den Bergh, R.C.N.; Yuan, C.Y.; Briers, E.; Bellmunt, J.; Bolla, M.; Cornford, P.; De Santis, M.; et al. The Benefits and Harms of Different Extents of Lymph Node Dissection During Radical Prostatectomy for Prostate Cancer: A Systematic Review. *Eur. Urol.* **2017**, *72*, 84–109. [CrossRef]
6. Lestingi, J.F.P.; Guglielmetti, G.B.; Trinh, Q.D.; Coelho, R.F.; Pontes, J., Jr.; Bastos, D.A.; Cordeiro, M.D.; Sarkis, A.S.; Faraj, S.F.; Mitre, A.I.; et al. Extended Versus Limited Pelvic Lymph Node Dissection During Radical Prostatectomy for Intermediate- and High-risk Prostate Cancer: Early Oncological Outcomes from a Randomized Phase 3 Trial. *Eur. Urol.* **2021**, *79*, 595–604. [CrossRef]
7. Gandaglia, G.; Ploussard, G.; Valerio, M.; Mattei, A.; Fiori, C.; Fossati, N.; Stabile, A.; Beauval, J.B.; Malavaud, B.; Roumiguié, M.; et al. A Novel Nomogram to Identify Candidates for Extended Pelvic Lymph Node Dissection among Patients with Clinically

Localized Prostate Cancer Diagnosed with Magnetic Resonance Imaging-targeted and Systematic Biopsies. *Eur. Urol.* **2019**, *75*, 506–514. [CrossRef]

8. Milonas, D.; Venclovas, Z.; Muilwijk, T.; Jievaltas, M.; Joniau, S. External validation of Memorial Sloan Kettering Cancer Center nomogram and prediction of optimal candidate for lymph node dissection in clinically localized prostate cancer. *Cent. Eur. J. Urol.* **2020**, *73*, 19–25. [CrossRef]
9. Hövels, A.M.; Heesakkers, R.A.; Adang, E.M.; Jager, G.J.; Strum, S.; Hoogeveen, Y.L.; Severens, J.L.; Barentsz, J.O. The diagnostic accuracy of CT and MRI in the staging of pelvic lymph nodes in patients with prostate cancer: A meta-analysis. *Clin. Radiol.* **2008**, *63*, 387–395. [CrossRef]
10. Van den Bergh, L.; Lerut, E.; Haustermans, K.; Deroose, C.M.; Oyen, R.; Isebaert, S.; Budiharto, T.; Ameye, F.; Mottaghy, F.M.; Bogaerts, K.; et al. Final analysis of a prospective trial on functional imaging for nodal staging in patients with prostate cancer at high risk for lymph node involvement. *Urol. Oncol.* **2015**, *33*, 109.e23–109.e31. [CrossRef]
11. Hinev, A.I.; Anakievski, D.; Kolev, N.H.; Hadjiev, V.I. Validation of nomograms predicting lymph node involvement in patients with prostate cancer undergoing extended pelvic lymph node dissection. *Urol. Int.* **2014**, *92*, 300–305. [CrossRef]
12. Bandini, M.; Marchioni, M.; Pompe, R.S.; Tian, Z.; Gandaglia, G.; Fossati, N.; Abdollah, F.; Graefen, M.; Montorsi, F.; Saad, F.; et al. First North American validation and head-to-head comparison of four preoperative nomograms for prediction of lymph node invasion before radical prostatectomy. *BJU Int.* **2018**, *121*, 592–599. [CrossRef] [PubMed]
13. Hueting, T.A.; Cornel, E.B.; Somford, D.M.; Jansen, H.; van Basten, J.A.; Pleijhuis, R.G.; Korthorst, R.A.; van der Palen, J.A.M.; Koffijberg, H. External Validation of Models Predicting the Probability of Lymph Node Involvement in Prostate Cancer Patients. *Eur. Urol. Oncol.* **2018**, *1*, 411–417. [CrossRef] [PubMed]
14. Diamand, R.; Oderda, M.; Albisinni, S.; Fourcade, A.; Fournier, G.; Benamran, D.; Iselin, C.; Fiard, G.; Descotes, J.L.; Assenmacher, G.; et al. External validation of the Briganti nomogram predicting lymph node invasion in patients with intermediate and high-risk prostate cancer diagnosed with magnetic resonance imaging-targeted and systematic biopsies: A European multicenter study. *Urol. Oncol.* **2020**, *38*, 847.e9–847.e16. [CrossRef] [PubMed]
15. Oderda, M.; Diamand, R.; Albisinni, S.; Calleris, G.; Carbone, A.; Falcone, M.; Fiard, G.; Gandaglia, G.; Marquis, A.; Marra, G.; et al. Indications for and complications of pelvic lymph node dissection in prostate cancer: Accuracy of available nomograms for the prediction of lymph node invasion. *BJU Int.* **2021**, *127*, 318–325, Erratum in *BJU Int.* **2022**, *129*, 777. [CrossRef]
16. Meijer, D.; van Leeuwen, P.J.; Roberts, M.J.; Siriwardana, A.R.; Morton, A.; Yaxley, J.W.; Samaratunga, H.; Emmett, L.; van de Ven, P.M.; van der Poel, H.G.; et al. External Validation and Addition of Prostate-specific Membrane Antigen Positron Emission Tomography to the Most Frequently Used Nomograms for the Prediction of Pelvic Lymph-node Metastases: An International Multicenter Study. *Eur. Urol.* **2021**, *80*, 234–242. [CrossRef]
17. Venclovas, Z.; Muilwijk, T.; Matjosaitis, A.J.; Jievaltas, M.; Joniau, S.; Milonas, D. Head-to-Head Comparison of Two Nomograms Predicting Probability of Lymph Node Invasion in Prostate Cancer and the Therapeutic Impact of Higher Nomogram Threshold. *J. Clin. Med.* **2021**, *10*, 999. [CrossRef]
18. Gandaglia, G.; Martini, A.; Ploussard, G.; Fossati, N.; Stabile, A.; De Visschere, P.; Borgmann, H.; Heidegger, I.; Steinkohl, F.; Kretschmer, A.; et al. EAU-YAU Prostate Cancer Working Group. External Validation of the 2019 Briganti Nomogram for the Identification of Prostate Cancer Patients Who Should Be Considered for an Extended Pelvic Lymph Node Dissection. *Eur. Urol.* **2020**, *78*, 138–142. [CrossRef]
19. Fukagawa, E.; Yamamoto, S.; Ohde, S.; Yoshitomi, K.K.; Hamada, K.; Yoneoka, Y.; Fujiwara, M.; Fujiwara, R.; Oguchi, T.; Komai, Y.; et al. External validation of the Briganti 2019 nomogram to identify candidates for extended pelvic lymph node dissection among patients with high-risk clinically localized prostate cancer. *Int. J. Clin. Oncol.* **2021**, *26*, 1736–1744. [CrossRef]
20. Frego, N.; Paciotti, M.; Buffi, N.M.; Maffei, D.; Contieri, R.; Avolio, P.P.; Fasulo, V.; Uleri, A.; Lazzeri, M.; Hurle, R.; et al. External Validation and Comparison of Two Nomograms Predicting the Probability of Lymph Node Involvement in Patients subjected to Robot-Assisted Radical Prostatectomy and Concomitant Lymph Node Dissection: A Single Tertiary Center Experience in the MRI-Era. *Front. Surg.* **2022**, *9*, 829515. [CrossRef]
21. Nason, G.J.; O'Connor, E.M.; MacMahon, D.; Moss, B.; Considine, S.W.; Cahill, A.; O'Rourke, C.; O'Brien, F.M. Comparison of nomograms predicting lymph node invasion in patients undergoing radical prostatectomy for prostate cancer. *Ir. J. Med. Sci.* **2018**, *187*, 33–37. [CrossRef]
22. Mattei, A.; Di Pierro, G.B.; Grande, P.; Beutler, J.; Danuser, H. Standardized and simplified extended pelvic lymph node dissection during robot-assisted radical prostatectomy: The monoblock technique. *Urology* **2013**, *81*, 446–450. [CrossRef] [PubMed]
23. Tay, K.J.; Gupta, R.T.; Brown, A.F.; Silverman, R.K.; Polascik, T.J. Defining the Incremental Utility of Prostate Multiparametric Magnetic Resonance Imaging at Standard and Specialized Read in Predicting Extracapsular Extension of Prostate Cancer. *Eur. Urol.* **2016**, *70*, 211–213. [CrossRef] [PubMed]
24. Budiharto, T.; Joniau, S.; Lerut, E.; Van den Bergh, L.; Mottaghy, F.; Deroose, C.M.; Oyen, R.; Ameye, F.; Bogaerts, K.; Haustermans, K.; et al. Prospective evaluation of 11C-choline positron emission tomography/computed tomography and diffusion-weighted magnetic resonance imaging for the nodal staging of prostate cancer with a high risk of lymph node metastases. *Eur. Urol.* **2011**, *60*, 125–130. [CrossRef] [PubMed]
25. Lucciola, S.; Pisciotti, M.L.; Frisenda, M.; Magliocca, F.; Gentilucci, A.; Del Giudice, F.; Canale, V.; Scarrone, E.; Busetto, G.M.; Carrieri, G.; et al. Predictive role of node-rads score in patients with prostate cancer candidates for radical prostatectomy with

extended lymph node dissection: Comparative analysis with validated nomograms. *Prostate Cancer Prostatic Dis.* **2022**. *epub ahead of print*. [CrossRef] [PubMed]
26. Hofman, M.S.; Lawrentschuk, N.; Francis, R.J.; Tang, C.; Vela, I.; Thomas, P.; Rutherford, N.; Martin, J.M.; Frydenberg, M.; Shakher, R.; et al. Prostate-specific membrane antigen PET-CT in patients with high-risk prostate cancer before curative-intent surgery or radiotherapy (proPSMA): A prospective, randomised, multicentre study. *Lancet* **2020**, *395*, 1208–1216. [CrossRef] [PubMed]
27. Franklin, A.; Yaxley, W.J.; Raveenthiran, S.; Coughlin, G.; Gianduzzo, T.; Kua, B.; McEwan, L.; Wong, D.; Delahunt, B.; Egevad, L.; et al. Histological comparison between predictive value of preoperative 3-T multiparametric MRI and 68 Ga-PSMA PET/CT scan for pathological outcomes at radical prostatectomy and pelvic lymph node dissection for prostate cancer. *BJU Int.* **2021**, *127*, 71–79. [CrossRef]
28. Sciarra, A.; Voria, G.; Monti, S.; Mazzone, L.; Mariotti, G.; Pozza, M.; D'Eramo, G.; Di Silverio, F. Clinical understaging in patients with prostate adenocarcinoma submitted to radical prostatectomy: Predictive value of serum chromogranin A. *Prostate* **2004**, *58*, 421–428. [CrossRef]
29. Cimino, S.; Reale, G.; Castelli, T.; Favilla, V.; Giardina, R.; Russo, G.I.; Privitera, S.; Morgia, G. Comparison between Briganti, Partin and MSKCC tools in predicting positive lymph nodes in prostate cancer: A systematic review and meta-analysis. *Scand. J. Urol.* **2017**, *51*, 345–350. [CrossRef]

cancers

MDPI

Article

Prognostic Significance of Amino Acid Metabolism-Related Genes in Prostate Cancer Retrieved by Machine Learning

Ivana Samaržija *, Koraljka Gall Trošelj and Paško Konjevoda

Laboratory for Epigenomics, Division of Molecular Medicine, Ruđer Bošković Institute, 10000 Zagreb, Croatia
* Correspondence: ivana.samarzija@irb.hr

Simple Summary: Prostate cancer is a highly heterogenous disease with respect to molecular, morphological and clinical features. Therefore, one of the major tasks in its management is to define the risk subgroups that would guide the treatment approach. Amino acid metabolism-related genes are involved in several aspects of prostate cancer progression. In this publication, we show that their expression is highly aberrant in prostate cancer, which could be potentially exploited for the establishment of disease progression parameters and therapeutic targets. We show that among the variables studied, the Gleason score was the strongest prognostic factor of progression-free survival in multivariate analysis. Additionally, the expression of *SERINC3* and *CSAD* genes strongly differentiated between better and worse prognosis (low and high risk) for high and low Gleason scores, respectively. These results offer a suggestion for potential biomarkers of prostate cancer progression in patients that are stratified by the Gleason score.

Abstract: Prostate cancer is among the leading cancers according to both incidence and mortality. Due to the high molecular, morphological and clinical heterogeneity, the course of prostate cancer ranges from slow growth that usually does not require immediate therapeutic intervention to aggressive and fatal disease that spreads quickly. However, currently available biomarkers cannot precisely predict the course of a disease, and novel strategies are needed to guide prostate cancer management. Amino acids serve numerous roles in cancers, among which are energy production, building block reservoirs, maintenance of redox homeostasis, epigenetic regulation, immune system modulation and resistance to therapy. In this article, by using The Cancer Genome Atlas (TCGA) data, we found that the expression of amino acid metabolism-related genes is highly aberrant in prostate cancer, which holds potential to be exploited in biomarker design or in treatment strategies. This change in expression is especially evident for catabolism genes and transporters from the solute carrier family. Furthermore, by using recursive partitioning, we confirmed that the Gleason score is strongly prognostic for progression-free survival. However, the expression of the genes *SERINC3* (phosphatidylserine and sphingolipids generation) and *CSAD* (hypotaurine generation) can refine prognosis for high and low Gleason scores, respectively. Therefore, our results hold potential for novel prostate cancer progression biomarkers.

Keywords: prostate cancer; prognosis; progression-free survival; recursive partitioning; Gleason score; CSAD; SERINC3; hypotaurine; phosphatidylserine and sphingolipids

Citation: Samaržija, I.; Trošelj, K.G.; Konjevoda, P. Prognostic Significance of Amino Acid Metabolism-Related Genes in Prostate Cancer Retrieved by Machine Learning. *Cancers* **2023**, *15*, 1309. https://doi.org/10.3390/cancers15041309

Academic Editor: Kouji Izumi

Received: 28 December 2022
Revised: 11 February 2023
Accepted: 16 February 2023
Published: 18 February 2023

1. Introduction

Prostate cancer is among the leading cancers according to both incidence and mortality. It is estimated that in 2020, there were 1,414,259 (7.3% of all sites) new cases diagnosed and 375,304 (3.8% of all sites) deaths from this disease [1]. Common treatment options for confined prostate cancer include surgical removal of the prostate (radical prostatectomy) and radiotherapy. However, biochemical recurrence, defined by a significant rise in blood levels of prostate specific antigen, occurs within approximately 10 years in 20–40% of patients after radical prostatectomy and 30–50% after radiotherapy [2]. The biochemical recurrence can lead to a progressive disease, which is accompanied by symptoms or evidence of disease progression on imaging [3]. One of the major problems in prostate cancer management is to predict the course of a disease, that is, to differentiate between the tumors that will grow slowly and require minimal or no treatment and those that are more aggressive and will progress fast. Therefore, novel treatment strategies and therapeutic targets are needed, as well as better biomarkers, which would guide prostate cancer management.

Metabolic rewiring is one of the hallmarks of cancer [4], through which the cancer cell satisfies its high demands for energy and biomass building blocks to sustain its rapid proliferation. In comparison to other solid cancer types, which largely rely on aerobic glycolysis (the Warburg effect), prostate cancer cells use oxidative phosphorylation more than non-transformed prostate cells [5–7]. However, in advanced stages of prostate cancer, an increased glycolytic phenotype has been observed. In addition to these specificities, a hallmark of the metastatic, castration-resistant prostate cancer (mCRPC) is lipid metabolism rewiring, which manifests as increased fatty acids and cholesterol synthesis, uptake and oxidation [8].

Along with carbohydrates and fatty acids, amino acids are among the main sources of nutrients for energy homeostasis (alternative fuels) and building blocks for macromolecular biosynthesis. Additionally, amino acids help to maintain the redox balance as they are the main elements for reduced glutathione (GSH) and nicotinamide adenine dinucleotide phosphate (NADPH) generation, which are among the key molecules involved in control of the cellular redox state. Amino acid derivatives contribute to epigenetic modifications and posttranscriptional regulation. Namely, one-carbon units from the methionine and folate cycle are methyl donors for DNA and histone methylation, while acetyl-CoA derived from a group of amino acids can be used for histone acetylation. Amino acids also largely influence immune system responses in tumorigenesis and metastasis formation by creating an immunosuppressive or immunoeffective microenvironment [9]. Moreover, amino acids enable cancer cells to circumvent anticancer therapies [10]. The metabolism and uptake of amino acids, therefore, are aberrantly upregulated in many cancer types, and some of those cancer types are characterized by addiction to particular amino acids [11]. For these reasons, amino acid depletion therapies are extensively being explored in the area of cancer research [12].

The amino acid profile in prostate cancer, unlike in other solid tumors, is characterized by their anaplerotic roles more than by energy-production roles. Anaplerotic reactions are chemical reactions that form intermediates of a metabolic pathway and fuel that certain pathway. Many of the amino acids are implicated in prostate cancer, and their involvement has been recently reviewed [13,14]. For example, amino acids commonly related to prostate cancer include glutamine, leucine, serine, glycine, sarcosine, proline and arginine. In the light of the results of this paper, we describe further the roles of serine and taurine in prostate cancer.

Serine/glycine biosynthesis and one-carbon metabolism are intertwined and essential in promoting cancer cell survival and rapid proliferation. The excessive activation of serine/glycine biosynthesis pathways drives tumorigenesis and provides a single carbon unit for one-carbon metabolism. One-carbon metabolism, which is based on the chemical reactions of methionine and folate compounds, is used for the de novo synthesis of nucleotides, polyamines, amino acids, creatine and phospholipids. Serine is also a precursor for the synthesis of glycine and cysteine, both of which contribute to the production of glutathione, which is essential for redox homeostasis [15,16]. In prostate cancer, it was recently shown that increased serine and one-carbon pathway metabolism promote a neuroendocrine phenotype, which is the most lethal subtype of castration-resistant prostate cancer [17]. This characteristic represents a targetable vulnerability for prostate cancer [18,19]. In line with these findings, the role of alanine-serine-cysteine transporter 2 (ASCT2, SLC1A5) was studied. ASCT2 is a Na+-dependent transporter involved in the cellular uptake of neutral amino acids, that is, amino acids with small, hydrophilic side chains, such as serine, cysteine, asparagine and glutamine, but also alanine with the nonpolar methyl side chain [20]. The inhibition of ASCT2 suppresses prostate cancer cell growth in vitro. However, the contribution of serine to this process was not delineated, and the preferred substrate for ASCT2 is the conditionally essential amino acid glutamine [21,22]. Along with ASCT2 and several other transporters, SERINC3 (Serine Incorporator 3) protein was predicted to enable L-serine transmembrane transporter activity.

Taurine was also suggested to be potentially involved in prostate cancer progression. Namely, taurine was shown to attenuate the expression of epithelial–mesenchymal transition-related genes in human prostate cancer cells [23]. It also promoted apoptosis and inhibited proliferation of the prostate cancer cell line DU145, probably through the MST1/Hippo signaling pathway [24]. In another paper, it was shown that taurine suppressed PSA and metastasis-related genes expression in the human prostate cancer cell lines LNCaP and PC-3. In addition, taurine inhibited the migration of LNCaP and PC-3 cells [25]. Hypotaurine is a sulfinic acid that is an intermediate in the biosynthesis of taurine. An important gene in the metabolism of (hypo)taurine is *CSAD* (cysteine sulfinic acid decarboxylase). Its protein product catalyzes the decarboxylation of L-aspartate, 3-sulfino-L-alanine and L-cysteate to beta-alanine, hypotaurine and taurine, respectively. The preferred CSAD substrate is 3-sulfino-L-alanine.

In this introductory part we aimed to briefly present the global metabolic changes in prostate cancer and to place the changes in specific amino acid metabolism-related genes into this big picture. Furthermore, in a search for biomarkers that could predict the course of prostate cancer, in this article, we analyzed The Cancer Genome Atlas (TCGA) prostate adenocarcinoma (PRAD) dataset for the expression of amino acid metabolism-related genes. We found that their expression is highly aberrant in prostate cancer. By using a machine learning approach, we found that the expression of the genes *CSAD* and *SERINC3* discriminates between better and worse prognosis (low and high risk) for progression-free survival (PFS) of prostate cancer patients when they are stratified according to the Gleason score. In brief, this article aimed at analyzing the expression and the prognostic significance of amino acid metabolism-related genes in prostate cancer. We believe that this publication (a) adds to the big picture of potential metabolic changes in prostate cancer and (b) suggests potential biomarkers for prostate cancer prognosis. Another value of this paper, in our opinion, is methodological, and that is because (c) we used machine learning techniques (recursive partitioning and survival tree) for the definition of prognostic subgroups, unlike many of the scientific papers with a similar topic that used Cox proportional hazards regression analysis for the definition of each gene's prognostic abilities. Considering the prostate cancer heterogeneity, we believe that our method better captures its complexity.

2. Materials and Methods

2.1. Data Preparation and Differential Gene Expression Analysis

Amino acid metabolism-related genes were retrieved from The Molecular Signatures Database (MSigDB) [26] by using Gene Ontology Biological Process (GOBP) categories. The genes that were used in our analyses are listed in the Supplementary Table S1. Briefly, the following categories were considered: amino acid activation, homeostasis, transport, salvage, biosynthesis, metabolism, catabolism, response to amino acid starvation and C- and N-terminal protein amino acid modification. The final list contained 518 genes.

The Cancer Genome Atlas [27] prostate adenocarcinoma (PRAD) dataset, containing gene expression data and clinical information for 497 prostate cancer patients and corresponding control (surrounding, non-transformed) tissues for a subset of 52 patients, was downloaded and analyzed using the TCGAbiolinks R package [28–30]. To obtain more thorough insight into differentially expressed amino acid metabolism-related genes and to search deeper for their transcriptional changes in prostate cancer in comparison to non-transformed prostate tissue, we chose the threshold of $|\log2FC| \geq 0.585$ ($|$fold change$| \geq 1.5$) and p adjusted < 0.01. The data based on differentially expressed amino acid metabolism-related genes obtained in this way (N = 121) are listed in Supplementary Table S2. The expression represents the value of normalized counts.

The clinical data shown in Table 1 were obtained from cBioPortal [31] and the NCI Genomic Data Commons (GDC, TCGA) portal [32]. In total, there were 493 patients with clinical information (age, Gleason score, TNM stage, information related to residual tumor and radiation therapy) available. The event that we analyzed was progression-free survival (93 patients with this event), since, fortunately, only a smaller subset of patients experienced an event needed for the overall survival calculation. Some variables contained missing data. However, decision trees that we obtained in survival analysis by using recursive partitioning method are not as adversely affected by missing data as traditional statistical methods [33].

Table 1. Clinical information of TCGA patients. The number (N) and the percentage (in parenthesis) of patients belonging to a certain category is shown. In some categories, there are unknowns (NAs).

		No Progression	Progression
N, total		400	93
Age, years	<60	166 (41.5%)	34 (36.6%)
	≥60	234 (58.5%)	59 (63.4%)
Gleason score	6	44 (11%)	1 (1.1%)
	7	221 (55.3%)	24 (25.8%)
	8	49 (12.3)	13 (14%)
	9	84 (21%)	53 (57%)
	10	2 (0.5%)	2 (2.2%)
Clinical T stage	cT1	158 (39.5%)	17 (18.3%)
	cT2	137 (34.3%)	35 (37.6%)
	cT3	28 (7%)	24 (25.8%)
	cT4	1 (0.3%)	1 (1.1%)
	NA	76 (19%)	16 (17.2%)
Clinical M stage	cM0	362 (90.5%)	89 (95.7%)
	cM1	2 (0.5%)	1 (1.1%)
	NA	36 (9%)	3 (3.2%)
Pathologic T stage	pT2	172 (43%)	14 (15.1%)
	pT3	215 (53.8%)	75 (80.7%)
	pT4	7 (1.8%)	3 (3.2%)
	NA	6 (1.5%)	1 (1.1%)
Pathologic N stage	pN0	280 (70%)	62 (66.7%)
	pN1	56 (14%)	22 (23.7%)
	NA	64 (16%)	9 (9.7%)
Residual tumor	R0	266 (66.5%)	46 (49.5%)
	R1	102 (25.5%)	44 (47.3%)
	R2	5 (1.3%)	0
	RX	13 (3.3%)	2 (2.2%)
	NA	14 (3.5%)	1 (1.1%)
Radiation therapy	Yes	48 (12%)	46 (49.5%)
	No	313 (78.3%)	43 (46.2%)
	NA	39 (9.8%)	4 (4.3%)

2.2. Functional Enrichment Analysis

The 121 differentially expressed amino acid metabolism-related genes (DEGs) from Supplementary Table S1 were subjected to a functional enrichment analysis, which was conducted by using the Enrichr web server [34,35]. The top 10 Gene Ontology Molecular Function (MF) and Biological Process (BP) terms are shown in Table 2. Table 3 lists the functional annotation of the solute carrier family genes with differential expression in prostate cancer retrieved from www.genecards.org [36]. Additionally, Table 4 lists the functional annotation of the catabolic genes from the category Cellular amino acid catabolic process (GO:0009063) with differential expression in prostate cancer. The functional information was also retrieved from www.genecards.org [36].

Table 2. Enrichment analysis for the differentially expressed amino acid metabolism-related genes (N = 121). The gene ontology (GO) Molecular Function (MF) and Biological Process (BP) categories are listed.

GO Molecular Function (First 10 Terms) and Biological Process (Last 10 Terms) Categories	Overlap	*p*-Value	Adj. *p*-Value	Genes
Amino acid transmembrane transporter activity (GO:0015171)	16/49	3.26×10^{-24}	6.98×10^{-22}	*SLC36A1; SLC6A19; SLC38A1; SLC47A1; SLC43A1; SLC3A1; SLC38A11; SLC7A11; SLC6A1; SLC7A1; SLC7A4; SLC7A5; SLC6A6; PDPN; SLC16A2; SLC38A5*
L-amino acid transmembrane transporter activity (GO:0015179)	13/53	5.15×10^{-18}	5.51×10^{-16}	*SLC36A1; SLC38A1; SLC47A1; SLC43A1; SLC1A3; SLC3A1; SLC7A11; SLC7A1; SLC7A5; SLC25A15; SLC25A12; SLC25A22; SLC38A5*
Organic anion transmembrane transporter activity (GO:0008514)	17/144	1.67×10^{-17}	1.19×10^{-15}	*SLC36A1; SLC38A1; SLC1A3; SLC3A1; SLC6A1; SLC7A1; SLC6A6; SLC25A15; SLC7A5; GJA1; PDPN; SFXN3; SLC25A21; SFXN2; SLC25A12; SLC25A22; SLC38A5*
Carboxylic acid transmembrane transporter activity (GO:0046943)	12/57	7.73×10^{-16}	4.14×10^{-14}	*SLC36A1; SLC7A4; SLC7A5; SLC6A6; SLC38A1; PDPN; SLC3A1; SLC6A11; SLC38A11; SLC16A2; SLC7A1; SLC38A5*
Neutral amino acid transmembrane transporter activity (GO:0015175)	9/32	2.00×10^{-13}	8.57×10^{-12}	*SLC36A1; SLC6A6; SLC7A5; SLC6A19; SLC38A1; SLC43A1; SFXN3; SFXN2; SLC38A5*
Cation transmembrane transporter activity (GO:0008324)	9/48	1.10×10^{-11}	3.94×10^{-10}	*SLC36A1; SLC6A6; SLC7A5; SLC25A15; SLC38A1; SFXN3; SFXN2; SLC7A1; SLC38A5*
Pyridoxal phosphate binding (GO:0030170)	6/21	2.18×10^{-9}	6.66×10^{-8}	*SDS; OAT; SHMT2; CBS; PSAT1; ACCS*
Amino acid: sodium symporter activity (GO:0005283)	5/12	3.35×10^{-9}	7.96×10^{-8}	*SLC38A1; SLC6A15; SLC1A3; SLC6A11; SLC6A1*
Transaminase activity (GO:0008483)	5/12	3.35×10^{-9}	7.96×10^{-8}	*OAT; AADAT; PSAT1; BCAT1; BCAT2*
Amino acid binding (GO:0016597)	6/32	3.45×10^{-8}	7.38×10^{-7}	*GRM7; SHMT2; NOS1; NAGS; ASS1; GNMT*
Cellular amino acid catabolic process (GO:0009063)	25/90	2.11×10^{-35}	2.40×10^{-32}	*SHMT2; HAAO; SDSL; DDO; GCSH; IL4I1; TDO2; CBS; SLC25A21; NOS1; PRODH; GLUL; HMGCLL1; ACAD8; MCCC2; SDS; AADAT; GAD1; AMT; PIPOX; GSTZ1; BCAT1; ASPA; IDO1; BCAT2*
Alpha-amino acid metabolic process (GO:1901605)	16/46	9.80×10^{-25}	5.57×10^{-22}	*OAT; AADAT; FOLH1B; ASNS; PYCR1; ASS1; GNMT; FOLH1; CPS1; CBS; NOX4; DPEP1; RIMKLA; SLC25A12; GLUL; ASPA*
Amino acid transport (GO:0006865)	16/50	4.77×10^{-24}	1.81×10^{-21}	*SLC36A1; SLC6A19; SLC38A1; SLC6A17; SLC6A15; SLC43A1; SLC3A1; SLC38A11; SLC16A10; SLC7A11; SLC7A1; SLC7A4; SLC7A5; SLC6A6; PDPN; SLC38A5*
Amino acid transmembrane transport (GO:0003333)	14/45	5.77×10^{-21}	1.64×10^{-18}	*SLC36A1; SLC38A1; SLC47A1; SLC38A11; SLC7A11; SLC7A1; SLC6A6; SLC7A5; SFXN3; SFXN2; SLC16A2; SLC25A12; SLC25A22; SLC38A5*
Amino acid import (GO:0043090)	10/22	2.73×10^{-17}	6.21×10^{-15}	*SLC36A1; SLC6A6; SLC7A5; SLC47A1; SFXN3; SLC1A3; SFXN2; SLC6A1; SLC16A2; SLC7A1*
Glutamine family amino acid metabolic process (GO:0009064)	11/37	1.87×10^{-16}	3.54×10^{-14}	*OAT; GLYATL1; CPS1; AADAT; PYCR1; NAGS; PRODH; RIMKLA; GLUL; NIT2; ART4*

Table 2. *Cont.*

GO Molecular Function (First 10 Terms) and Biological Process (Last 10 Terms) Categories	Overlap	*p*-Value	Adj. *p*-Value	Genes
Nitrogen compound transport (GO:0071705)	15/143	8.73×10^{-15}	1.42×10^{-12}	*SLC36A1; SLC6A19; SLC38A1; SLC11A1; SLC6A15; SLC43A1; SLC3A1; SLC16A10; SLC7A11; SLC7A1; SLC7A4; SLC6A6; SLC7A5; PDPN; SLC38A5*
Organic acid transport (GO:0015849)	13/100	3.43×10^{-14}	4.88×10^{-12}	*SLC36A1; SLC6A19; SLC38A1; SLC6A15; SLC43A1; SLC3A1; SLC16A10; SLC7A11; SLC7A1; SLC7A4; SLC6A6; PDPN; SLC38A5*
Import into cell (GO:0098657)	10/41	4.3×10^{-14}	5.44×10^{-12}	*SLC36A1; SLC6A6; SLC7A5; SLC38A1; SLC47A1; SLC1A3; ATP1A2; SLC16A2; SLC7A1; GLUL*
Aspartate family amino acid metabolic process (GO:0009066)	9/30	1.01×10^{-13}	1.07×10^{-11}	*FOLH1; FOLH1B; SMS; ASNS; SLC25A12; ASPA; NIT2; ASS1*

Table 3. Functional annotation of solute carrier (SLC) family genes for which expression changes were observed in prostate cancer. The up- and down-regulated genes are listed separately. FC indicates fold change (tumor, T vs. normal, N), and FDR is the false discovery rate.

Gene	Function	FC (T/N)	FDR
SLC3A1	Transports neutral and basic amino acids in the renal tubule and intestinal tract.	2.72	2.93×10^{-5}
SLC6A11	Sodium-dependent transporter that uptakes gamma-aminobutyric acid (GABA), an inhibitory neurotransmitter, which ends the GABA neurotransmission.	3.72	7.57×10^{-13}
SLC6A15	Encodes a member of the solute carrier family 6 protein family, which transports neutral amino acids.	2.15	0.003273
SLC6A17	Responsible for the presynaptic uptake of neurotransmitters. The encoded vesicular transporter is selective for proline, glycine, leucine and alanine.	3.61	8.27×10^{-10}
SLC6A19	Encodes a system B(0) transmembrane protein that actively transports most neutral amino acids across the apical membrane of epithelial cells.	6.40	0.000127
SLC7A1	Enables L-arginine transmembrane transporter activity and L-histidine transmembrane transporter activity.	1.52	9.93×10^{-8}
SLC7A11	Encodes a member of a heteromeric, sodium-independent, anionic amino acid transport system that is highly specific for cysteine and glutamate.	3.67	6.95×10^{-22}
SLC11A1	Member of the proton-coupled divalent metal ion transporters family; encodes a multi-pass membrane protein that functions as a divalent transition metal (iron and manganese) transporter involved in iron metabolism.	1.79	2.91×10^{-11}
SLC16A10	Member of a family of plasma membrane amino acid transporters that mediate the Na(+)-independent transport of aromatic amino acids across the plasma membrane.	1.56	0.000213
SLC25A15	Member of the mitochondrial carrier family. The encoded protein transports ornithine across the inner mitochondrial membrane from the cytosol to the mitochondrial matrix. The protein is an essential component of the urea cycle and functions in ammonium detoxification and biosynthesis of the amino acid arginine.	1.74	3.49×10^{-14}
SLC25A21	Mitochondrial carrier that transports C5-C7 oxodicarboxylates across inner mitochondrial membranes.	1.98	5.81×10^{-12}
SLC25A22	Encodes a mitochondrial glutamate carrier.	1.88	1.43×10^{-24}

Table 3. *Cont.*

Gene	Function	FC (T/N)	FDR
SLC36A1	The encoded protein functions as a proton-dependent, small amino acid transporter.	1.80	3.82×10^{-6}
SLC38A11	Predicted to enable amino acid transmembrane transporter activity.	2.45	1.02×10^{-6}
SLC43A1	Belongs to the system L family of plasma membrane carrier proteins that transports large neutral amino acids.	2.72	2.92×10^{-17}
SLC1A3	Member of a high affinity glutamate transporter family.	0.55	1.63×10^{-12}
SLC6A1	The protein encoded by this gene is a gamma-aminobutyric acid (GABA) transporter that localizes to the plasma membrane.	0.65	3.31×10^{-5}
SLC6A6	This gene encodes a multi-pass membrane protein that is a member of a family of sodium and chloride-ion-dependent transporters. The encoded protein transports taurine and beta-alanine.	0.64	1.32×10^{-9}
SLC7A4	Predicted to enable amino acid transmembrane transporter activity. Predicted to be involved in amino acid transport.	0.53	0.001077
SLC7A5	Enables L-leucine transmembrane transporter activity, L-tryptophan transmembrane transporter activity and thyroid hormone transmembrane transporter activity.	0.31	2.00×10^{-26}
SLC16A2	Encodes an integral membrane protein that functions as a transporter of thyroid hormone.	0.58	1.00×10^{-17}
SLC25A12	Encodes a calcium-binding mitochondrial carrier protein. The encoded protein localizes to the mitochondria and is involved in the exchange of aspartate for glutamate across the inner mitochondrial membrane.	0.64	3.29×10^{-24}
SLC38A1	An important transporter of glutamine, an intermediate in the detoxification of ammonia and the production of urea.	0.64	9.92×10^{-14}
SLC38A5	The encoded protein transports glutamine, asparagine, histidine, serine, alanine and glycine across the cell membrane, but does not transport charged amino acids, imino acids, or N-alkylated amino acids.	0.45	3.30×10^{-16}
SLC47A1	Among its related pathways are the transport of inorganic cations/anions and amino acids/oligopeptides.	0.39	6.09×10^{-29}

Table 4. Functional annotation of Cellular amino acid catabolic process (GO:0009063) genes from Table 2 for which expression changes were observed in prostate cancer. The up- and down-regulated genes are listed separately. FC indicates fold change (tumor, T vs. normal, N), and FDR is the false discovery rate.

Gene	Function	FC (T/N)	FDR
AADAT	Aminoadipate aminotransferase. Highly similar to mouse and rat kynurenine aminotransferase II. The rat protein is a homodimer with two transaminase activities. One activity is the transamination of alpha-aminoadipic acid, a final step in the saccaropine pathway, which is the major pathway for L-lysine catabolism. The other activity involves the transamination of kynurenine to produce kynurenine acid, the precursor of kynurenic acid.	2.01	6.04×10^{-12}
ACAD8	Acyl-CoA dehydrogenase family member 8. This gene encodes a member of the acyl-CoA dehydrogenase family of enzymes that catalyzes the dehydrogenation of acyl-CoA derivatives in the metabolism of fatty acids or branch-chained amino acids. The encoded protein is a mitochondrial enzyme that functions in catabolism of the branched-chain amino acid valine.	1.67	2.96×10^{-5}
BCAT1	Branched chain amino acid transaminase 1. This gene encodes the cytosolic form of the enzyme branched-chain amino acid transaminase. This enzyme catalyzes the reversible transamination of branched-chain alpha-keto acids to branched-chain L-amino acids essential for cell growth.	1.71	0.00045

Table 4. *Cont.*

Gene	Function	FC (T/N)	FDR
BCAT2	Branched chain amino acid transaminase 2. This gene encodes a branched-chain aminotransferase found in mitochondria. The encoded protein forms a dimer that catalyzes the first step in the production of the branched-chain amino acids leucine, isoleucine and valine.	1.51	3.01×10^{-12}
CBS	Cystathionine beta-synthase. The protein encoded by this gene acts as a homotetramer to catalyze the conversion of homocysteine to cystathionine, the first step in the transsulfuration pathway.	2.23	2.09×10^{-14}
GAD1	Glutamate decarboxylase 1. This gene encodes one of several forms of glutamic acid decarboxylase, identified as a major autoantigen in insulin-dependent diabetes. The enzyme encoded is responsible for catalyzing the production of gamma-aminobutyric acid from L-glutamic acid.	3.07	4.07×10^{-13}
GCSH	Glycine cleavage system protein H. The degradation of glycine is brought about by the glycine cleavage system, which is composed of four mitochondrial protein components: P protein (a pyridoxal phosphate-dependent glycine decarboxylase), H protein (a lipoic acid-containing protein), T protein (a tetrahydrofolate-requiring enzyme), and L protein (a lipoamide dehydrogenase). The protein encoded by this gene is the H protein, which transfers the methylamine group of glycine from the P protein to the T protein.	1.62	1.98×10^{-5}
GSTZ1	Glutathione S-transferase zeta 1. This gene is a member of the glutathione S-transferase (GST) super-family that encodes multifunctional enzymes important in the detoxification of electrophilic molecules, including carcinogens, mutagens and several therapeutic drugs, via conjugation with glutathione. This enzyme catalyzes the conversion of maleylacetoacetate to fumarylacetoacatate, which is one of the steps in the phenylalanine/tyrosine degradation pathway.	1.51	1.98×10^{-9}
IDO1	Indoleamine 2,3-dioxygenase 1. This gene encodes indoleamine 2,3-dioxygenase (IDO)—a heme enzyme that catalyzes the first and rate-limiting step in tryptophan catabolism to N-formyl-kynurenine. This enzyme acts on multiple tryptophan substrates, including D-tryptophan, L-tryptophan, 5-hydroxy-tryptophan, tryptamine, and serotonin.	1.51	0.009556
IL4I1	Interleukin 4 induced 1. This gene encodes a secreted L-amino acid oxidase protein, which primarily catabolizes L-phenylalanine and, to a lesser extent, L-arginine.	1.81	5.50×10^{-10}
MCCC2	Methylcrotonyl-CoA carboxylase subunit 2. This gene encodes the small subunit of 3-methylcrotonyl-CoA carboxylase. This enzyme functions as a heterodimer and catalyzes the carboxylation of 3-methylcrotonyl-CoA to form 3-methylglutaconyl-CoA.	2.45	5.63×10^{-12}
SDS	Serine dehydratase. This gene encodes one of three enzymes that are involved in metabolizing serine and glycine. L-serine dehydratase converts L-serine to pyruvate and ammonia and requires pyridoxal phosphate as a cofactor. The encoded protein can also metabolize threonine to NH4+ and 2-ketobutyrate.	3.32	1.36×10^{-14}
SDSL	Serine dehydratase like. Predicted to be involved in the isoleucine biosynthetic process and threonine catabolic process.	1.52	3.11×10^{-10}
SHMT2	Serine hydroxymethyltransferase 2. This gene encodes the mitochondrial form of a pyridoxal phosphate-dependent enzyme that catalyzes the reversible reaction of serine and tetrahydrofolate to glycine and 5,10-methylene tetrahydrofolate. The encoded product is primarily responsible for glycine synthesis. The activity of the encoded protein has been suggested to be the primary source of intracellular glycine.	1.69	7.99×10^{-17}

Table 4. *Cont.*

Gene	Function	FC (T/N)	FDR
SLC25A21	Solute carrier family 25 member 21. Homolog of the S. cerevisiae ODC proteins, mitochondrial carriers that transport C5-C7 oxodicarboxylates across inner mitochondrial membranes. One of the species transported by ODC is 2-oxoadipate, a common intermediate in the catabolism of lysine, tryptophan and hydroxylysine in mammals.	1.98	5.81×10^{-12}
TDO2	Tryptophan 2,3-dioxygenase. This gene encodes a heme enzyme that plays a critical role in tryptophan metabolism by catalyzing the first and rate-limiting step of the kynurenine pathway.	3.45	0.0044
AMT	Aminomethyltransferase. This gene encodes one of four critical components of the glycine cleavage system.	0.52	7.11×10^{-13}
ASPA	Aspartoacylase. This gene encodes an enzyme that catalyzes the conversion of N-acetyl-L-aspartic acid (NAA) to aspartate and acetate.	0.24	6.87×10^{-31}
DDO	D-aspartate oxidase. The protein encoded by this gene is a peroxisomal flavoprotein that catalyzes the oxidative deamination of D-aspartate and N-methyl D-aspartate.	0.50	1.01×10^{-15}
GLUL	Glutamate-ammonia ligase. The protein encoded by this gene belongs to the glutamine synthetase family. It catalyzes the synthesis of glutamine from glutamate and ammonia in an ATP-dependent reaction.	0.64	7.49×10^{-16}
HAAO	3-Hydroxyanthranilate 3,4-dioxygenase is a monomeric cytosolic protein belonging to the family of intramolecular dioxygenases containing nonheme ferrous iron. HAAO catalyzes the synthesis of quinolinic acid (QUIN) from 3-hydroxyanthranilic acid.	0.45	2.36×10^{-19}
HMGCLL1	3-Hydroxymethyl-3-methylglutaryl-CoA lyase like 1. Non-mitochondrial 3-hydroxymethyl-3-methylglutaryl-CoA lyase that catalyzes the cation-dependent cleavage of (S)-3-hydroxy-3-methylglutaryl-CoA into acetyl-CoA and acetoacetate, a key step in ketogenesis.	0.32	5.18×10^{-15}
NOS1	Nitric oxide synthase 1. The protein encoded by this gene belongs to the family of nitric oxide synthases, which synthesize nitric oxide from L-arginine.	0.28	2.12×10^{-14}
PIPOX	Pipecolic acid and sarcosine oxidase. Enables L-pipecolate oxidase activity and sarcosine oxidase activity. Involved in L-lysine catabolic process to acetyl-CoA via L-pipecolate.	0.39	3.84×10^{-24}
PRODH	Proline dehydrogenase 1. This gene encodes a mitochondrial protein that catalyzes the first step in proline degradation.	0.35	1.70×10^{-24}

2.3. Survival Analysis

Pre-processed and normalized, but un-filtered, TCGA [27] expression data for the amino acid metabolism-related genes were obtained through the TCGAbiolinks R package [28–30]. The clinical data were added to expression data, organized in a data matrix and analyzed using the data analysis software R [37], version 4.2.1.

For the survival analysis, we used rpart module [38,39] in the programming language R [37]. rpart stands for Recursive PARTitioning and is the most used application for the construction of survival trees. Survival trees obtained via this method enable visual identification and comparisons of prognostic factors in a simple and straightforward manner [40,41]. The method is insensitive to missing data, in contrast to classical statistical methods, and gives reliable and robust conclusions in most clinical scenarios. The method is described in more detail in our previous publications [42]. Briefly, at the beginning of the analysis, all patients are included and in subsequent steps, they are divided into prognostic subgroups in a survival tree. At the first split (root node), a logical check is performed. If the criterion of that node is met, the left side of the tree is approached; otherwise it is the right. This is repeated at each stage (decision node) until the terminal node is reached. Therefore, a survival tree obtained in this way is composed of decision nodes and terminal nodes (leaves). Each decision node uses a provided variable to subdivide patients into two subgroups with a maximum difference in hazard ratios (HRs). The terminal nodes are reached when no further improvement in subdivision is possible. Patients in the first decision node have hazard ratio of 1. The hazard ratio for patients in each node is expressed in comparison to this value. To avoid overfitting, that is, an extensive fragmentation of the tree for which it would be hard to infer a biological meaning, we set the complexity parameter CP to 0.0373.

2.4. Kaplan–Meier Survival Estimate

The difference in survival between patients in terminal nodes was analyzed using a log-rank test and is presented as survival curves based on the Kaplan–Meier survival estimate [43]. This part of the analysis was based on the EZR package [44] in programming language R. Data were considered statistically significant if the p value of the log-rank test was ≤ 0.05.

3. Results

3.1. Prostate Cancer Amino Acid Metabolism-Related Gene Expression Appears to Be Highly Aberrant

As elaborated previously, amino acid metabolism-related genes play important roles in prostate cancer. To search for amino acid metabolism-related genes that are specifically changed in prostate cancer, we conducted differential gene expression analysis. The results with thresholds $|\log 2FC| > 0.585$ and p adjusted < 0.01 revealed 4215 differentially expressed genes (DEGs) in total. Among them, there were 121 differentially expressed amino acid metabolism-related genes, which are listed in Supplementary Table S2. The enrichment analysis conducted on those 121 differentially expressed genes (Table 2) showed that the expression of genes involved in amino acid transmembrane transport (mainly of the solute carrier family) is highly perturbed. The functional annotation of the solute carrier family genes listed in Supplementary Table S2 is provided in Table 3.

Table 4 lists the roles of Cellular amino acid catabolic process (GO:0009063) genes from Table 2 for which expression changes were observed in prostate cancer. Some important genes involved, for example, in the synthesis of glycine from serine, such as *SHMT2* (serine hydroxymethyltransferase 2), showed increased expression in tumor tissue. The activity of SHMT2 has been suggested to be the primary source of intracellular glycine. Genes that encode proteins involved in the catabolism of L-lysine (AADAT), valine (ACAD8), glycine (GCSH), phenylalanine/tyrosine (GSTZ1), tryptophan (IDO1, TDO2), L-phenylalanine and L-arginine (IL4I1) and serine and glycine (SDS) also showed increased expression. The genes encoding proteins involved in production of the branched-chain amino acids leucine, isoleucine and valine (BCAT2, BCAT1) were also increased in tumor vs. non-transformed tissue. On the other hand, genes with decreased expression in tumor tissue were *AMT*, which is involved in glycine cleavage system; *GLUL*, which catalyzes the synthesis of glutamine from glutamate and ammonia; *NOS1*, nitric oxide synthase, which synthesizes nitric oxide from L-arginine; *PIPOX*, which is involved in L-lysine catabolic process; and *PRODH*, which catalyzes the first step in proline degradation.

For the genes that we show are involved in prostate cancer prognosis (see further section), *CSAD* had increased expression in prostate cancer (fold-change = 1.61, FDR < 0.001, Supplementary Table S2), while the expression of *SERINC3* did not change according to the criteria used.

3.2. *CSAD and SERINC3 Genes Further Refine the Prognostic Value of the Gleason Score in Prostate Cancer*

Prognostic values of variables listed in Table 1 (age, Gleason score, TNM staging, residual tumor information and radiation therapy) supplemented with gene expression data for amino acid metabolism-related genes were determined using recursive partitioning, the recommended method by the AJCC (American Joint Committee on Cancer) for the analysis of prognostic studies [40,41]. The importance of individual variables is shown in Figure 1. The four most informative variables were the Gleason score and the expression of *CSAD*, *GABBR1* and *SERINC3* genes. Among them, only GABBR1 did not appear in multivariate analysis. The *GABBR1* gene encodes a receptor for gamma-aminobutyric acid (GABA), which is the main inhibitory neurotransmitter in the mammalian central nervous system. Its role in the progression of prostate cancer has been documented [45].

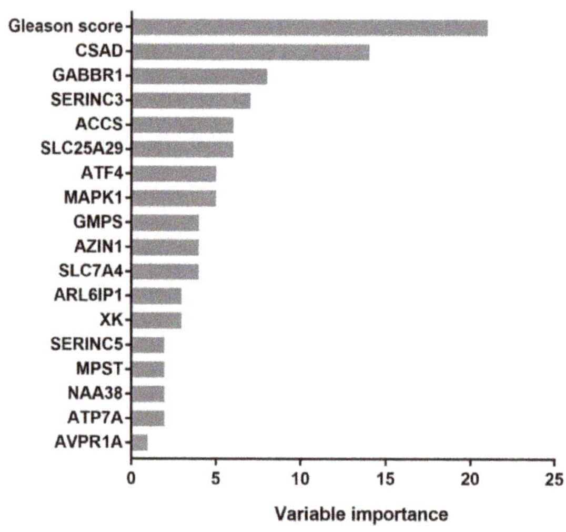

Figure 1. Variable importance determined via the rpart method. CSAD, cysteine sulfinic acid decarboxylase; GABBR1, gamma-aminobutyric acid type B receptor subunit 1; SERINC3, serine incorporator 3; ACCS, 1-aminocyclopropane-1-carboxylate synthase homolog (inactive); SLC25A29, solute carrier family 25 member 29; ATF4, activating transcription factor 4; MAPK1, mitogen-activated protein kinase 1; GMPS, guanine monophosphate synthase; AZIN1, antizyme inhibitor 1; SLC7A4, solute carrier family 7 member 4; ARL6IP1, ADP ribosylation factor-like GTPase 6 interacting protein 1; XK, X-linked Kx blood group antigen, Kell and VPS13A-binding protein; SERINC5, serine incorporator 5; MPST, mercaptopyruvate sulfurtransferase; NAA38, N-alpha-acetyltransferase 38, NatC auxiliary subunit; ATP7A, ATPase copper transporting alpha; AVPR1A, arginine vasopressin receptor 1A.

However, AJCC criteria for prognostic studies require that a prognostic value of a variable must be always assessed in the context of other variables [40,41]. The rpart algorithm obeys this criterion since rpart uses all variables (multivariate approach) in the analysis. The rpart results are presented on a survival tree (Figure 2). Figure 2 shows that by using three variables, patients could be subdivided into three decision nodes and four terminal nodes (leaves). Variables used in the decision nodes were as follows: (1) the Gleason score, (2) *CSAD* gene expression (for Gleason score < 9), and (3) *SERINC3* gene expression (for Gleason score ≥ 9). The importance of variables was determined by their position in the survival tree: the topmost variable (Gleason score) is the most informative, the variable below topmost is the second one by information value, and so on. The first number in a decision node rectangle denotes the hazard ratio (HR) and the numbers in the second row denote patients with the event (progression) vs. the total number of patients. The number in a third row denotes the percentage of patients in that node. Therefore, it is evident that, while the analysis starts with all patients included in the study (decision node 1; N = 493; N with progression = 93), decision node 2 is based on 71% and decision node 3 on 29% of patients. Further refinement of survival data revealed four prognostic groups: low Gleason score, low *CSAD* expression (28% of patients); low Gleason score, high *CSAD* expression (43%); high Gleason score, low *SERINC3* expression (6%); and finally, high Gleason score, high *SERINC3* expression (23%). The leftmost terminal node represents the group of patients at a very low risk (HR = 0.088), and the second represents patients at a medium risk (HR = 0.97). The second terminal node from the right represent patients at a low risk (HR = 0.48) and the right-most terminal node describes patients at a high risk of prostate cancer progression (HR = 2.9) (Table 5). To emphasize once again, patients in the first decision node have a hazard ratio of 1. The hazard ratio for patients in each node is expressed in comparison to this value. In conclusion, by using the information based on the Gleason score and the expression of *CSAD* and *SERINC3* genes, a subdivision of prostate cancer patients into four prognostic groups with substantially different HRs was achieved.

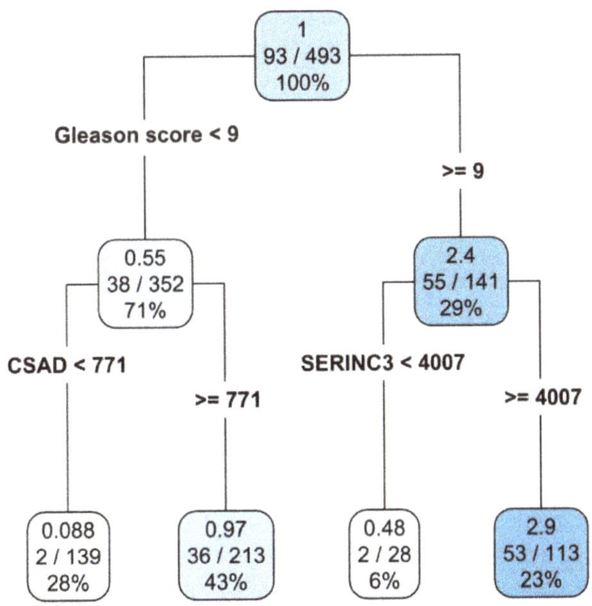

Figure 2. Survival tree constructed using the rpart method identifies four terminal subgroups of patients. The shading of the color denotes the risk group (darker color stands for a higher risk).

Table 5. Risk subgroups extracted via rpart analysis.

Risk Subgroup	Hazard Ratio	Rule
Very low risk	0.088	Gleason score < 9 AND *CSAD* < 771
Low risk	0.480	Gleason score $\geq$ 9 AND *SERINC3* < 4007
Medium risk	0.974	Gleason score < 9 AND *CSAD* $\geq$ 771
High risk	2.923	Gleason score $\geq$ 9 AND *SERINC3* $\geq$ 4007

3.3. Kaplan–Meier Estimate on Prostate Cancer Patients Stratified According to Gleason Score and CSAD and SERINC3 Expression

The results of recursive partitioning (Figure 2) were further supplemented by survival curves (Kaplan–Meier method) for subgroups defined in each decision node. The difference for subgroups defined by the left and right branches of decision node 1 is shown in Figure 3, and it was statistically significant (log-rank test, $p < 0.001$). The subgroups defined by the left and right branches of node 2 are shown in Figure 4 (log-rank test, $p < 0.001$). Figure 5 shows that the difference between subgroups of node 3 was also statistically significant (log-rank test, $p < 0.001$).

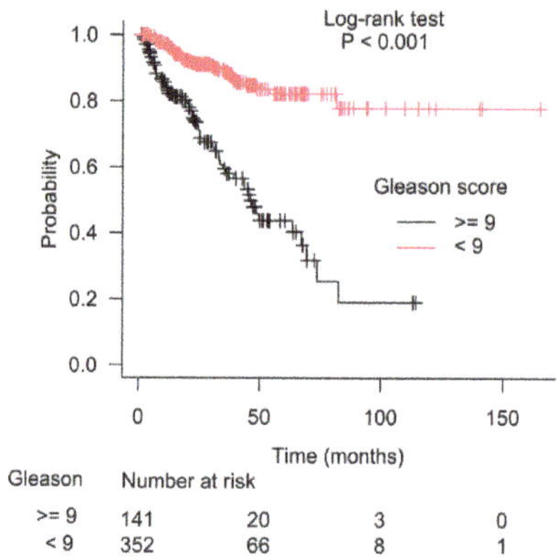

Figure 3. Difference in patients' survival for the left and the right branches of the starting decision node (node 1), which used the Gleason score as a separation criterion.

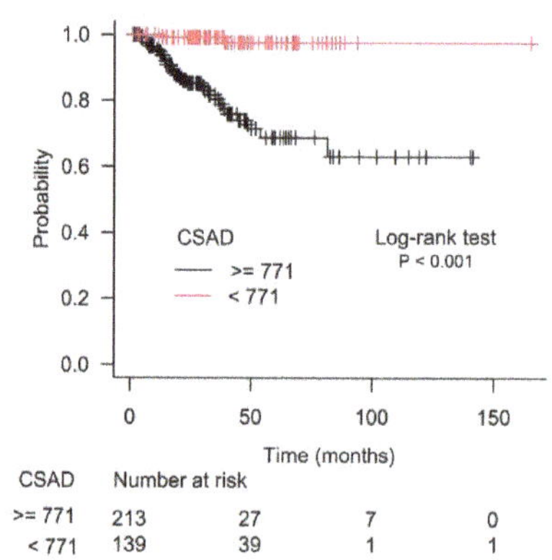

Figure 4. Difference in patients' survival for the left and the right branches of the second decision node (node 2), which used *CSAD* gene expression as a separation criterion.

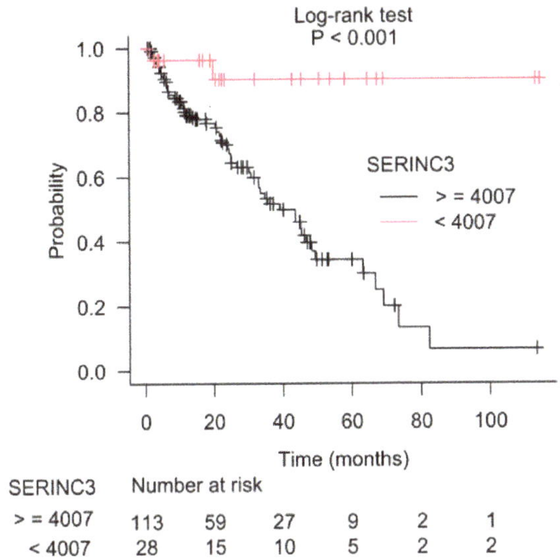

Figure 5. Difference in patients' survival for the left and the right branches of the third decision node (node 3), which used *SERINC3* gene expression as a separation criterion.

4. Discussion

4.1. Metabolites and Metabolism-Related Genes in the Prognosis of Prostate Cancer

The driving events in prostate cancer progression include entangled actions of several signaling pathways that are potentiated by changes in gene expression, genetic and epigenetic alterations [46] and post-transcriptional and post-translational modifications [47]. However, although a substantial amount of information is gathered in regard to the mentioned processes, one of the major obstacles in prostate cancer management is still the inability to predict the course of a disease, that is, to differentiate between slowly growing cancers that do not require immediate treatment and those that are more aggressive and will progress fast.

The metabolic landscape in cancers is highly perturbed in comparison to that in healthy tissue and metabolic genes and molecules, therefore, hold potential to be exploited in a search for disease biomarkers and novel therapeutic targets. This is especially the case since, not only primary tumors, but also metastases from certain tissues (e.g., liver and some other sites [48,49]), acquire changes in metabolism-related gene expression profiles. Metabolic profiles in prostate cancer have been thoroughly studied and reviewed by Kelly et al. [50] who analyzed the articles reporting metabolites in prostate tissue, blood, urine and prostatic secretions. They showed that amino acids are among the most promising metabolic diagnostic biomarkers and biomarkers of tumor aggressiveness. Some amino acids (e.g., glutamine) were also used in terms of predicting disease recurrence [5]. In addition to metabolites themselves, the repertoire of metabolic genes as a source of prostate cancer biomarkers has already been studied. Namely, Zhang et al. identified three metabolism-associated prostate cancer clusters that were characterized by significantly different outcomes in disease-free survival (DFS), clinical stage, stemness index, tumor microenvironment (including stromal and immune cells), presence of DNA mutation (TP53 and SPOP), copy number variation and microsatellite instability [51]. In a further paper, they established metabolism-scores of tumors to predict the prognosis of prostate cancer. This metabolic score was closely related to the tumor microenvironment, presence of DNA mutations and drug sensitivity [52]. Feng et al. studied energy metabolism-related genes in prostate cancer and defined an energy metabolism-related gene prognostic index, which proved to predict biochemical recurrence for patients with prostate cancer that were undergoing radical prostatectomy [53]. Finally, Zhao et al. were able to predict biochemical-recurrence-free survival (BRFS) using a three-metabolic-gene risk score model in prostate cancer patients [2].

4.2. Differentially Expressed Amino Acid Metabolism-Related Genes in Prostate Cancer

Although, as elaborated, several papers already dealt with the potential of metabolic genes in predicting the outcome of prostate cancer patients, none of them, to the best of our knowledge, analyzed the amino-acid metabolism-related genes separately. Since amino acids themselves, as already mentioned [50], are involved in the prognosis for prostate cancer patients, it is to be expected that the genes encoding proteins that participate in their metabolism would also show prognostic capabilities. In very recent papers, the amino acid metabolism genes already showed good performance in the prognosis of e.g., colorectal cancer [54], hepatocellular carcinoma [55], clear cell renal cell carcinoma [56], glioma [57] and head and neck squamous cell carcinomas [58]. In this research, we studied the potential of amino acid metabolism-related genes to predict progression-free survival (PFS) using The Cancer Genome Atlas prostate adenocarcinoma (PRAD) dataset.

The first relevant finding of this paper is that the expression of the genes encoding proteins that are involved in amino acid transport across both the cellular (majority) and the mitochondrial (to a lesser extent) membrane show changed expression. Namely, the solute carrier (SLC) family genes were among the top terms in functional enrichment analysis of both Gene Ontology (GO) Molecular Function and GO Biological Process categories of differentially expressed genes (DEGs) (Tables 2 and 3). The SLC group of membrane transport proteins include over 400 members organized into 66 families. Solutes that are transported by the various SLC proteins are extremely diverse and include charged and uncharged organic molecules, inorganic ions and the gas ammonia. However, most of the SLC group members listed in Table 3 are involved in amino acid transport as they were selected because of their connection with amino acid metabolism. Although more of the SLCs are up-regulated (15) than down-regulated (10) in prostate cancer, it is hard to speculate about the 'big picture', that is, to establish which of the amino acids are largely influenced by these changes in the expression of SLCs. What is known is that some of these gene products were shown to be implicated in prostate cancer progression, such as, for example, SLC7A5 [59], SLC7A11 [60], SLC11A1 [61], SLC43A1 [62] and SLC1A3 [63]. Although not listed in the Table 3, a recent paper documented metabolic reprogramming and the predominance of several solute carrier genes (*SLC12A5*, *SLC25A17* and *SLC27A6*) during acquired enzalutamide resistance in prostate cancer [64], emphasizing the importance of the SLC family members in prostate cancer.

Another group of genes with changed expression in prostate cancer includes the genes coding for proteins that are involved in the catabolism of different amino acids, as elaborated in the Results section and shown in Tables 2 and 4.

4.3. Prognostic Value of Amino Acid Metabolism-Related Genes in Prostate Cancer

To get back to the primary question of this publication, which would be the prediction of prostate cancer outcomes, several publications already used gene expression profiles to foresee the prostate cancer prognosis (e.g., [65–72]). However, as already mentioned, those still did not make it to the clinics; that is, the course of prostate cancer remains mainly unpredictable. Therefore, in this paper, we extended the knowledge on potential prostate cancer progression-free survival biomarkers to amino acid metabolism-related genes. The changes in expression of those genes are extensive in prostate cancer and therefore hold potential for biomarkers and therapeutic targets. We found that the Gleason score is the strongest variable influencing prostate cancer progression-free survival in a multivariate analysis. This is to be expected, since the Gleason score is highly informative of the characteristics of tumor cells that constitute the tumor tissue. However, when the patients were stratified according to a low/high Gleason score, the genes *CSAD* (for the low Gleason score) and *SERINC3* (for the high Gleason score) differentiated the risk of progression. That is, patients with higher *CSAD* and higher *SERINC3* expression are at a higher risk of progression (Figure 2).

CSAD protein is involved in the generation of beta-alanine, hypotaurine and taurine. Although papers suggest that taurine has a beneficial role in prostate cancer (see Introduction), it needs to be emphasized that hypotaurine is the preferential product of the biochemical reaction involving CSAD. It was shown that hypotaurine potentiates a malignant phenotype in glioma through aberrant hypoxic signaling. The authors show that taurine, the oxidation metabolite of hypotaurine, decreased intracellular hypotaurine and resulted in glioma cell growth arrest [73]. Therefore, the ratio of hypotaurine/taurine could play a role in prostate cancer as well. Additionally, long non-coding RNA TUG1 (taurine up-regulated 1) was originally identified in a genomic screen of taurine-treated mouse retinal cells [74]. TUG1 accelerates prostate cancer progression [75,76]. Its knockdown inhibits the tumorigenesis and progression of prostate cancer in vitro and in vivo [77] and enhances radiosensitivity [78]. Finally, high expression of TUG1 correlates with progression of the disease and less favorable survival profiles in prostate cancer patients [79]. To emphasize that CSAD plays versatile roles in different cancer types, data from The Human Protein Atlas [80,81] state that *CSAD* is an unfavorable prognostic marker in renal and colorectal cancer, which would agree with our study. However, it is favorable in urothelial, liver, pancreatic and head and neck cancer. To add more complexity to the potential mechanisms of action involving hypotaurine/taurine, CSAD also catalyzes the generation of beta-alanine. It would be interesting to further detangle these complex relationships (hypotaurine–taurine–beta–alanine), of which taurine is the most studied, and define their impact on prostate cancer.

As elaborated in an introductory part, serine metabolism potentiates the malignancy of prostate cancer. The serine incorporator (SERINC) proteins are a family of multipass transmembrane proteins associated with the biosynthesis of serine-containing phospholipids and sphingolipids [82]. More precisely, SERINC2–4 are carrier proteins that incorporate the polar amino acid serine into membranes to facilitate the synthesis of phosphatidylserine and sphingolipids [83]. SERINC proteins were most studied in the context of viral infections during which they are constitutive host resistance factors, which suppress viral infection by incorporating into virus particles [83]. Phosphatidylserine (PS) is a serine-containing phospholipid and a component of the cell membrane. It plays a key role in cell cycle signaling, specifically in relation to apoptosis. Studies using pre-clinical models of prostate cancer showed that antibody-mediated PS blockade reprograms the innate immune system to promote anti-tumor responses. Therefore, bavituximab, a PS-targeting antibody, is being assessed in multiple clinical trials, including those for prostate cancer [84]. Sphingolipids are synthesized from serine and palmitoyl-CoA. Inhibitors of sphingolipid metabolism were shown to antagonize pro-survival responses. Moreover, cancer cells use sphingolipid-driven escape mechanisms to evade therapies. Sphingolipids have also been implicated in prostate cancer, as recently reviewed [85]. This brief overview of the promoting roles of phosphatidylserine and sphingolipids in prostate tumorigenesis agrees with our findings that the increased expression of *SERINC3*, which potentiates their biosynthesis, represents a higher risk of disease progression for prostate cancer patients that are stratified according to the Gleason score. In addition to *SERINC3*, *SERINC5*, for which the gene product has a similar function to SERINC3, is present on the list of genes implicated by our univariate analysis (Figure 1). This further indicates that the processes conducted by proteins encoded by these genes are potentially critically involved in prostate tumorigenesis.

4.4. Methodological Considerations

Besides dealing with biological processes involved in prostate cancer progression, our paper differs from those with a similar topic in that we used machine learning to define prognostic subgroups instead of using Cox proportional hazards regression analysis to define gene-based prognosis. From the technical point of view, the recursive partitioning method used has the advantage in that it establishes the hierarchy of the variables studied;

that is, this method lists the variables by their importance for prognosis. In this way, subgroups of patients are defined, and the knowledge on their specificities is refined. Given the heterogeneity of prostate cancer, we believe that this method is more suitable to define gene expression-specific prostate cancer characteristics. Additionally, the survival tree, generated through recursive partitioning, is easier to interpret than the Cox regression results.

5. Conclusions

In our study, we analyzed differentially expressed genes between prostate cancer and surrounding non-transformed prostate tissue by using TCGA data. We found that the expression of amino acid metabolism-related genes is highly aberrant in prostate cancer. The groups of genes that are the most affected include solute carrier family of amino acid transporters and the genes involved in the catabolism of amino acids, which are mainly up-regulated. Furthermore, we found that the Gleason score is the strongest prognostic factor for progression-free survival in prostate cancer patients, which is expected given the amount of information provided by this parameter. However, when the patients are stratified according to the Gleason score, the genes *CSAD* (low Gleason score) and *SERINC3* (high Gleason score) further refine the prognosis. The high expression of both *CSAD* and *SERINC3* is correlated with worse outcomes. The *CSAD* gene product is involved in hypotaurine generation, and the *SERINC3* gene product is involved in the generation of phosphatidylserine and sphingolipids. There are indications that hypotaurine, phosphatidylserine and sphingolipids promote prostate cancer progression. We believe that our results hold potential for the future design of prognostic biomarkers in prostate cancer, which is an intensive field of research, considering that the progression of prostate cancer is currently hard to predict. Functional studies on *CSAD* and *SERINC3* genes and their regulators are needed to further delineate their roles in prostate cancer, which would reveal their potential for further interventions.

Supplementary Materials: The following supporting information can be downloaded at: https://www.mdpi.com/article/10.3390/cancers15041309/s1, Table S1: Human amino-acid metabolism-related genes categorized through Gene Ontology Biological Processes (GOBPs; retrieved from https://www.gsea-msigdb.org/gsea/msigdb/index.jsp (accessed on 1 November 2022)); Table S2: Differentially expressed amino-acid metabolism-related genes between prostate cancer tumor and non-tumor tissue with a threshold $|\log2FC| \geq 0.585$ and FDR < 0.01.

Author Contributions: Conceptualization, I.S. and P.K.; methodology, I.S. and P.K.; formal analysis, I.S. and P.K.; investigation, I.S., P.K. and K.G.T.; data curation, I.S. and P.K.; writing—original draft preparation, I.S.; writing—review and editing, I.S., P.K. and K.G.T.; supervision, P.K. All authors have read and agreed to the published version of the manuscript.

Funding: This research was funded by a MY ZABA START 2019 donation from Zagrebačka banka (I.S.).

Institutional Review Board Statement: Not applicable.

Informed Consent Statement: Not applicable (this study uses publicly available data).

Data Availability Statement: In this article, we used The Cancer Genome Atlas (TCGA) prostate adenocarcinoma (PRAD) dataset available at https://gdc.cancer.gov/ (accessed on 1 November 2022).

Conflicts of Interest: The authors declare no conflict of interest.

References

1. Sung, H.; Ferlay, J.; Siegel, R.L.; Laversanne, M.; Soerjomataram, I.; Jemal, A.; Bray, F. Global Cancer Statistics 2020: GLOBOCAN Estimates of Incidence and Mortality Worldwide for 36 Cancers in 185 Countries. *CA Cancer J. Clin.* **2021**, *71*, 209–249. [CrossRef]
2. Zhao, Y.; Tao, Z.; Li, L.; Zheng, J.; Chen, X. Predicting Biochemical-Recurrence-Free Survival Using a Three-Metabolic-Gene Risk Score Model in Prostate Cancer Patients. *BMC Cancer* **2022**, *22*, 239. [CrossRef]
3. van den Broeck, T.; van den Bergh, R.C.N.; Briers, E.; Cornford, P.; Cumberbatch, M.; Tilki, D.; de Santis, M.; Fanti, S.; Fossati, N.; Gillessen, S.; et al. Biochemical Recurrence in Prostate Cancer: The European Association of Urology Prostate Cancer Guidelines Panel Recommendations. *Eur. Urol. Focus* **2020**, *6*, 231–234. [CrossRef]

4. Hanahan, D.; Weinberg, R.A. Hallmarks of Cancer: The next Generation. *Cell* **2011**, *144*, 646–674. [CrossRef]
5. Zadra, G.; Loda, M. Metabolic Vulnerabilities of Prostate Cancer: Diagnostic and Therapeutic Opportunities. *Cold Spring Harb Perspect Med* **2018**, *8*, a030569. [CrossRef]
6. Eidelman, E.; Twum-Ampofo, J.; Ansari, J.; Siddiqui, M.M. The Metabolic Phenotype of Prostate Cancer. *Front. Oncol.* **2017**, *7*, 131. [CrossRef]
7. Ahmad, F.; Cherukuri, M.K.; Choyke, P.L. Metabolic Reprogramming in Prostate Cancer. *Br. J. Cancer* **2021**, *125*, 1185–1196. [CrossRef]
8. Chetta, P.; Zadra, G. Metabolic Reprogramming as an Emerging Mechanism of Resistance to Endocrine Therapies in Prostate Cancer. *Cancer Drug Resist.* **2021**, *4*, 143–162. [CrossRef]
9. Lieu, E.L.; Nguyen, T.; Rhyne, S.; Kim, J. Amino Acids in Cancer. *Exp. Mol. Med.* **2020**, *52*, 15–30. [CrossRef]
10. Yoo, H.C.; Han, J.M. Amino Acid Metabolism in Cancer Drug Resistance. *Cells* **2022**, *11*, 140. [CrossRef]
11. Wei, Z.; Liu, X.; Cheng, C.; Yu, W.; Yi, P. Metabolism of Amino Acids in Cancer. *Front. Cell Dev. Biol.* **2021**, *8*, xxx. [CrossRef]
12. Butler, M.; van der Meer, L.T.; van Leeuwen, F.N. Amino Acid Depletion Therapies: Starving Cancer Cells to Death. *Trends Endocrinol. Metab.* **2021**, *32*, 367–381. [CrossRef]
13. Strmiska, V.; Michalek, P.; Eckschlager, T.; Stiborova, M.; Adam, V.; Krizkova, S.; Heger, Z. Prostate Cancer-Specific Hallmarks of Amino Acids Metabolism: Towards a Paradigm of Precision Medicine. *Biochim. Biophys. Acta Rev. Cancer* **2019**, *1871*, 248–258. [CrossRef]
14. Schcolnik-Cabrera, A.; Juárez-López, D. Dual Contribution of the MTOR Pathway and of the Metabolism of Amino Acids in Prostate Cancer. *Cell Oncol.* **2022**, *45*, 831–859. [CrossRef]
15. Yang, M.; Vousden, K.H. Serine and One-Carbon Metabolism in Cancer. *Nat. Rev. Cancer* **2016**, *16*, 650–662. [CrossRef]
16. Pan, S.; Fan, M.; Liu, Z.; Li, X.; Wang, H. Serine, Glycine and One-Carbon Metabolism in Cancer (Review). *Int. J. Oncol.* **2021**, *58*, 158–170. [CrossRef]
17. Reina-Campos, M.; Linares, J.F.; Duran, A.; Cordes, T.; L'Hermitte, A.; Badur, M.G.; Bhangoo, M.S.; Thorson, P.K.; Richards, A.; Rooslid, T.; et al. Increased Serine and One-Carbon Pathway Metabolism by PKCλ/ι Deficiency Promotes Neuroendocrine Prostate Cancer. *Cancer Cell* **2019**, *35*, 385–400.e9. [CrossRef]
18. Gao, X.; Locasale, J.W.; Reid, M.A. Serine and Methionine Metabolism: Vulnerabilities in Lethal Prostate Cancer. *Cancer Cell* **2019**, *35*, 339–341. [CrossRef]
19. Ganini, C.; Amelio, I.; Bertolo, R.; Candi, E.; Cappello, A.; Cipriani, C.; Mauriello, A.; Marani, C.; Melino, G.; Montanaro, M.; et al. Serine and One-Carbon Metabolisms Bring New Therapeutic Venues in Prostate Cancer. *Discov. Oncol.* **2021**, *12*, 45. [CrossRef]
20. Ndaru, E.; Garibsingh, R.A.A.; Shi, Y.Y.; Wallace, E.; Zakrepine, P.; Wang, J.; Schlessinger, A.; Grewer, C. Novel Alanine Serine Cysteine Transporter 2 (ASCT2) Inhibitors Based on Sulfonamide and Sulfonic Acid Ester Scaffolds. *J. Gen. Physiol.* **2019**, *151*, 357–368. [CrossRef]
21. Saruta, M.; Takahara, K.; Yoshizawa, A.; Niimi, A.; Takeuchi, T.; Nukaya, T.; Takenaka, M.; Zennami, K.; Ichino, M.; Sasaki, H.; et al. Alanine-Serine-Cysteine Transporter 2 Inhibition Suppresses Prostate Cancer Cell Growth In Vitro. *J. Clin. Med.* **2022**, *11*, 5466. [CrossRef]
22. Scalise, M.; Pochini, L.; Console, L.; Losso, M.A.; Indiveri, C. The Human SLC1A5 (ASCT2) Amino Acid Transporter: From Function to Structure and Role in Cell Biology. *Front. Cell Dev. Biol.* **2018**, *6*, 96. [CrossRef]
23. Tang, Y.; Kim, Y.S.; Choi, E.J.; Hwang, Y.J.; Yun, Y.S.; Bae, S.M.; Park, P.J.; Kim, E.K. Taurine Attenuates Epithelial-Mesenchymal Transition-Related Genes in Human Prostate Cancer Cells. *Adv. Exp. Med. Biol.* **2017**, *975*, 1203–1212. [CrossRef]
24. Song, X.; Yuan, B.; Zhao, S.; Zhao, D. Effect of Taurine on the Proliferation, Apoptosis and MST1/Hippo Signaling in Prostate Cancer Cells. *Transl. Cancer Res.* **2022**, *11*, 1705–1712. [CrossRef]
25. Tang, Y.; Choi, E.J.; Cheong, S.H.; Hwang, Y.J.; Arokiyaraj, S.; Park, P.J.; Moon, S.H.; Kim, E.K. Effect of Taurine on Prostate-Specific Antigen Level and Migration in Human Prostate Cancer Cells. *Adv. Exp. Med. Biol.* **2015**, *803*, 203–214. [CrossRef]
26. Liberzon, A.; Birger, C.; Thorvaldsdóttir, H.; Ghandi, M.; Mesirov, J.P.; Tamayo, P. The Molecular Signatures Database Hallmark Gene Set Collection. *Cell Syst.* **2015**, *1*, 417–425. [CrossRef]
27. Weinstein, J.N.; Collisson, E.A.; Mills, G.B.; Shaw, K.R.M.; Ozenberger, B.A.; Ellrott, K.; Sander, C.; Stuart, J.M.; Chang, K.; Creighton, C.J.; et al. The Cancer Genome Atlas Pan-Cancer Analysis Project. *Nat. Genet.* **2013**, *45*, 1113–1120. [CrossRef]
28. Silva, T.C.; Colaprico, A.; Olsen, C.; D'Angelo, F.; Bontempi, G.; Ceccarelli, M.; Noushmehr, H. TCGA Workflow: Analyze Cancer Genomics and Epigenomics Data Using Bioconductor Packages. *F1000 Res.* **2016**, *5*, 1542. [CrossRef]
29. Colaprico, A.; Silva, T.C.; Olsen, C.; Garofano, L.; Cava, C.; Garolini, D.; Sabedot, T.S.; Malta, T.M.; Pagnotta, S.M.; Castiglioni, I.; et al. TCGAbiolinks: An R/Bioconductor Package for Integrative Analysis of TCGA Data. *Nucleic Acids Res.* **2016**, *44*, e17. [CrossRef]
30. Mounir, M.; Lucchetta, M.; Silva, T.C.; Olsen, C.; Bontempi, G.; Chen, X.; Noushmehr, H.; Colaprico, A.; Papaleo, E. New Functionalities in the TCGAbiolinks Package for the Study and Integration of Cancer Data from GDC and GTEX. *PLoS Comput. Biol.* **2019**, *15*. [CrossRef]
31. Gao, J.; Aksoy, B.A.; Dogrusoz, U.; Dresdner, G.; Gross, B.; Sumer, S.O.; Sun, Y.; Jacobsen, A.; Sinha, R.; Larsson, E.; et al. Integrative Analysis of Complex Cancer Genomics and Clinical Profiles Using the CBioPortal. *Sci. Signal* **2013**, *6*, pl1. [CrossRef]
32. Heath, A.P.; Ferretti, V.; Agrawal, S.; An, M.; Angelakos, J.C.; Arya, R.; Bajari, R.; Baqar, B.; Barnowski, J.H.B.; Burt, J.; et al. The NCI Genomic Data Commons. *Nat. Genet.* **2021**, *53*, 257–262. [CrossRef]

33. Narayanachar Tattar, P.; Vaman, H.J. *Survival Analysis*; CRC Press: Boca Raton, FL, USA, 2023.
34. Chen, E.Y.; Tan, C.M.; Kou, Y.; Duan, Q.; Wang, Z.; Meirelles, G.V.; Clark, N.R.; Ma'ayan, A. Enrichr: Interactive and Collaborative HTML5 Gene List Enrichment Analysis Tool. *BMC Bioinform.* **2013**, *14*, 128. [CrossRef]
35. Kuleshov, M.V.; Jones, M.R.; Rouillard, A.D.; Fernandez, N.F.; Duan, Q.; Wang, Z.; Koplev, S.; Jenkins, S.L.; Jagodnik, K.M.; Lachmann, A.; et al. Enrichr: A Comprehensive Gene Set Enrichment Analysis Web Server 2016 Update. *Nucleic Acids Res.* **2016**, *44*, W90–W97. [CrossRef]
36. Stelzer, G.; Rosen, N.; Plaschkes, I.; Zimmerman, S.; Twik, M.; Fishilevich, S.; Iny Stein, T.; Nudel, R.; Lieder, I.; Mazor, Y.; et al. The GeneCards Suite: From Gene Data Mining to Disease Genome Sequence Analyses. *Curr. Protoc. Bioinform.* **2016**, *2016*. [CrossRef]
37. R Core Team. *R Core Team*; R: A Language and Environment for Statistical Computing; R Foundation for Statistical Computing: Vienna, Austria, 2017. Available online: http://www.R-project.org/ (accessed on 1 November 2022).
38. Atkinson, E.J.; Therneau, T.M. An Introduction to Recursive Partitioning Using the RPART Routines. *Mayo Clin.* **2000**, *61*, xxx.
39. Therneau, T.; Atkinson, B. Rpart: Recursive Partitioning and Regression Trees. R Package Version 4.1-15. 2019. Available online: https://CRAN.R-project.org/package=rpart (accessed on 1 November 2022).
40. Ulm, K.; Kriner, M.; Eberle, S.; Reck, M.; Hessler, S. Statistical Methods to Identify Predictive Factors. In *Handbook of Statistics in Clinical Oncology*; Crowley, J., Ankerst, D., Eds.; Chapman & Hall/CRC: Boca Raton, FL, USA, 2006; pp. 335–345.
41. Schumacher, M.; Hollander, N.; Schwarzer, G.; Sauerbrei, W. Prognostic Factor Studies. In *Handbook of Statistics in Clinical Oncology*; Crowley, J., Ankerst, D., Eds.; Chapman & Hall/CRC: Boca Raton, FL, USA, 2006; pp. 289–333.
42. Aralica, G.; Šarec Ivelj, M.; Pačić, A.; Baković, J.; Milković Periša, M.; Krištić, A.; Konjevoda, P. Prognostic Significance of Lacunarity in Preoperative Biopsy of Colorectal Cancer. *Pathol. Oncol. Res.* **2020**, *26*, 2567–2576. [CrossRef]
43. Rowe, P. *Essential Statistics for the Pharmaceutical Sciences*; Wiley Online Library: Hoboken, NJ, USA, 2015.
44. Kanda, Y. Investigation of the Freely Available Easy-to-Use Software "EZR" for Medical Statistics. *Bone Marrow Transpl.* **2013**, *48*, 452–458. [CrossRef]
45. Solorzano, S.R.; Imaz-Rosshandler, I.; Camacho-Arroyo, I.; García-Tobilla, P.; Morales-Montor, G.; Salazar, P.; Arena-Ortiz, M.L.; Rodríguez-Dorantes, M. GABA Promotes Gastrin-Releasing Peptide Secretion in NE/NE-like Cells: Contribution to Prostate Cancer Progression. *Sci. Rep.* **2018**, *8*, 10272. [CrossRef]
46. Testa, U.; Castelli, G.; Pelosi, E. Cellular and Molecular Mechanisms Underlying Prostate Cancer Development: Therapeutic Implications. *Medicines* **2019**, *6*, 82. [CrossRef]
47. Samaržija, I. Post-Translational Modifications That Drive Prostate Cancer Progression. *Biomolecules* **2021**, *11*, 247. [CrossRef]
48. Samaržija, I. Site-Specific and Common Prostate Cancer Metastasis Genes as Suggested by Meta-Analysis of Gene Expression Data. *Life* **2021**, *11*, 636. [CrossRef]
49. Samaržija, I. A Need for Stratification of Metastasis Samples According to Secondary Site in Gene Expression Studies. *Biocell* **2022**, *46*, 1747–1750. [CrossRef]
50. Kelly, R.S.; Heiden, M.G.V.; Giovannucci, E.; Mucci, L.A. Metabolomic Biomarkers of Prostate Cancer: Prediction, Diagnosis, Progression, Prognosis, and Recurrence. *Cancer Epidemiol. Biomark. Prev.* **2016**, *25*, 887–906. [CrossRef]
51. Zhang, Y.; Zhang, R.; Liang, F.; Zhang, L.; Liang, X. Identification of Metabolism-Associated Prostate Cancer Subtypes and Construction of a Prognostic Risk Model. *Front Oncol.* **2020**, *10*. [CrossRef]
52. Zhang, Y.; Liang, X.; Zhang, L.; Wang, D. Metabolic Characterization and Metabolism-Score of Tumor to Predict the Prognosis in Prostate Cancer. *Sci. Rep.* **2021**, *11*, 22486. [CrossRef]
53. Feng, D.; Shi, X.; Zhang, F.; Xiong, Q.; Wei, Q.; Yang, L. Energy Metabolism-Related Gene Prognostic Index Predicts Biochemical Recurrence for Patients With Prostate Cancer Undergoing Radical Prostatectomy. *Front. Immunol.* **2022**, *13*. [CrossRef]
54. Peng, X.; Zheng, T.; Guo, Y.; Zhu, Y. Amino Acid Metabolism Genes Associated with Immunotherapy Responses and Clinical Prognosis of Colorectal Cancer. *Front Mol. Biosci.* **2022**, *9*. [CrossRef]
55. Zhao, Y.; Zhang, J.; Wang, S.; Jiang, Q.; Xu, K. Identification and Validation of a Nine-Gene Amino Acid Metabolism-Related Risk Signature in HCC. *Front Cell Dev. Biol.* **2021**, *9*. [CrossRef]
56. Zhang, F.; Lin, J.; Zhu, D.; Tang, Y.; Lu, Y.; Liu, Z.; Wang, X. Identification of an Amino Acid Metabolism-Associated Gene Signature Predicting the Prognosis and Immune Therapy Response of Clear Cell Renal Cell Carcinoma. *Front. Oncol.* **2022**, *12*. [CrossRef]
57. Liu, Y.Q.; Chai, R.C.; Wang, Y.Z.; Wang, Z.; Liu, X.; Wu, F.; Jiang, T. Amino Acid Metabolism-Related Gene Expression-Based Risk Signature Can Better Predict Overall Survival for Glioma. *Cancer Sci.* **2019**, *110*, 321–333. [CrossRef]
58. Li, W.; Zou, Z.; An, N.; Wang, M.; Liu, X.; Mei, Z. A Multifaceted and Feasible Prognostic Model of Amino Acid Metabolism-Related Genes in the Immune Response and Tumor Microenvironment of Head and Neck Squamous Cell Carcinomas. *Front. Oncol.* **2022**, *12*. [CrossRef]
59. Xu, M.; Sakamoto, S.; Matsushima, J.; Kimura, T.; Ueda, T.; Mizokami, A.; Kanai, Y.; Ichikawa, T. Up-Regulation of LAT1 during Antiandrogen Therapy Contributes to Progression in Prostate Cancer Cells. *J. Urol.* **2016**, *195*, 1588–1597. [CrossRef]
60. Cordova, R.A.; Misra, J.; Amin, P.H.; Klunk, A.J.; Damayanti, N.P.; Carlson, K.R.; Elmendorf, A.J.; Kim, H.-G.; Mirek, E.T.; Elzey, B.D.; et al. GCN2 EIF2 Kinase Promotes Prostate Cancer by Maintaining Amino Acid Homeostasis. *Elife* **2022**, *11*, e81083. [CrossRef]
61. Zhu, Q.; Meng, Y.; Li, S.; Xin, J.; Du, M.; Wang, M.; Cheng, G. Association of Genetic Variants in Autophagy Lysosome Pathway Genes with Susceptibility and Survival to Prostate Cancer. *Gene* **2022**, *808*, 145953. [CrossRef]

62. Rii, J.; Sakamoto, S.; Sugiura, M.; Kanesaka, M.; Fujimoto, A.; Yamada, Y.; Maimaiti, M.; Ando, K.; Wakai, K.; Xu, M.; et al. Functional Analysis of LAT3 in Prostate Cancer: Its Downstream Target and Relationship with Androgen Receptor. *Cancer Sci.* **2021**, *112*, 3871–3883. [CrossRef]
63. Sun, J.; Nagel, R.; Zaal, E.A.; Ugalde, A.P.; Han, R.; Proost, N.; Song, J.; Pataskar, A.; Burylo, A.; Fu, H.; et al. SLC 1A3 Contributes to L-asparaginase Resistance in Solid Tumors. *EMBO J.* **2019**, *38*, e102147. [CrossRef]
64. Verma, S.; Shankar, E.; Chan, E.R.; Gupta, S. Metabolic Reprogramming and Predominance of Solute Carrier Genes during Acquired Enzalutamide Resistance in Prostate Cancer. *Cells* **2020**, *9*, 2535. [CrossRef]
65. Zhang, L.; Li, Y.; Wang, X.; Ping, Y.; Wang, D.; Cao, Y.; Dai, Y.; Liu, W.; Tao, Z. Five-Gene Signature Associating with Gleason Score Serve as Novel Biomarkers for Identifying Early Recurring Events and Contributing to Early Diagnosis for Prostate Adenocarcinoma. *J. Cancer* **2021**, *12*, 3626–3647. [CrossRef]
66. Meng, J.; Guan, Y.; Wang, B.; Chen, L.; Chen, J.; Zhang, M.; Liang, C. Risk Subtyping and Prognostic Assessment of Prostate Cancer Based on Consensus Genes. *Commun. Biol.* **2022**, *5*, 233. [CrossRef]
67. Wu, X.; Lv, D.; Lei, M.; Cai, C.; Zhao, Z.; Eftekhar, M.; Gu, D.; Liu, Y. A 10-Gene Signature as a Predictor of Biochemical Recurrence after Radical Prostatectomy in Patients with Prostate Cancer and a Gleason Score ≥ 7. *Oncol. Lett.* **2020**, *20*, 2906–2918. [CrossRef]
68. Glinsky, G.V.; Glinskii, A.B.; Stephenson, A.J.; Hoffman, R.M.; Gerald, W.L. Gene Expression Profiling Predicts Clinical Outcome of Prostate Cancer. *J. Clin. Investig.* **2004**, *113*, 913–923. [CrossRef]
69. Mou, Z.; Spencer, J.; Knight, B.; John, J.; McCullagh, P.; McGrath, J.S.; Harries, L.W. Gene Expression Analysis Reveals a 5-Gene Signature for Progression-Free Survival in Prostate Cancer. *Front. Oncol.* **2022**, *12*. [CrossRef]
70. Zhou, R.; Feng, Y.; Ye, J.; Han, Z.; Liang, Y.; Chen, Q.; Xu, X.; Huang, Y.; Jia, Z.; Zhong, W. Prediction of Biochemical Recurrence-Free Survival of Prostate Cancer Patients Leveraging Multiple Gene Expression Profiles in Tumor Microenvironment. *Front. Oncol.* **2021**, *11*. [CrossRef]
71. Lu, G.; Cai, W.; Wang, X.; Huang, B.; Zhao, Y.; Shao, Y.; Wang, D. Identifying Prognostic Signatures in the Microenvironment of Prostate Cancer. *Transl. Androl. Urol.* **2021**, *10*. [CrossRef]
72. Wang, Y.; Yang, Z. A Gleason Score-Related Outcome Model for Human Prostate Cancer: A Comprehensive Study Based on Weighted Gene Co-Expression Network Analysis. *Cancer Cell Int.* **2020**, *20*, 159. [CrossRef]
73. Gao, P.; Yang, C.; Nesvick, C.L.; Feldman, M.J.; Sizdahkhani, S.; Liu, H.; Chu, H.; Yang, F.; Tang, L.; Tian, J.; et al. Hypotaurine Evokes a Malignant Phenotype in Glioma through Aberrant Hypoxic Signaling. *Oncotarget* **2016**, *7*, 15200–15214. [CrossRef]
74. Zhou, H.; Sun, L.; Wan, F. Molecular Mechanisms of TUG1 in the Proliferation, Apoptosis, Migration and Invasion of Cancer Cells (Review). *Oncol. Lett.* **2019**, *18*, 4393–4402. [CrossRef]
75. Hao, S.D.; Ma, J.X.; Liu, Y.; Liu, P.J.; Qin, Y. Long Non-Coding TUG1 Accelerates Prostate Cancer Progression through Regulating MiR-128-3p/YES1 Axis. *Eur. Rev. Med. Pharmacol. Sci.* **2020**, *24*, 619–632. [CrossRef]
76. Yang, B.; Tang, X.; Wang, Z.; Sun, D.; Wei, X.; Ding, Y. TUG1 Promotes Prostate Cancer Progression by Acting as a CeRNA of MiR-26a. *Biosci. Rep.* **2018**, *38*, BSR20180677. [CrossRef]
77. Li, G.; Yang, J.; Chong, T.; Huang, Y.; Liu, Y.; Li, H. TUG1 Knockdown Inhibits the Tumorigenesis and Progression of Prostate Cancer by Regulating MicroRNA-496/Wnt/β-Catenin Pathway. *Anticancer Drugs* **2020**, *31*, 592–600. [CrossRef]
78. Xiu, D.; Liu, L.; Cheng, M.; Sun, X.; Ma, X. Knockdown of LncRNA TUG1 Enhances Radiosensitivity of Prostate Cancer via the TUG1/MiR-139-5p/SMC1A Axis. *Onco. Targets Ther.* **2020**, *13*, 2319–2331. [CrossRef]
79. Yu, J.; Wang, Y.; Peng, S. The High Expression of LncRNA TUG1 Correlates with Progressive Tumor Condition and Less Satisfying Survival Profiles in Prostate Cancer Patients. *Transl. Cancer Res.* **2019**, *8*. [CrossRef]
80. Uhlén, M.; Fagerberg, L.; Hallström, B.M.; Lindskog, C.; Oksvold, P.; Mardinoglu, A.; Sivertsson, Å.; Kampf, C.; Sjöstedt, E.; Asplund, A.; et al. Tissue-Based Map of the Human Proteome. *Science* **2015**, *347*. [CrossRef]
81. Uhlén, M.; Björling, E.; Agaton, C.; Szigyarto, C.A.K.; Amini, B.; Andersen, E.; Andersson, A.C.; Angelidou, P.; Asplund, A.; Asplund, C.; et al. A Human Protein Atlas for Normal and Cancer Tissues Based on Antibody Proteomics. *Mol. Cell. Proteom.* **2005**, *4*, 1920–1932. [CrossRef]
82. Tu, M.; Saputo, S. From Beginning to End: Expanding the SERINC3 Interactome Through an in Silico Analysis. *Bioinform. Biol. Insights* **2022**, *16*. [CrossRef]
83. Xu, S.; Zheng, Z.; Pathak, J.L.; Cheng, H.; Zhou, Z.; Chen, Y.; Wu, Q.; Wang, L.; Zeng, M.; Wu, L. The Emerging Role of the Serine Incorporator Protein Family in Regulating Viral Infection. *Front. Cell Dev. Biol.* **2022**, *10*, 856468. [CrossRef]
84. Birge, R.B.; Boeltz, S.; Kumar, S.; Carlson, J.; Wanderley, J.; Calianese, D.; Barcinski, M.; Brekken, R.A.; Huang, X.; Hutchins, J.T.; et al. Phosphatidylserine Is a Global Immunosuppressive Signal in Efferocytosis, Infectious Disease, and Cancer. *Cell Death Differ.* **2016**, *23*, 962–978. [CrossRef]
85. Voelkel-Johnson, C.; Norris, J.S.; White-Gilbertson, S. Interdiction of Sphingolipid Metabolism Revisited: Focus on Prostate Cancer. *Adv. Cancer Res.* **2018**, *140*, 265–293. [CrossRef]

cancers

Article

Dosimetric Impact of Intrafraction Prostate Motion and Interfraction Anatomical Changes in Dose-Escalated Linac-Based SBRT

Valeria Faccenda [1], Denis Panizza [1,2], Martina Camilla Daniotti [1,3], Roberto Pellegrini [4], Sara Trivellato [1], Paolo Caricato [1], Raffaella Lucchini [2], Elena De Ponti [1,2] and Stefano Arcangeli [2,5,*]

1 Medical Physics Department, Fondazione IRCCS San Gerardo dei Tintori, 20900 Monza, Italy
2 School of Medicine and Surgery, University of Milan Bicocca, 20126 Milan, Italy
3 Department of Physics, University of Milan, 20133 Milan, Italy
4 Elekta AB, 113 57 Stockholm, Sweden
5 Radiation Oncology Department, Fondazione IRCCS San Gerardo dei Tintori, 20900 Monza, Italy
* Correspondence: stefano.arcangeli@unimib.it

Simple Summary: With an ever-growing acceptance by the radiation oncology community, stereotactic body radiation therapy (SBRT) has become an increasingly common option for localized prostate cancer in recent years. However, such high doses per fraction require the specific management of the inter- and intrafraction movements of the target. In this work, synchronized motion-inclusive dose distributions using intrafraction motion data provided by a novel electromagnetic transmitter-based device were reconstructed and recomputed on deformed CTs reflecting the CBCT daily anatomy to represent the actual delivered dose. To our knowledge, there have been no previously published studies where the dosimetric impact on the target and organs at risk (OARs) of both intrafraction prostate motion and interfraction anatomical changes was investigated together in dose-escalated linac-based SBRT. Moreover, treatments that would have been delivered without any organ motion management (non-gated) were simulated to also evaluate the dosimetric benefit of employing continuous monitoring, beam gating, and motion correction strategies.

Abstract: The dosimetric impact of intrafraction prostate motion and interfraction anatomical changes and the effect of beam gating and motion correction were investigated in dose-escalated linac-based SBRT. Fifty-six gated fractions were delivered using a novel electromagnetic tracking device with a 2 mm threshold. Real-time prostate motion data were incorporated into the patient's original plan with an isocenter shift method. Delivered dose distributions were obtained by recalculating these motion-encoded plans on deformed CTs reflecting the patient's CBCT daily anatomy. Non-gated treatments were simulated using the prostate motion data assuming that no treatment interruptions have occurred. The mean relative dose differences between delivered and planned treatments were −3.0% [−18.5–2.8] for CTV D99% and −2.6% [−17.8–1.0] for PTV D95%. The median cumulative CTV coverage with 93% of the prescribed dose was satisfactory. Urethra sparing was slightly degraded, with the maximum dose increased by only 1.0% on average, and a mean reduction in the rectum and bladder doses was seen in almost all dose metrics. Intrafraction prostate motion marginally contributed in gated treatments, while in non-gated treatments, further deteriorations in the minimum target coverage and bladder dose metrics would have occurred on average. The implemented motion management strategy and the strict patient preparation regimen, along with other treatment optimization strategies, ensured no significant degradations of dose metrics in delivered treatments.

Keywords: prostate cancer; stereotactic body radiotherapy; intrafraction motion management; daily anatomy; delivered dose assessment

Citation: Faccenda, V.; Panizza, D.; Daniotti, M.C.; Pellegrini, R.; Trivellato, S.; Caricato, P.; Lucchini, R.; De Ponti, E.; Arcangeli, S. Dosimetric Impact of Intrafraction Prostate Motion and Interfraction Anatomical Changes in Dose-Escalated Linac-Based SBRT. *Cancers* **2023**, *15*, 1153. https://doi.org/10.3390/cancers15041153

Academic Editor: Kouji Izumi

Received: 20 December 2022
Revised: 23 January 2023
Accepted: 9 February 2023
Published: 10 February 2023

1. Introduction

Due to the unusual radiobiology of prostate cancer, with a low α/β ratio estimated to be ~1.5 Gy [1–3], ultra-hypofractionated, or stereotactic body radiation therapy (SBRT), treatments have become a standard option for localized prostate cancer in recent years [4–7]. In view of the decreased margins for the planning target volume (PTV), the reduced statistical averaging of setup errors (low number of fractions), and the longer delivery fraction time, such protocols require that higher doses per fraction are delivered with much greater accuracy and precision than conventional treatments in order not to jeopardize the target coverage and the sparing of surrounding organs at risk (OARs).

Since different studies [8–13] have recognized significant and unpredictable prostate motion during delivery, devices that provide real-time prostate monitoring and can be used for beam gating and patient position correction have increasingly been implemented. Among the available technologies, a novel electromagnetic (EM) transmitter-based device without surgical intervention has been shown to be a reliable and safe option to localize and monitor the prostate and the urethra during SBRT [13,14]. To limit prostate mobility and assess anatomical reproducibility throughout the treatment, strict preparation of the patient is usually necessary as well. Nevertheless, slow drifts or sudden transient movements of the prostate, as well as daily bladder and rectum volume modifications, are expected, and both may strongly affect the target coverage and OARs sparing [15–22]. Hence, their dosimetric effects should be investigated to fully understand the feasibility and safety of such extreme treatment schedules and the benefit of online motion management strategies.

Several methods have been applied to evaluate the impact of intrafraction prostate motion on dose distributions [16,23–30]. The first used approach involved the convolution of the static 3D dose matrix with probability density functions of the target motion [24]. Disregarding time information, this method cannot account for the interplay effect between the target motion and multileaf collimator (MLC) motion during beam delivery, which is characteristic of dynamic treatments such as volumetric arc therapy (VMAT) [21]. Synchronized dose reconstruction methods that establish the temporal correspondence between the target and MLC motion by incorporating real-time target motion data into the treatment plan recomputation need to be employed to achieve accurate motion-inclusive dose distributions [23,25,26,29,31].

Dose-of-the-day evaluations have been enabled by the increased availability of daily patient images; cone-beam computed tomography (CBCT) acquired before each SBRT fraction to check the actual status of the bladder and rectum and to adjust the position of the prostate gland with respect to the planned position may serve this purpose. However, an accurate dose calculation on CBCT is challenging due to the reduced image contrast, artifacts, CT Hounsfield Units (HU) fluctuations, the dependence on acquisition parameters and patient size, and smaller field-of-view (FOV) dimensions [17,32–35]. When images were not cropped and no missing patient tissue was observed, some studies [19,36] overcame these issues by obtaining the HU-to-electron density (ED) calibration curve for the specific CBCT system's properties. In the case of a large patient size or too small FOV, methods that use synthetic CT images obtained by deforming the planning CT into the daily CBCT frame-of-reference have instead been proposed [30,37,38]. In this way, the FOV remains the same as in the planning CT, and so does the HU, thus not requiring the configuration of a different HU-to-ED curve in the treatment planning system (TPS).

In this work, synchronized motion inclusive dose distributions using intrafraction motion data provided by the RayPilot system with RayPilot HypoCath (Micropos Medical AB, Gothenburg, Sweden) were reconstructed and recomputed on deformed CTs reflecting the CBCT daily anatomy to represent the actual delivered dose. To our knowledge, there have been no previously published studies where the dosimetric impacts on the target and OARs of both intrafraction prostate motion and interfraction anatomical changes were investigated together in dose-escalated linac-based SBRT. Moreover, treatments that would have been delivered without any organ motion management (non-gated) were simulated to also evaluate the dosimetric benefit of employing continuous monitoring, beam gating, and motion correction strategies.

2. Materials and Methods

2.1. Patient Cohort and Treatment Protocol

Thirteen patients (56 fractions) with organ-confined prostate cancer between June 2020 and May 2021 received 40 Gy in 5 fractions (n = 4) or 38 Gy in 4 fractions (n = 9) on consecutive days. Patients lay in the supine position with their arms over their chest and straight knees, and the FeetFix (CIVCO Medical Solutions, IA, USA) was the only immobilization system used for ankle fixation. A 16-French Foley catheter was used to fill the bladder with 100 cc of saline solution before the simulation and before each fraction, and a rectal micro-enema was administered as well. The PTV was obtained by applying a 2 mm isotropic expansion of the clinical target volume (CTV), defined as the prostate gland plus seminal vesicles. Treatments were planned with the Monte Carlo algorithm (1 mm grid spacing and 1% statistical uncertainty for calculation) of the Monaco TPS (Elekta AB, Stockholm, Sweden) on a VersaHD linear accelerator (Elekta AB, Stockholm, Sweden) using the VMAT technique with two 6 MV (n = 6) or 10 MV (n = 7) flattening-filter-free (FFF) arcs, and it was ensured that at least 95% of the PTV received 95% of the prescription dose. An accurate patient setup was achieved by using initial CBCT soft tissue matching. CBCT images were acquired using the fast prostate preset of 120 kV, 850 mAs, full scan, 60 s acquisition time, and FOV medium. The EM device consisted of a wired transmitter integrated into a dedicated lumen of the RayPilot HypoCath, a Foley catheter inserted into the patient's urethra, and it provided real-time 3D prostate motion data. The shift of the transmitter was used as a surrogate for prostate motion [13]. Treatment was interrupted whenever the transmitter exceeded a 2 mm threshold in any of the three spatial directions. If the position of the prostate did not return within tolerances, the couch position was corrected after the matching of a new CBCT. The prostate trajectories resulting from this clinically implemented strategy of beam gating and motion correction are listed below as "case A".

2.2. Intrafraction Prostate Trajectories and Simulation of Non-Gated Treatments

RayPilot data processing has been detailed elsewhere [13]. In short, prostate trajectories with and without beam gating and motion correction events with an update rate of 15 Hz were reconstructed and analyzed with an in-house C++ code. The trajectories that would have occurred without any organ motion management were simulated by removing all resets of the transmitter position with the acquisition of a new CBCT and by adjusting the setup and delivery duration. To this aim, a fixed duration of 3.5 min to account for image acquisition and matching on the planning CT and the real delivery time of each treatment plan were used for the setup and delivery, respectively. The prostate trajectories from this simulated scenario of non-gated treatments are referenced as "case B" hereafter. For fractions in which no interventions were required, the observed prostate trajectory data were also considered non-gated treatments. In Figure 1, examples of the prostate trajectories in case A and case B for the same treatment fraction is reported.

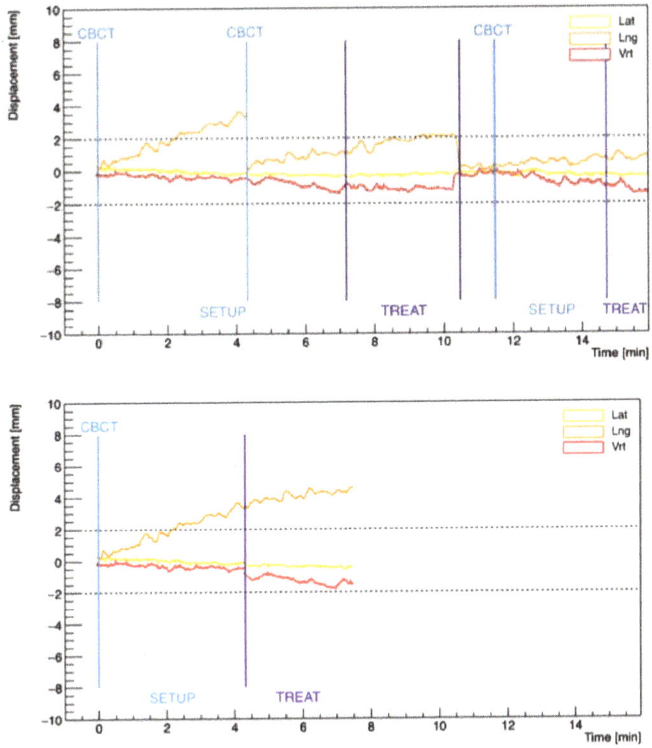

Figure 1. Examples of prostate trajectories in the three spatial directions obtained from case A (gated) (**top**) and case B (non-gated) (**bottom**) motion data for the same treatment fraction. The first light-blue vertical line highlights the tracking starting point (zero position) corresponding to the acquisition of the first CBCT. The following lines indicate every other acquisition of a new CBCT due to prostate displacements beyond the 2 mm threshold. The dark-blue lines separate the setup and delivery phases.

2.3. Motion-Inclusive Reconstruction Method and Dose Calculation

To evaluate the intrafraction prostate motion during SBRT delivery, synchronized motion-inclusive dose distributions were reconstructed using an isocenter shift method developed and validated by Poulsen et al. [31] and then used in other studies [21,39,40]. This method consists of dividing the patient's original Dicom RT plan into several sub-beams formed by a certain number of control points and displacing the beam isocenter at each sub-beam according to the 3D prostate motion observed during beam delivery for each fraction. Sub-beams were created using an in-house MATLAB program (MathWorks Inc, Natick, MA, USA) to represent the part of the treatment delivery synchronized with each prostate position bin extracted from the recorded trajectories [31]. In this work, two different motion-encoded plans using data from prostate trajectories in case A and case B were reconstructed for each fraction.

To include the impact of the anatomy-of-the-day on dose distributions, synthetic CT (dCT) scans were created by deforming the planning CT on the first daily CBCT acquired during each fraction. All 56 CBCTs were exported from the X-ray Volume Imaging XVI software (Elekta AB, Stockholm, Sweden) to the Monaco TPS with the coordinate frame after registration with planning CT. Adapted contours of the main structures (i.e., CTV, urethra, rectum, bladder, and femoral heads) were checked and manually adjusted on each CBCT by an expert physician. The external structure also took into account the patient's surface variations due to the slightly different setup positions. Deformable fusion was then performed on the CT FOV using external software (ADMIRE, research version 3.13, Elekta AB, Stockholm, Sweden), with the structures used as constraints to drive the deformation in the region of interest. In this way, inside the CBCT FOV, the resulting dCTs have the soft tissue geometry detected in the CBCT, while outside, the tissue density distributions of the planning CT were used. The accuracy of the deformation was qualitatively analyzed by evaluating the correspondence of the structure positions between dCT and CBCT and the absence of unrealistic deformations. The HU transfer between the CT and the dCT was also checked for each relevant structure. The reconstructed fraction motion-inclusive plans for case A were recalculated on the corresponding dCT using the same algorithm and calculation properties as in the original plan. The resulting dose distributions, including the contribution of both intrafraction motion and anatomical changes, were considered a good estimation of the daily dose delivered to the patients.

2.4. *Data Analysis and Statistical Tests*

Intrafraction prostate motion metrics during beam delivery were calculated in lateral, longitudinal, and vertical directions and in 3D in both case A and case B. The prostate displacements were all calculated relative to the tracking starting point position, defined at the beginning of the acquisition of the first daily CBCT.

The volumes of CTV, rectum, and bladder contoured on each daily CBCT were recorded and compared to the simulation and in between the different treatment fractions. The coefficient of variation (CV) of these structure volumes over the different treatment fractions of the same patient was also calculated.

Differences between planned and delivered doses to the target and OARs were evaluated by comparing daily fraction dose–volume histograms (DVHs) obtained from case A motion-encoded plans recomputed on each dCT with the values predicted by the original plan. The total effect of motion and anatomical changes throughout the course of treatment was also estimated by taking into account the average of the reconstructed dose parameters from all fractions of each patient. The dose-volume parameters analyzed for target structures, i.e., CTV, PTV, and the PTV shell volume around the CTV (PTV-CTV), were the mean dose, minimum dose to 99% (D99%) or 95% (D95%) of the volume and maximum dose to 2% (D2%) of the volume. For the OARs structures, the dose constraints [14] were extracted and used to assess the protocol compliance and to compare the delivered plans. This first analysis is also referenced as "comparison I" hereafter.

Moreover, case A and case B motion-inclusive plans were recomputed on the planning CT images for each fraction. A direct comparison between the individual fraction and patient cumulative DVHs of the two plans was used to quantify any variation only due to the implementation (or not) of an online target motion management strategy. Thus, an estimate of which dose distributions would have been delivered to the patients if beam gating and motion correction were not employed was available. Afterward, this dosimetric analysis is referenced as "comparison II". Figure 2 summarizes the data reconstruction process and the dosimetric comparisons performed in the study.

The Wilcoxon–Mann–Whitney signed-rank test was performed to assess the significance level, and only p-values less than 0.05 were considered statistically significant. The Bonferroni correction factor was also used to account for multiple testing.

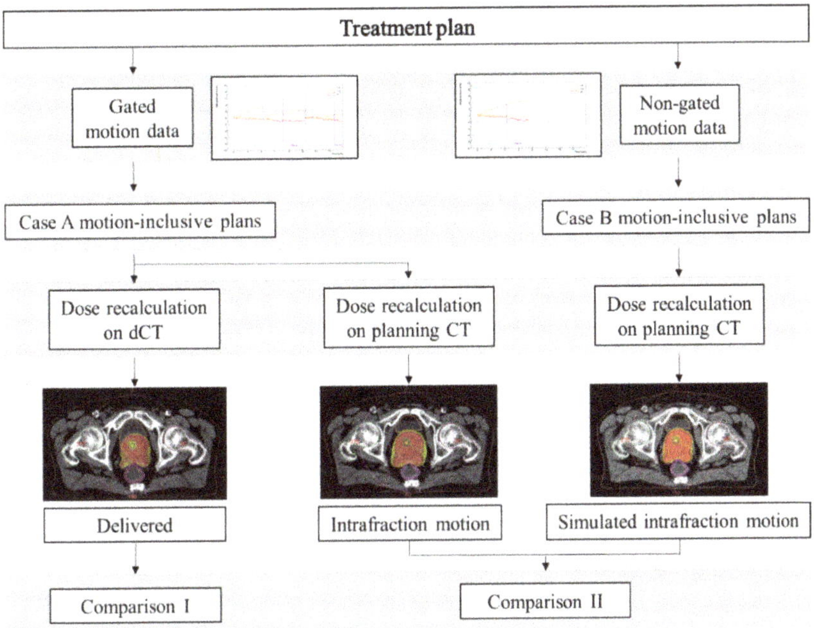

Figure 2. Overview of the data reconstruction process and dosimetric comparisons performed in the study.

3. Results

3.1. Intrafraction Prostate Motion

The prostate motion detected during beam delivery was modest in both case A and case B. Averaged over all 56 fractions, the mean [range] of the fraction mean prostate displacements were −0.2 mm [−1.5–0.8], 0.1 mm [−1.4–1.5], and −0.3 mm [−1.7–1.4] for case A and −0.3 mm [−3.1–0.8], 0.0 mm [−4.2–3.7], and −0.7 mm [−3.5–1.9] for case B in the lateral, longitudinal, and vertical directions, respectively. Positive signs indicate anterior, superior, and left displacements. The mean absolute displacements in each translational direction were 0.4 mm, 0.6 mm, and 0.7 mm in case A and 0.5 mm, 0.9 mm, and 1 mm in case B. The mean values of 3D prostate motion in the two cases were 1.1 mm [0.2–2.3] and 1.7 mm [0.2–5.1], respectively. However, the prostate would have exceeded the 2 mm margins during beam delivery in at least one spatial direction in 60% of the 25 fractions that required an intervention due to an out-of-tolerance shift. The mean prostate motion metrics over only these 25 fractions are presented in Table 1. The differences from the real shifts (case A) observed in the corresponding fractions are also reported.

Table 1. Mean, mean absolute "abs", and range of intrafraction prostate displacements during beam delivery in case B averaged over the 25 fractions that required an intervention due to excessive prostate motion. Values are provided in each of the three spatial directions and in 3D and are all expressed in mm. Mean differences from real shifts observed in the corresponding fractions are indicated by "diff".

Direction	Mean [Range]	Mean Abs	Mean Diff [Range]	Mean Abs Diff
Lateral	−0.5 [−3.1–0.8]	0.7	−0.3 [−1.6–0.3]	0.3
Longitudinal	−0.4 [−4.2–3.7]	1.4	−0.4 [−2.8–2.4]	0.7
Vertical	−1.2 [−3.5–1.9]	1.6	−0.7 [−1.8–0.7]	0.7
3D	2.6 [0.7–5.1]		1.3 [0.3–2.8]	

3.2. CTV, Rectum, and Bladder Volume Changes

The median CTV volume was 47.1 cc [32.1–96.7] in the simulation and 47.8 cc [34.5–97.8] during treatment. Median volumes in the simulation were 60.9 cc [34.5–91.6] for the rectum and 131.4 cc [93.8–304.5] for the bladder, while at the time of treatment, median volumes of 61.3 cc [32.8–95.3] and 154.1 cc [86.7–335.1] were observed, respectively. Table 2 shows the mean, SD, median, and range over all patients and fractions of the percentage differences of the CTV, rectum, and bladder volumes on daily CBCTs as compared to planning CT. The average intrapatient CVs of the structure volumes with the corresponding minimum and maximum variations were also reported. None of the volume variations were statistically significant ($p > 0.05$).

Table 2. Mean, standard deviation (SD), median, and range of percentage differences in CTV, rectum, and bladder volumes between daily fraction CBCTs and planning CTs. The values were averaged over the means of each patient for CTV and over all 56 fractions for rectum and bladder. Average intrapatient CV and range of the structure volumes are also reported.

	Mean (SD)	Median [Range]	CV [Range]
CTV	−1.3% (4.0)	−0.1% [−12.6–2.2]	2.3% [0.4–4.2]
Rectum	−3.5% (10.1)	−3.8% [−19.9–27.3]	5.7% [2.3–8.5]
Bladder	+8.9% (42.0)	+8.7% [−60.9–117.6]	19.6% [13.5–28.3]

The rectum and bladder showed larger variations both between the simulation and treatment and between the different treatment fractions of the same patient. Figure 3 shows the changes in the rectum and bladder volumes between planning and the five treatment fractions for the two patients who had the minimum and maximum bladder volumes at simulation.

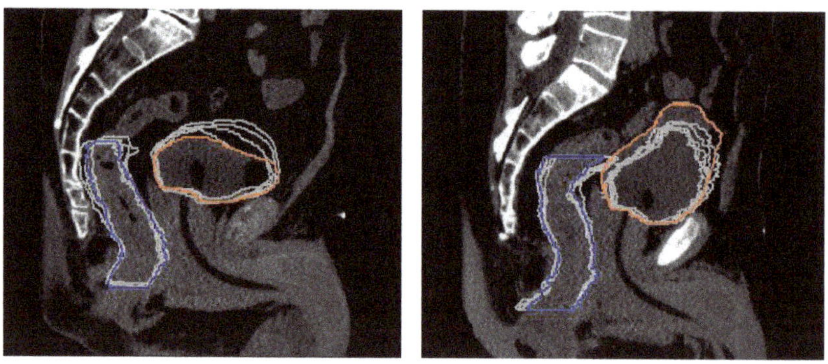

Figure 3. Superposition of rectum and bladder contours from the planning CT (colored lines) and each treatment fraction (gray lines) for the two patients who had the minimum (**left**) and maximum (**right**) bladder volume in the simulation.

3.3. Dosimetric Analysis

Table 3 provides the mean and range (over all fractions and patients) of the percentage differences in dosimetric parameters of delivered vs. planned dose distributions (comparison I) and between the two motion-inclusive dose distributions reconstructed using simulated case B vs. observed case A prostate motion data (comparison II). p-values according to the Wilcoxon signed-rank test are also reported.

Table 3. Mean and range (over all fractions and patients) of the percentage differences in target and OARs dosimetric parameters between the delivered and planned dose distributions (comparison I) and between the two motion-inclusive dose distributions reconstructed from case B and case A prostate motion data (comparison II). In the latter, for the individual fractions, only the 25 fractions that required an intervention due to prostate motion outside the tolerances were considered, while the cumulative mean differences were obtained by summing the gated and non-gated fractions as required. Statistically significant differences ($p < 0.05$) are highlighted.

		Comparison I			Comparison II		
	Metrics	**Individual Fractions**	***p*-Value**	**Cumulative Treatments**	**Individual Fractions**	***p*-Value**	**Cumulative Treatments**
CTV	Dmean	−0.5% [−2.0–1.2]	0.416	−0.5% [−1.4–0.2]	−0.2% [−2.3–0.8]	0.312	0.0% [−0.5–1.2]
	D99%	−3.0% [−18.5–2.8]	0.001	−3.1% [−13.2–0.5]	−2.8% [−16.3–1.1]	0.020	−1.3% [−8.3–0.2]
	D2%	−0.4% [−1.6–2.8]	0.028	−0.4% [−1.2–0.1]	−0.1% [−4.2–0.6]	1.000	+0.1% [−0.7–1.3]
						0.284	
PTV	Dmean	−0.7% [−2.9–1.2]	0.059	−0.6% [−1.9–0.2]	−0.4% [−2.1–0.8]	0.284	−0.1% [−0.6–1.4]
	D95%	−2.6% [−17.8–1.0]	0.000	−2.7% [−11.9–−0.2]	−2.4% [−11.9–0.9]	0.002	−1.0% [−5.3–0.6]
	D2%	−0.4% [−1.5–2.7]	0.074	−0.3% [−1.1–0.2]	−0.4% [−4.1–0.6]	0.926	+0.1% [−0.8–1.4]
PTV—CTV	Dmean	−1.2% [−5.8–1.3]	0.059	−1.2% [−3.9–0.5]	−0.8% [−3.6–0.6]	0.270	−0.2% [−1.5–1.8]
	D95%	−4.8% [−27.3–6.4]	0.001	−4.9% [−19.3–3.6]	−5.6% [−23.7–1.9]	0.013	−2.0% [−8.9–1.1]
Urethra PRV	D0.035 cc	+1.0% [−1.6–5.6]	0.046	+1.1% [−0.7–2.2]	+0.4% [−5.3–2.9]	0.333	+0.2% [−0.6–0.8]
	D10%	+0.7% [−1.2–4.9]	0.158	+0.7% [−0.6–1.3]	+0.6% [−5.0–6.3]	0.312	+0.2% [−0.7–1.0]
Rectum	D5%	−4.7% [−35.9–24.6]	0.163	−4.7% [−27.7–12.0]	−4.3% [−30.8–13.0]	0.240	−1.8% [−9.6–5.7]
	D10%	−5.0% [−41.7–31.7]	0.371	−5.1% [−33.5–14.6]	−4.6% [−33.8–27.5]	0.248	−2.0% [−10.5–6.6]
	D20%	−3.6% [−38.4–39.0]	0.514	−3.7% [−31.3–15.5]	−4.8% [−31.2–38.0]	0.343	−2.0% [−11.5–7.3]
	D50%	−1.5% [−24.1–38.8]	0.792	−1.5% [−18.9–16.1]	−1.9% [−22.1–25.1]	0.742	−0.9% [−8.8–8.2]
Rectum wall	D0.035 cc	−0.8% [−13.5–12.6]	0.921	−0.5% [−5.9–8.7]	−3.0% [−25.2–4.7]	0.177	−1.4% [−12.0–3.3]
Rectum mucosa	D0.035 cc	+0.8% [−27.1–33.9]	0.560	+1.0% [−10.5–22.6]	−3.9% [−30.3–8.6]	0.338	−1.8% [−10.9–4.7]
Bladder	D0.035 cc	−0.8% [−7.0–1.2]	0.123	−0.8% [−2.4–0.4]	+0.3% [−6.3–3.0]	0.445	+0.3% [−1.2–3.2]
	D10%	−4.6% [−44.6–38.0]	0.077	−4.6% [−27.6–20.5]	+3.1% [−13.8–24.6]	0.421	+0.9% [−4.2–5.4]
	D40%	+2.6% [−74.0–319.9]	0.019	−0.9% [−52.7–234.4]	+11.6% [−22.8–83.5]	0.680	+3.2% [−9.8–17.7]

3.3.1. Comparison I: Delivered vs. Planned Dose Distributions

Consistent dose deficits were seen in the minimum coverage of CTV, PTV, and PTV-CTV, and the largest deviations were observed in the PTV peripheral zone; mean and maximum doses to these target structures were instead minimally affected. A median coverage of at least 93% of the prescribed dose to 99% of the CTV was achieved during treatment fractions. Considering the cumulative patient dose over the 4–5 fractions, the median CTV D99% degraded from 94% [86–96%] of the prescribed dose at planning to 93% [77–95%] at treatment. The rate of target coverage violations (D95% < 95%), along with the number of patients who did not meet the constraints in planning and treatment, is reported in Table 4. Urethra planning organ at risk volume (PRV) sparing was slightly degraded, with >1% increases in D0.035 cc and D10% observed in 48% and 36% of the fractions, respectively. In eight and three patients, at least one dose metric at the end of the treatment exceeded the planned dose to the rectum and bladder, respectively. However, only a deterioration in the protocol constraint violation rate for rectum wall D0.035 cc and two major deviations in rectum mucosa D0.035 cc were noticed at treatment completion (Table 4).

Table 4. Protocol dose constraint infringement rate for target and OARs, along with the number of patients who failed in planning and treatment, for the delivered treatments.

	Planning			Treatment		
Dose Constraints	**Patients Failing**	**Infringement Rate**	**Major Deviations**	**Patients Failing**	**Infringement Rate**	**Major Deviations**
PTV D95% < 95%	0	0%	-	7	54%	1
CTV D95% < 95%	-	-	-	4	31%	-
Rectum wall D0.035 cc	0	0%	-	2	15%	-
Rectum mucosa D0.035 cc	6	46%	-	5	38%	2
Bladder D40%	1	8%	1	1	8%	1

3.3.2. Comparison II: Case B vs. Case A Motion-Inclusive Dose Distributions

In the motion-inclusive plans, the target dose deficits, as well as the degradations in OAR dose metrics, were marginal. None of the dosimetric parameters significantly differed from the planned values (Table A1). However, without an organ motion management strategy, significant dose reductions for CTV D99%, PTV D95%, and PTV-CTV D95% would have additionally occurred in 54%, 50%, and 70% of the fractions. For the cumulative treatments, the contribution of fractions in which prostate motion remained within the 2 mm gating threshold diminished the deterioration in the dose metrics (Table 3). Additional target coverage losses > 1% would have been experienced by four patients. Similarly, further overdoses > 1% to the urethra, rectum, and bladder would have been delivered to one, three, and seven patients, respectively. The target D95% > 95% criteria would not have been achieved in the same patients of comparison I (Table 4), but undetected out-of-tolerance prostate motion would have led to decreased minimum PTV coverage values, passing from 85% to 81% of the prescription dose in the worst case. Compared to the values presented in Table 4, one additional patient would have had a minor violation in the rectum wall D0.035 cc constraint (infringement rate equal to 23%).

4. Discussion

The actual delivered dose, including the contribution of both intrafraction motion and interfraction anatomical changes, was estimated by recalculating motion-encoded plans on synthetic CT deformed on the CBCT daily anatomy for dose-escalated linac-based prostate SBRT.

The motion-inclusive dose reconstruction method assumed that all target motion is due to the rigid motion of the whole patient. Small changes in the radiological path length due to changes in tissue density and the amount of tissue along the beam path were ignored, but they were not expected to compromise the accuracy of the target dose calculation in such a treatment modality. In this study, possible deformations of adjacent OARs occurring between each treatment fraction were considered to provide an accurate estimation of the effects in rectum and bladder doses [20,21,25,31]. Organ-filling variations occurring within the same daily fraction were not investigated. However, since the treatment duration was about 10 min on average, not taking into account these changes did not prevent a fair assessment of the dose delivered to OARs. It also has to be highlighted that the deformable image registration process to create the dCTs has several weaknesses itself, starting from the use of software in an undesirable "black-box" mode. According to AAPM TG-132 [41], other potential drawbacks due to different extensions, scan parameters, and image quality of the two studies being registered exist. Nevertheless, these related uncertainties are common to any commercial software and image registration process, and thus, the obtained dCTs, after being qualitatively validated, were deemed a reasonable representation of the daily organ morphology.

Our findings showed that the CTV largely differed from the simulation in only one patient, for whom a mean volume reduction of −12.6% was observed. This may be due to the cytoreductive effect of the androgen deprivation therapy (ADT) started by the patient almost six weeks before the treatment. Deformation and swelling in the prostate gland during extremely hypofractionated regimens have been observed [42,43], but our clinical schedule of 4 or 5 fractions delivered on consecutive days with ADT, received as per the standard of care [44] by 77% of the patients, seemed to have no relevant effect on prostate size. Gunnlauggsson et al. [42] found a 14% mean relative volume increase after three treatment fractions, while our mean increase at the same point was about 1%, although the different fractionation (6.1 Gy × 7), the use of magnetic resonance imaging (MRI) for the determination of prostate volume variations, and the use of ADT as exclusion criteria make these results not directly comparable. In keeping with previous experiences [15,17,19,22,36], large variations in rectum and bladder volumes likely occurred between the simulation and the daily treatment fractions. In the present study, the rectal micro-enema administered in the department shortly before each fraction appeared to be more effective than the procedure of filling the bladder with 100 cc of saline solution through the catheter in ensuring anatomical reproducibility. This may be related to the user-dependent bladder-filling procedure and the different positions that the catheter may take during its insertion on the first treatment day compared to the simulation.

A possible weakness of the current analysis is related to the challenges and thus possible uncertainties in CBCT contouring due to the poor image quality and the reduced contrast with respect to conventional CT images. We tried to minimize the inter-observer variability by leaving the contouring to the discretion of a single radiation oncologist experienced in the field. Pawloswki et al. [45] demonstrated that even though the prostate and the rectum were very sensitive to the uncertainties of CBCT contours, with volume variations up to 41% and 50%, respectively, in extreme cases, the effect on the calculated dose distributions was modest when image guidance was used. Hatton et al. [46], instead, by directly investigating the contouring accuracy between fan-beam and cone-beam CT scans, found no systematic differences in contour sizes and shapes.

Our dosimetric results from the delivered vs. planned dose distributions (Table 3, comparison I) showed that both intrafraction prostate motion and daily anatomical deformations minimally affected the mean and maximum doses to the target structures. The minimum doses, instead, more largely and frequently differed from the planned values. However, it must be pointed out that the results were a function of the chosen dosimetric endpoints: D99% of the CTV and D95% of the PTV were considered surrogates of the minimum target coverage in this study since they are already used as the treatment plan acceptability criteria at our institution. Moreover, since no other studies have performed dose recalculations accounting for both motion and daily anatomy in such treatments to our knowledge, these findings are difficult to compare to the existing literature. Langen et al. [25] investigated only the effect of motion during tomotherapy treatments and found an unexpected similarity between the observed D95% changes in the prostate and PTV, suggesting that the effects of motion are not necessarily restricted to the periphery of the PTV and, thus, that margins may not completely protect the target from a geographic miss. Conversely, we found that major degradations in the minimum but also the mean dose occurred in the PTV shell around the CTV, indicating the positive impact of the margins on ensuring the target coverage.

Margins were not the only implemented strategy to minimize a potential target miss: a strict patient preparation regimen, soft-tissue CBCT matching, intrafraction organ motion management, robust treatment planning, and fast FFF-beam delivery also played a crucial role. The registrations were focused on the prostate gland and were always performed to obtain the best overlap between the HypoCath and the urethra PRV delineated in the planning CT. This refinement allowed us to achieve the urethral sparing at which our plans aimed and to prevent a possible underdose to the surrounding CTV due to the lower prescribed dose to the urethra. Our findings showing no relevant differences in urethra dosimetry confirm the efficacy of this strategy.

Still, it is noteworthy that only translational errors in the target position were corrected, while rotations were not. Ma et al. [43] investigated the dosimetric impact of uncorrected interfraction rotations in the prostate and proximal seminal vesicles separately and found that the seminal vesicles exhibited inferior target dosimetry results to those of the prostate due to their considerable variations in the relative angle, both between the two lobes and relative to the vertical axis. By including the seminal vesicles in CTVs, target coverage reductions might have been at least partly affected by their rotational shifts. However, although severe target degradations as large as about 15–20% were observed in some individual fractions, they were infrequent, and their effect on the cumulative dose was smoothed with the number of fractions. The DVH analysis showed that the coverage of the prostate gland was satisfactory, with a median cumulative CTV coverage of 93% of the prescribed dose and only two patients who experienced a CTV dose deficit of more than 5%.

Due to the consistent daily variations in bladder and rectal volumes, the delivered doses to these OARs did not meet the treatment plan provisions in most fractions, as reported by many other studies [15,19,20,22]. The pattern of these differences, however, is hard to explain and to compare to the literature since the synergic effects of random volume and shape variations, organ motion, and changes in dynamic beam parameters may cause unpredictable differences in dose distributions and have never been explored. Wahl et al. [20] demonstrated that significantly higher doses during prostate SBRT were received by the rectum, while the bladder modestly differed from the original plan's dose. Instead, for our patient cohort and treatment delivery technique, the rectum received higher-than-planned doses in less than 40% of the fractions, and the bladder doses exhibited the largest and most frequent variations.

The minimal differences resulting from the motion-inclusive plans using case A prostate trajectories compared to the planned values implied that the intrafraction prostate motion marginally contributed in the scenario of gated treatments with a 2 mm threshold (Table A1). In our treatments, even with an accurate correction strategy using continuous tracking, beam gating, and target repositioning, the dosimetric variability was still not completely compensated, as similarly reported by two other works [15,20], indicating that the major contribution to both target and OARs discrepancies came from interfraction anatomical deformations. This emphasizes the importance of assessing the effects of daily variations in non-rigid body anatomy and led us to work toward especially improving the bladder preparation procedure through more specific instructions and different filling modalities. The current study determined that only a few patients failed at least one of the rectum and bladder constraints at treatment completion (Table 4). However, the larger doses delivered to the rectum and the bladder did not necessarily correlate with increased toxicity. The early treatment outcomes for this patient group were previously published [14], showing that no Grade 2 or higher gastrointestinal (rectal) or genitourinary side effects occurred within 90 days from the end of the treatment. At a median follow-up of 18 months, only two late Grade 2 side effects were observed. Those differences slightly affected the target coverage, and indeed, biochemical control was not compromised.

The recent randomized trial MIRAGE [47] reported a significantly lower toxicity profile with MR-guided daily adaptive RT (MRgRT) vs. CT-guided SBRT in prostate cancer. The 4 mm margins and delivery without intrafraction monitoring used in the CT arm, however, make a direct comparison with the current study findings difficult. Moreover, Nicosia et al. [36], evaluating the dosimetric differences between MRgRT and image-guided SBRT with or without fiducial markers, found the highest accuracy of MRgRT as compared to SBRT without fiducials but minimal or absent differences with fiducials. Interfraction anatomical variation issues may be better overcome in an online adaptive setting, but the use of internal markers, fiducials, or transmitters, along with the other abovementioned planning and delivery techniques, keeps linac-based prostate SBRT valid and suitable. Similar results in terms of a reduction in the target coverage and an increase in the OAR constraint violation rate in a recent dosimetric analysis for 15 patients by Brennan et al. [48], using different real-time MRI scans to estimate the true delivered dose, support this conclusion.

A direct comparison between case B and case A motion-inclusive dose distributions showed that the implemented strategy of organ motion mitigation was effective at preventing larger target dose deficits and bladder overdoses for fractions that would have had higher prostate displacements. Similarly, Colvill et al. [16] demonstrated that gated dose calculations with a 3 mm–5 s threshold would have led to improvements in all CTV D99% and PTV D95% values with respect to delivered non-gated treatments. The results of the current study, however, showed that even in non-gated treatments, deteriorations in dose parameters would not have been as relevant, with only one additional patient experiencing a constraint violation for the rectum wall. This is explained by the fact that prostate motion beyond the tolerances would have been rare even in case B due to the short treatment times enabled by VMAT-FFF plans. Indeed, the likelihood of prostate motion has been demonstrated to increase with increasing treatment time. Vanhanen et al. [21] also concluded that continuous motion monitoring and gating may have a greater beneficial effect with treatment techniques associated with a longer beam delivery time. However, intratreatment position correction, along with accurate CBCT-based interfraction motion correction, ensured superior results for every fraction and patient. Hence, they are recommended to use in dose-escalated treatments with an increased risk of OARs adverse events and a further reduction in PTV margins.

5. Conclusions

For the first time, the dosimetric impacts of intrafraction motion and interfraction changes have been investigated together in dose-escalated linac-based prostate SBRT. The implemented organ motion management strategy and the strict patient preparation regimen, along with current PTV margins, the robustness of the original treatment plans, soft-tissue CBCT matching, and fast FFF-beam delivery, ensured there were no significant degradations of target and OARs dose metrics. Non-gated treatments would have resulted in larger target dose deficits and bladder overdoses in some fractions. Thus, continuous monitoring, beam gating, and motion correction are recommended to safely deliver such extreme hypofractionated treatments.

Author Contributions: Conceptualization, D.P.; investigation, V.F. and D.P.; methodology, D.P. and V.F.; resources, M.C.D., P.C., S.T. and R.L.; software, M.C.D. and R.P.; validation, R.P., E.D.P. and S.A.; formal analysis, V.F., D.P. and E.D.P.; data curation, M.C.D., P.C., S.T. and R.L.; writing—original draft preparation, V.F.; writing—review and editing, D.P. and S.A.; visualization, V.F. and D.P.; supervision, D.P.; project administration, E.D.P. and S.A. All authors have read and agreed to the published version of the manuscript.

Funding: This research received no external funding.

Institutional Review Board Statement: The study was conducted in accordance with the Declaration of Helsinki. Ethical review and approval were waived because the study shows results on a retrospective analysis of treated patients as part of routine care, according to national and international guidelines and agreements.

Informed Consent Statement: Informed consent was obtained from all subjects involved in the study.

Data Availability Statement: Research data are stored in an institutional repository and can be shared upon reasonable request to the corresponding author.

Conflicts of Interest: The authors declare no conflict of interest.

Appendix A

Table A1. Mean and range (over all fractions and patients) of the percentage differences in target and OARs dosimetric parameters between intrafraction motion-inclusive recalculations considering the observed case A prostate motion data and the planned dose distributions. *p*-values ($p < 0.05$) for the individual fractions' dose parameters are also reported.

	Metric	Individual Fractions	*p*-Value	Cumulative Treatments
CTV	Dmean	+0.1% [−0.7–2.3]	0.522	+0.1% [−0.1–0.5]
	D99%	−0.2% [−5.1–5.1]	0.392	+0.0% [−1.8–1.1]
	D2%	+0.3% [−0.4–4.4]	0.086	−0.4% [−0.7–0.1]
PTV	Dmean	0.0% [−0.7–2.0]	0.875	0.0% [−0.4–0.4]
	D95%	−0.4% [−3.7–1.4]	0.136	−0.2% [−1.6–0.8]
	D2%	+0.4% [−0.4–4.3]	0.056	−0.4% [−0.7–0.1]
PTV—CTV	Dmean	−0.1% [−1.5–1.0]	0.907	−0.1% [−1.0–0.3]
	D95%	−1.0% [−12.1–7.1]	0.337	−1.1% [−7.8–2.5]
Urethra PRV	D0.035 cc	+0.7% [−0.8–6.4]	0.168	−0.2% [−0.6–0.4]
	D10%	+0.6% [−0.9–5.4]	0.175	+0.1% [−0.3–0.9]

Table A1. *Cont.*

	Metric	Individual Fractions	p-Value	Cumulative Treatments
Rectum	D5%	−1.7% [−14.4–11.5]	0.419	−2.5% [−8.8–3.1]
	D10%	−2.3% [−16.7–14.2]	0.526	−2.9% [−9.7–3.8]
	D20%	−2.9% [−39.8–13.6]	0.592	−3.1% [−10.4–4.9]
	D50%	−1.3% [−12.5–6.2]	0.852	−1.8% [−7.6–2.2]
Rectum wall	D0.035 cc	−0.6% [−7.9–5.3]	0.584	−1.6% [−4.8–1.7]
Rectum mucosa	D0.035 cc	−1.1% [−13.5–14.0]	0.507	−2.3% [−8.3–3.3]
Bladder	D0.035 cc	+0.3% [−1.9–3.3]	0.580	−0.2% [−1.1–1.1]
	D10%	+0.2% [−11.7–11.4]	0.926	+1.2% [−4.9–7.5]
	D40%	+1.4 [−18.7–37.7]	0.907	+5.1% [−7.8–25.1]

Only in 25% of all fractions did the PTV coverage drop below 95% of the prescribed dose, with a minimum coverage value of 92%. The percentage of fractions with more than 90% minimum CTV coverage was 95%. Degradations larger than 1% in CTV D99% and PTV D95% were seen only for three patients. The cumulative effect of intrafraction prostate motion would have caused violations of the minimum PTV coverage requirement (D95% > 95%) in only one patient, whose target would have been covered by 94% of the prescribed dose at minimum. Overdoses >5% to the urethra, rectum, and bladder were observed in some treatment fractions. In the motion-inclusive cumulative plans, differences no larger than 1% with respect to planned values would have been observed for the urethra. Only three patients would have had rectum dose increases >1% in at least one parameter at the end of treatment, while for the bladder, the same occurred in nine patients. With a 2 mm threshold beam gating strategy implemented, no differences in the OARs protocol dose constraint violation rate would have been observed due to the intrafraction motion of the prostate.

References

1. Proust-Lima, C.; Taylor, J.M.; Sécher, S.; Sandler, H.; Kestin, L.; Pickles, T.; Bae, K.; Allison, R.; Williams, S. Confirmation of a Low α/β Ratio for Prostate Cancer Treated by External Beam Radiation Therapy Alone Using a Post-Treatment Repeated-Measures Model for PSA Dynamics. *Int. J. Radiat. Oncol. Biol. Phys.* **2011**, *79*, 195–201. [CrossRef] [PubMed]
2. Miralbell, R.; Roberts, S.A.; Zubizarreta, E.; Hendry, J.H. Dose-Fractionation Sensitivity of Prostate Cancer Deduced from Radiotherapy Outcomes of 5969 Patients in Seven International Institutional Datasets: α/β = 1.4 (0.9–2.2) Gy. *Int. J. Radiat. Oncol. Biol. Phys.* **2012**, *82*, e17–e24. [CrossRef] [PubMed]
3. Dasu, A.; Toma-Dasu, I. Prostate alpha/beta revisited—An analysis of clinical results from 14 168 patients. *Acta Oncol.* **2012**, *51*, 963–974. [CrossRef] [PubMed]
4. Morgan, S.C.; Hoffman, K.; Loblaw, D.A.; Buyyounouski, M.K.; Patton, C.; Barocas, D.; Bentzen, S.; Chang, M.; Efstathiou, J.; Greany, P.; et al. Hypofractionated radiation therapy for localized prostate cancer: An ASTRO, ASCO, and AUA evidence-based guideline. *Pract. Radiat. Oncol.* **2018**, *8*, 354–360. [CrossRef]
5. King, C.R.; Freeman, D.; Kaplan, I.; Fuller, D.; Bolzicco, G.; Collins, S.; Meier, R.; Wang, J.; Kupelian, P.; Steinberg, M.; et al. Stereotactic body radiotherapy for localized prostate cancer: Pooled analysis from a multi-institutional consortium of prospective phase II trials. *Radiother. Oncol.* **2013**, *109*, 217–221. [CrossRef]
6. Katz, A.J.; Kang, J. Stereotactic Body Radiotherapy as Treatment for Organ Confined Low- and Intermediate-Risk Prostate Carcinoma, a 7-Year Study. *Front. Oncol.* **2014**, *4*, 240. [CrossRef]
7. Alayed, Y.; Cheung, P.; Pang, G.; Mamedov, A.; D'Alimonte, L.; Deabreu, A.; Commisso, K.; Commisso, A.; Zhang, L.; Quon, H.C.; et al. Dose escalation for prostate stereotactic ablative radiotherapy (SABR): Late outcomes from two prospective clinical trials. *Radiother. Oncol.* **2018**, *127*, 213–218. [CrossRef]
8. Langen, K.; Jones, D. Organ motion and its management. *Int. J. Radiat. Oncol. Biol. Phys.* **2001**, *50*, 265–278. [CrossRef]
9. Kron, T.; Thomas, J.; Fox, C.; Thompson, A.; Owen, R.; Herschtal, A.; Haworth, A.; Tai, K.-H.; Foroudi, F. Intra-fraction prostate displacement in radiotherapy estimated from pre- and post-treatment imaging of patients with implanted fiducial markers. *Radiother. Oncol.* **2010**, *95*, 191–197. [CrossRef]
10. Ballhausen, H.; Li, M.; Hegemann, N.-S.; Ganswindt, U.; Belka, C. Intra-fraction motion of the prostate is a random walk. *Phys. Med. Biol.* **2015**, *60*, 549–563. [CrossRef]
11. Legge, K.; Nguyen, D.; Ng, J.A.; Wilton, L.; Richardson, M.; Booth, J.; Keall, P.; O'Connor, D.J.; Greer, P.; Martin, J. Real-time intrafraction prostate motion during linac based stereotactic radiotherapy with rectal displacement. *J. Appl. Clin. Med. Phys.* **2017**, *18*, 130–136. [CrossRef] [PubMed]

12. Gorovets, D.; Burleson, S.; Jacobs, L.; Ravindranath, B.; Tierney, K.; Kollmeier, M.; McBride, S.; Happersett, L.; Hunt, M.; Zelefsky, M. Prostate SBRT With Intrafraction Motion Management Using a Novel Linear Accelerator–Based MV-kV Imaging Method. *Pract. Radiat. Oncol.* **2020**, *10*, e388–e396. [CrossRef] [PubMed]
13. Panizza, D.; Faccenda, V.; Lucchini, R.; Daniotti, M.C.; Trivellato, S.; Caricato, P.; Pisoni, V.; De Ponti, E.; Arcangeli, S. Intrafraction Prostate Motion Management During Dose-Escalated Linac-Based Stereotactic Body Radiation Therapy. *Front. Oncol.* **2022**, *12*, 883725. [CrossRef] [PubMed]
14. Lucchini, R.; Panizza, D.; Colciago, R.R.; Vernier, V.; Daniotti, M.C.; Faccenda, V.; Arcangeli, S. Treatment outcome and compliance to dose-intensified linac-based SBRT for unfavorable prostate tumors using a novel real-time organ-motion tracking. *Radiat. Oncol.* **2021**, *16*, 180. [CrossRef] [PubMed]
15. Kupelian, P.A.; Langen, K.M.; Zeidan, O.A.; Meeks, S.L.; Willoughby, T.R.; Wagner, T.H.; Jeswani, S.; Ruchala, K.J.; Haimerl, J.; Olivera, G.H. Daily variations in delivered doses in patients treated with radiotherapy for localized prostate cancer. *Int. J. Radiat. Oncol. Biol. Phys.* **2006**, *66*, 876–882. [CrossRef] [PubMed]
16. Colvill, E.; Poulsen, P.R.; Booth, J.T.; O'Brien, R.T.; Ng, J.A.; Keall, P.J. DMLC tracking and gating can improve dose coverage for prostate VMAT. *Med. Phys.* **2014**, *41*, 091705. [CrossRef]
17. McParland, N.; Pearson, M.; Wong, J.; Sigur, I.; Stenger, C.; Tyldesley, S. Quantifying daily variation in volume and dose to the prostate, rectum and bladder using cone-beam computerised tomography. *J. Radiother. Pract.* **2014**, *13*, 79–86. [CrossRef]
18. Lovelock, D.M.; Messineo, A.P.; Cox, B.W.; Kollmeier, M.A.; Zelefsky, M.J. Continuous Monitoring and Intrafraction Target Position Correction During Treatment Improves Target Coverage for Patients Undergoing SBRT Prostate Therapy. *Int. J. Radiat. Oncol. Biol. Phys.* **2015**, *91*, 588–594. [CrossRef]
19. Pearson, D.; Gill, S.K.; Campbell, N.; Reddy, K. Dosimetric and volumetric changes in the rectum and bladder in patients receiving CBCT-guided prostate IMRT: Analysis based on daily CBCT dose calculation. *J. Appl. Clin. Med. Phys.* **2016**, *17*, 107–117. [CrossRef]
20. Wahl, M.; Descovich, M.; Shugard, E.; Pinnaduwage, D.; Sudhyadhom, A.; Chang, A.; Roach, M.; Gottschalk, A.; Chen, J. Interfraction Anatomical Variability Can Lead to Significantly Increased Rectal Dose for Patients Undergoing Stereotactic Body Radiotherapy for Prostate Cancer. *Technol. Cancer Res. Treat.* **2017**, *16*, 178–187. [CrossRef]
21. Vanhanen, A.; Poulsen, P.; Kapanen, M. Dosimetric effect of intrafraction motion and different localization strategies in prostate SBRT. *Phys. Med.* **2020**, *75*, 58–68. [CrossRef] [PubMed]
22. Devlin, L.; Dodds, D.; Sadozye, A.; McLoone, P.; MacLeod, N.; Lamb, C.; Currie, S.; Thomson, S.; Duffton, A. Dosimetric impact of organ at risk daily variation during prostate stereotactic ablative radiotherapy. *Br. J. Radiol.* **2020**, *93*, 20190789. [CrossRef]
23. Litzenberg, D.W.; Hadley, S.W.; Tyagi, N.; Balter, J.M.; Haken, R.K.T.; Chetty, I.J. Synchronized dynamic dose reconstruction. *Med. Phys.* **2007**, *34*, 91–102. [CrossRef]
24. Li, H.S.; Chetty, I.J.; Enke, C.A.; Foster, R.D.; Willoughby, T.R.; Kupellian, P.A.; Solberg, T.D. Dosimetric Consequences of Intrafraction Prostate Motion. *Int. J. Radiat. Oncol. Biol. Phys.* **2008**, *71*, 801–812. [CrossRef] [PubMed]
25. Langen, K.M.; Lü, W.; Ngwa, W.; Willoughby, T.R.; Chauhan, B.; Meeks, S.L.; Kupelian, A.P.; Olivera, G. Correlation between dosimetric effect and intrafraction motion during prostate treatments delivered with helical tomotherapy. *Phys. Med. Biol.* **2008**, *53*, 7073–7086. [CrossRef] [PubMed]
26. Zhang, P.; Mah, D.; Happersett, L.; Cox, B.; Hunt, M.; Mageras, G. Determination of action thresholds for electromagnetic tracking system-guided hypofractionated prostate radiotherapy using volumetric modulated arc therapy. *Med. Phys.* **2011**, *38*, 4001–4008. [CrossRef] [PubMed]
27. Adamson, J.; Wu, Q.; Yan, D. Dosimetric Effect of Intrafraction Motion and Residual Setup Error for Hypofractionated Prostate Intensity-Modulated Radiotherapy with Online Cone Beam Computed Tomography Image Guidance. *Int. J. Radiat. Oncol. Biol. Phys.* **2011**, *80*, 453–461. [CrossRef]
28. van de Water, S.; Valli, L.; Aluwini, S.; Lanconelli, N.; Heijmen, B.; Hoogeman, M. Intrafraction Prostate Translations and Rotations During Hypofractionated Robotic Radiation Surgery: Dosimetric Impact of Correction Strategies and Margins. *Int. J. Radiat. Oncol. Biol. Phys.* **2014**, *88*, 1154–1160. [CrossRef]
29. Azcona, J.D.; Xing, L.; Chen, X.; Bush, K.; Li, R. Assessing the Dosimetric Impact of Real-Time Prostate Motion During Volumetric Modulated Arc Therapy. *Int. J. Radiat. Oncol. Biol. Phys.* **2014**, *88*, 1167–1174. [CrossRef]
30. Russo, S.; Ricotti, R.; Molinelli, S.; Patti, F.; Barcellini, A.; Mastella, E.; Pella, A.; Paganelli, C.; Marvaso, G.; Pepa, M.; et al. Dosimetric Impact of Inter-Fraction Anatomical Changes in Carbon Ion Boost Treatment for High-Risk Prostate Cancer (AIRC IG 14300). *Front. Oncol.* **2021**, *11*, 740661. [CrossRef]
31. Poulsen, P.R.; Schmidt, M.L.; Keall, P.; Worm, E.S.; Fledelius, W.; Hoffmann, L. A method of dose reconstruction for moving targets compatible with dynamic treatments. *Med. Phys.* **2012**, *39*, 6237–6246. [CrossRef] [PubMed]
32. Richter, A.; Hu, Q.; Steglich, D.; Baier, K.; Wilbert, J.; Guckenberger, M.; Flentje, M. Investigation of the usability of conebeam CT data sets for dose calculation. *Radiat. Oncol.* **2008**, *3*, 42. [CrossRef] [PubMed]
33. Hatton, J.; McCurdy, B.; Greer, P. Cone beam computerized tomography: The effect of calibration of the Hounsfield unit number to electron density on dose calculation accuracy for adaptive radiation therapy. *Phys. Med. Biol.* **2009**, *54*, N329–N346. [CrossRef] [PubMed]
34. Varadhan, R.; Hui, S.K.; Way, S.; Nisi, K. Assessing prostate, bladder and rectal doses during image guided radiation therapy-need for plan adaptation? *J. Appl. Clin. Med. Phys.* **2009**, *10*, 56–74. [CrossRef]

35. Fotina, I.; Hopfgartner, J.; Stock, M.; Steininger, T.; Lütgendorf-Caucig, C.; Georg, D. Feasibility of CBCT-based dose calculation: Comparative analysis of HU adjustment techniques. *Radiother. Oncol.* **2012**, *104*, 249–256. [CrossRef]
36. Nicosia, L.; Sicignano, G.; Rigo, M.; Figlia, V.; Cuccia, F.; De Simone, A.; Giaj-Levra, N.; Mazzola, R.; Naccarato, S.; Ricchetti, F.; et al. Daily dosimetric variation between image-guided volumetric modulated arc radiotherapy and MR-guided daily adaptive radiotherapy for prostate cancer stereotactic body radiotherapy. *Acta Oncol.* **2020**, *60*, 215–221. [CrossRef]
37. Chen, S.; Quan, H.; Qin, A.; Yee, S.; Yan, D. MR image-based synthetic CT for IMRT prostate treatment planning and CBCT image-guided localization. *J. Appl. Clin. Med. Phys.* **2016**, *17*, 236–245. [CrossRef]
38. Imae, T.; Haga, A.; Watanabe, Y.; Takenaka, S.; Shiraki, T.; Nawa, K.; Ogita, M.; Takahashi, W.; Yamashita, H.; Nakagawa, K.; et al. Retrospective dose reconstruction of prostate stereotactic body radiotherapy using cone-beam CT and a log file during VMAT delivery with flattening-filter-free mode. *Radiol. Phys. Technol.* **2020**, *13*, 238–248. [CrossRef]
39. Juneja, P.; Colvill, E.; Kneebone, A.; Eade, T.; Ng, J.A.; Thwaites, D.I.; Keall, P.; Kaur, R.; Poulsen, P.R.; Booth, J.T. Quantification of intrafraction prostate motion and its dosimetric effect on VMAT. *Australas. Phys. Eng. Sci. Med.* **2017**, *40*, 317–324. [CrossRef]
40. Jaccard, M.; Ehrbar, S.; Miralbell, R.; Hagen, T.; Koutsouvelis, N.; Poulsen, P.; Rouzaud, M.; Tanadini-Lang, S.; Tsoutsou, P.; Guckenberger, M.; et al. Single-fraction prostate stereotactic body radiotherapy: Dose reconstruction with electromagnetic intrafraction motion tracking. *Radiother. Oncol.* **2021**, *156*, 145–152. [CrossRef]
41. Brock, K.K.; Mutic, S.; McNutt, T.R.; Li, H.; Kessler, M.L. Use of image registration and fusion algorithms and techniques in radiotherapy: Report of the AAPM Radiation Therapy Committee Task Group No. 132. *Med. Phys.* **2017**, *44*, e43–e76. [CrossRef]
42. Gunnlaugsson, A.; Kjellén, E.; Hagberg, O.; Thellenberg-Karlsson, C.; Widmark, A.; Nilsson, P. Change in prostate volume during extreme hypo-fractionation analysed with MRI. *Radiat. Oncol.* **2014**, *9*, 22. [CrossRef]
43. Ma, T.M.; Neylon, J.; Casado, M.; Sharma, S.; Sheng, K.; Low, D.; Yang, Y.; Steinberg, M.L.; Lamb, J.; Cao, M.; et al. Dosimetric impact of interfraction prostate and seminal vesicle volume changes and rotation: A post-hoc analysis of a phase III randomized trial of MRI-guided versus CT-guided stereotactic body radiotherapy. *Radiother. Oncol.* **2021**, *167*, 203–210. [CrossRef] [PubMed]
44. Schaeffrer, E.; Srinivas, S.; Adra, N.; An, Y.; Barocas, D.; Bitting, R.; Bryce, A.; Chapin, B.; Cheng, H.H.; D'Amico, A.V.; et al. Prostate cancer, version 1.2023 featured updates to the NCCN guidelines. *J. Natl. Compr. Cancer Netw.* **2022**, *20*, 1288–1298. [CrossRef]
45. Pawlowski, J.M.; Yang, E.S.; Malcolm, A.W.; Coffey, C.W.; Ding, G.X. Reduction of Dose Delivered to Organs at Risk in Prostate Cancer Patients via Image-Guided Radiation Therapy. *Int. J. Radiat. Oncol. Biol. Phys.* **2010**, *76*, 924–934. [CrossRef]
46. Hatton, J.A.; Greer, P.B.; Tang, C.; Wright, P.; Capp, A.; Gupta, S.; Parker, J.; Wratten, C.; Denham, J.W. Does the planning dose–volume histogram represent treatment doses in image-guided prostate radiation therapy? Assessment with cone-beam computerised tomography scans. *Radiother. Oncol.* **2011**, *98*, 162–168. [CrossRef] [PubMed]
47. Kishan, A.U.; Ma, T.M.; Lamb, J.M.; Casado, M.; Wilhalme, H.; Low, D.A.; Sheng, K.; Sharma, S.; Nickols, N.G.; Pham, J.; et al. Magnetic Resonance Imaging–Guided vs Computed Tomography–Guided Stereotactic Body Radiotherapy for Prostate Cancer: The MIRAGE Randomized Clinical Trial. *JAMA Oncol.* **2023**. [CrossRef]
48. Brennan, V.S.; Burleson, S.; Kostrzewa, C.; Scripes, P.G.; Subashi, E.; Zhang, Z.; Tyagi, N.; Zelefsky, M.J. SBRT focal dose intensification using an MR-Linac adaptive planning for intermediate-risk prostate cancer: An analysis of the dosimetric impact of intra-fractional organ changes. *Radiother. Oncol.* **2022**, *179*, 109441. [CrossRef] [PubMed]

cancers

Article

Three Months' PSA and Toxicity from a Prospective Trial Investigating STereotactic sAlvage Radiotherapy for Macroscopic Prostate Bed Recurrence after Prostatectomy—STARR (NCT05455736)

Giulio Francolini [1], Pietro Garlatti [1], Vanessa Di Cataldo [1], Beatrice Detti [1], Mauro Loi [1], Daniela Greto [1], Gabriele Simontacchi [1], Ilaria Morelli [2], Luca Burchini [2], Andrea Gaetano Allegra [2], Giulio Frosini [2], Michele Ganovelli [2], Viola Salvestrini [3], Emanuela Olmetto [1], Luca Visani [3], Carlotta Becherini [1], Marianna Valzano [2], Maria Grazia Carnevale [2], Manuele Roghi [2], Sergio Serni [4], Chiara Mattioli [2], Isacco Desideri [2] and Lorenzo Livi [2,*]

1 Radiation Oncology Unit, Oncology Department, Azienda Ospedaliero Universitaria Careggi, 50134 Firenze, Italy
2 Department of Biomedical, Experimental and Clinical Sciences "M. Serio", University of Florence, 50121 Firenze, Italy
3 CyberKnife Center, Istituto Fiorentino di Cura e Assistenza (IFCA), 50134 Firenze, Italy
4 Department of Urologic Robotic Surgery and Renal Transplantation, Careggi Hospital, University of Florence, 50121 Firenze, Italy
* Correspondence: lorenzo.livi@unifi.it; Tel.: +39-055-7947719

Citation: Francolini, G.; Garlatti, P.; Di Cataldo, V.; Detti, B.; Loi, M.; Greto, D.; Simontacchi, G.; Morelli, I.; Burchini, L.; Allegra, A.G.; et al. Three Months' PSA and Toxicity from a Prospective Trial Investigating STereotactic sAlvage Radiotherapy for Macroscopic Prostate Bed Recurrence after Prostatectomy—STARR (NCT05455736). *Cancers* **2023**, *15*, 992. https://doi.org/10.3390/cancers15030992

Academic Editor: Kouji Izumi

Received: 22 December 2022
Revised: 27 January 2023
Accepted: 30 January 2023
Published: 3 February 2023

Simple Summary: This article is a report about early toxicity and biochemical outcomes after stereotactic salvage radiotherapy for macroscopic recurrence within prostate bed after radical prostatectomy. Data reported suggest optimal tolerability profile and promising oncologic outcomes after this approach within a prospective multicentric trial.

Abstract: Biochemical recurrences after radical prostatectomy (RP) can be managed with curative purpose through salvage radiation therapy (SRT). RT dose escalation, such as stereotactic RT (SSRT), may improve relapse-free survival in this setting. STARR trial (NCT05455736) is a prospective multicenter study including patients affected by macroscopic recurrence within the prostate bed after RP treated with SSRT. Recurrence was detected with a Choline or PSMA CT-PET. In the current analysis, the early biochemical response (BR) rate and toxicity profile after three months of follow-up were assessed. Twenty-five patients were enrolled, and data about BR and toxicity at three months after treatment were available for 19 cases. Overall, BR was detected after three months in 58% of cases. Four G1–G2 adverse events were recorded; no G $\geq$ 3 adverse events were detected. SSRT appears feasible and safe, with more than half of patients experiencing BR and an encouraging toxicity profile. The STARR trial is one of the few prospective studies aimed at implementing this promising treatment strategy in this scenario.

Keywords: radical prostatectomy; adjuvant therapy; local invasion

1. Introduction

Radical Prostatectomy (RP) is one of the preferred treatment approaches for localized prostate cancer (pCA). However, up to 29% of men undergoing RP eventually develop recurrence within 10 years of surgery [1]. Prostate bed salvage radiotherapy (SRT) is a widely accepted treatment option for this scenario [2]; nonetheless, the outcome after salvage treatment is significantly worse in patients with positive metabolic imaging detecting nodal or distant macroscopic recurrences [3]. In this scenario, RT dose escalation aimed at improving disease control is advocated by some authors [4,5], but no consensus exists on the management of macroscopic relapse detected within the prostate bed. According to European Association of Urology (EAU) guidelines, given the variations of techniques and dose-constraints, a satisfactory agreement about target volume definition and optimal SRT dose has not been well defined [6]. Modern imaging methods (e.g., Choline or PSMA PET/CT and Magnetic resonance imaging-MRI) allowed the precise definition of the extent and location of recurrence within the prostate bed, and prompted the use of tailored treatment approaches including Stereotactic SRT (SSRT) on macroscopic relapse. Currently, SSRT is considered experimental and should be restricted to clinical trials [7], but promising results have been reported in preliminary experiences, even in comparison to conventional SRT [8]. SSRT yields potential advantages if compared to conventional SRT considering the dose-escalated approach on a limited treatment volume, deliverable in a lower number of fractions (usually 3–5). Given the lack of prospective evidence about this issue, a prospective trial was designed, enrolling patients affected by macroscopic prostate bed relapse undergoing SSRT (STereotactic sAlvage Radiotherapy for macroscopic prostate bed Recurrence after prostatectomy, STARR trial, NCT05455736). STARR trial is aimed at prospectively assessing the rate of biochemical relapse and adverse events after SSRT in this setting. In the present work, we present an analysis of the first cohort enrolled within the trial, focusing on early biochemical outcomes and acute toxicity.

2. Materials and Methods

2.1. Study Population

STARR (NCT05455736) is a prospective multicenter study including patients treated with RP for localized prostate cancer and affected by macroscopic recurrence within the prostate bed. Recurrence was detected with a Choline or PSMA CT PET performed at biochemical recurrence (PSA > 0.2 ng/mL) after surgery, and confirmed with MRI (except for patients in whom MRI was contraindicated). No imaging after surgery and before biochemical relapse was routinely performed to rule out the presence of residual prostate gland tissue. All patients with evidence of regional or distant metastatic disease were excluded from the trial. All patients in whom any contraindication to SSRT was detected (e.g., chronic bowel inflammatory disease, relevant toxicity after surgery) were excluded from the trial. Patients reporting urethral stenosis after surgery or relevant incontinence were not deemed fit for SSRT and were excluded from the trial.

2.2. Study Procedures

All patients underwent Cyberknife^{R} SSRT for a total dose of 35 Gy in 5 fractions. Treatment was administered with an every-other-day schedule. Use of different techniques (e.g., Volumetric Modulated Arc Therapy-VMAT or MR based SSRT) was allowed within the protocol, provided that the treatment respected doses and fractionation indicated per protocol (35 Gy in 5 fractions) and that dose constraints to organs at risk were observed. However, first, patients were enrolled in the promoting institution, where CyberknifeR SSRT is used for this kind of treatment. PSMA or choline CT-PET and MRI were co-registered with the planning CT scan for target volume delineation purposes. The Gross Target Volume (GTV) corresponded to macroscopic neoplastic tissue within the prostate bed. Clinical Target Volume (CTV) was obtained, adding a 2 mm margin to GTV. A margin of 3 mm (1 mm in the posterior direction) was added to CTV to obtain the final Planning Target Volume (PTV) (Figure 1). Patient alignment and target tracking were performed through implanted fiducials. During delivery, radiographic images were acquired using the InTempo^{TM} System (AccurayInc.), which alters imaging frequency between 15 and 60 s depending on the magnitude of the prostate or recurrence on prostatic bed motion detected. Bladder catheter placement was not performed for planning and delivery procedures. The following organs at risk were contoured: rectum, bladder, bowel, urethra, penile bulb, femoral heads, and bowel. The main dose constraints used are reported in Table 1. Concomitant Androgen Deprivation Therapy (ADT) was not allowed (patients should be free from ADT from at least 12 months before enrollment). All patients were evaluated every three months with a PSA and a clinical examination. The first treatment response evaluation was performed at 3 months after end of treatment with serum PSA. No protocol assessments were performed before 3 months from end of treatment. Re-staging was performed in case of biochemical or clinical progression of disease.

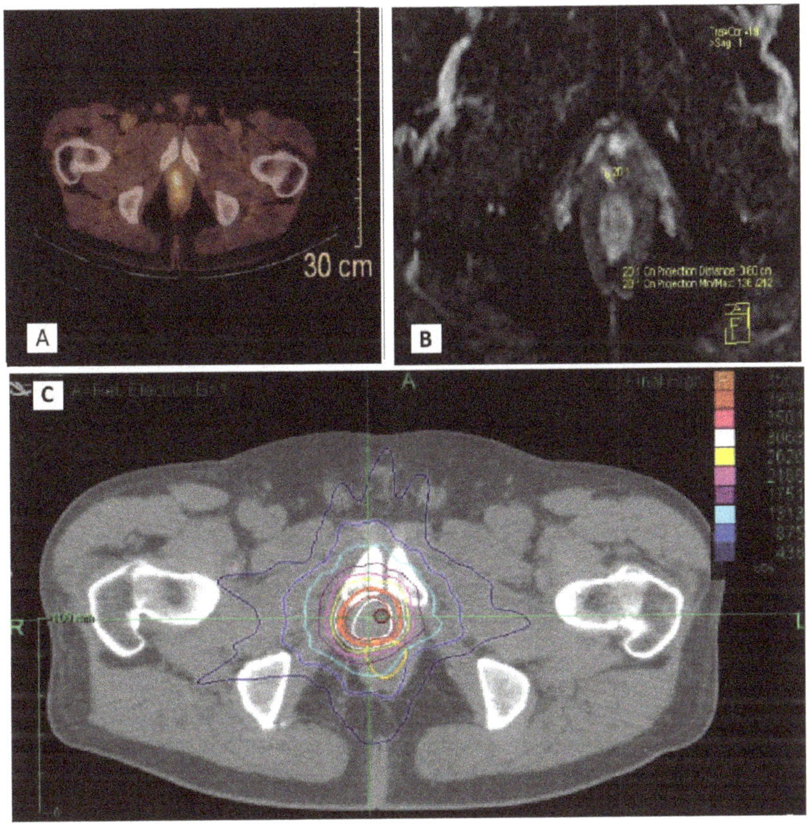

Figure 1. An example of radiotherapy treatment plan with PSMA imaging (**A**), MRI imaging (**B**) and Cyberknife^{R} treatment volumes and isodose lines (**C**).

Table 1. Main dose constraints used.

Organ at Risk	Dose Constraint	Aim
Rectum	V18.1 Gy V29 Gy V36 Gy	<50% <20% <1 cc
Bladder	V18.1 Gy V37 Gy	<40% <10 cc
Urethra	V42 Gy	<50% (not mandatory)
Femoral heads	V14.5 Gy	<5%
Penile bulb	V29.5 Gy	<50%
Bowel	V18.1 Gy V30 Gy	<5 cc <1 cc

2.3. Outcomes

Complete biochemical response and biochemical response were defined as aPSA nadir ≤ 0.2 ng/mL and ≤50% of baseline, respectively. Biochemical relapse was defined as a PSA increase above 0.2 ng/mL for patients with a PSA nadir ≤ 0.2 ng/mL (or 2 consecutive PSA increases > 25% if compared to nadir in patients with a PSA nadir > 0.2 ng/mL). These definitions were adapted from the Prostate Cancer Working Group 3 recommendations [9]. A PSA was defined as stable if neither a biochemical response nor biochemical relapse could be defined. Acute Gastrointestinal (GI) and Genitourinary (GU) Toxicity was assessed every 3 months after treatment according to the Common Terminology Criteria for Adverse Events (CTCAE) score v.4.03 [10].

2.4. Statistical Analysis

Primary endpoint of the trial will be to assess rate of biochemical relapse free patients after 2 years of follow up. Considering previous reported data about use of SSRT in this setting [11], a sample size of 90 patients will be needed to assess with a +/−9% margin of error the biochemical relapse free survival rate in this population. In this work, we present early results in terms of acute toxicity and early biochemical outcomes after 3 months from treatment in the first cohort of enrolled patients.

3. Results

As of 25 September 2022, twenty-five pts have been enrolled from March 2021. Data about biochemical response and toxicity at 3 months after treatment were available for 19 of these patients, included in the current analysis. The main features of the included population are summarized in Table 2. The median time from surgery to recurrence was 37 months (IQR 21.7–124.5). The median PSA at recurrence was 1.13 ng/mL (IQR 0.43–2.3 ng/mL). Macroscopic recurrence was detected by PSMA PET/CT or Choline PET/CT in fifteen (79%) and four (21%) patients, respectively. Five patients did not perform MRI confirmation. PET/CT and MRI imaging were reviewed by nuclear medicine and a dedicated radiologist with more than 5 years of experience in genitourinary cancers.

Table 2. Principal baseline features of included patients.

Age (Median Value, IQR)	74 (IQR 69–80)
Baseline T stage (%)	T2b-c: 8 (42%) T3a-b: 11 (58%)
Baseline N stage	N0: 12 (63%) N1: 0 (0) Nx: 7 (37%)
Margin status	R0: 7(37%) R1: 12 (63%)
Baseline ISUP pattern	≤3: 14 (74%) Gleason 3 + 3:1 Gleason 3 + 4: 8 Gleason 4 + 3: 5 >3: 5 (26%) Gleason 4 + 4:4 Gleason 4 + 5:1
Baseline PSA (median, IQR)	1.13 ng/mL (IQR 0.4–2.3)
Baseline NCCN risk category	Low: 0 (0) Intermediate: 6 (32%) High: 13 (68%)

Note: Nx is defined as no lymph nodes removed.

Overall, complete biochemical response and biochemical response were detected after 3 months in five (26.3%) and eleven (58%) of cases, respectively. One biochemical relapse at first evaluation has been registered and the patient started ADT; seven patients had stable PSA if compared to baseline and continued observation. A PSA reduction was detected in 17 patients, with a median PSA drop (defined as difference between PSA at baseline and PSA after 3 months from treatment) of 0.53 ng/mL (IQR 0.17–1.59) (Figure 2). None of the patients reported GI or GU symptoms at baseline (after surgery and before SSRT). Adverse events were recorded in two patients, one patient reported G2 GI and G1 GU toxicity, and G2 GU and GI toxicity were reported in another case.

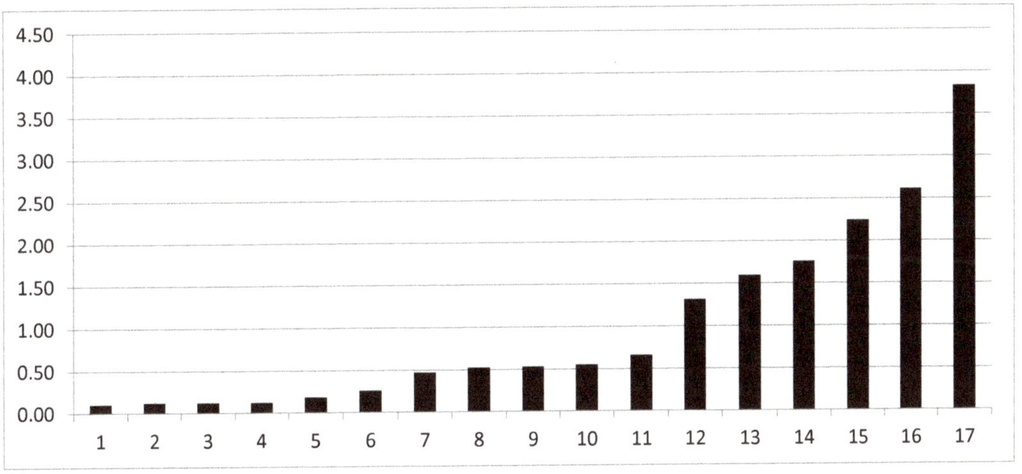

Figure 2. PSA drop for the 17 patients reporting any reduction in PSA. On the vertical axis, absolute values of PSA in ng/mL are reported.

4. Discussion

4.1. Clinical Outcomes

In the current analysis, promising biochemical results after SSRT in patients affected by macroscopic recurrence were evidenced, with a favorable toxicity profile. Biochemical response was reported in more than half of patients, and 26% of them reached a complete biochemical response within 3 months of treatment. These promising results in terms of biochemical outcomes, despite the unfavorable prognostic impact of macroscopic disease within the prostate bed [3], may have been related to the possibility of a dose escalated treatment. Indeed, considering an alpha/beta ratio for prostate cancer of 1.5 or 3 Gy [12], the dose fractionation schedule in the used STARR trial would correspond to a 2 Gy equivalent dose (EQD2) of 85 or 70 Gy, respectively, which is considerably higher if compared to a standard conventional postoperative treatment delivering 64–66 Gy [2].

4.2. ADT Administration

ADT was not allowed by protocol, meaning that biochemical outcome was related to local treatment alone. Of course, some clinicians may feel that short course concomitant ADT should be performed in a similar scenario. However, trials suggesting benefits of concomitant administration of ADT in this setting (e.g., GETUG AFU 16 or RTOG 9601 [13,14]) were conducted in patients in whom metabolic imaging was not performed before salvage treatment, suggesting that part of the benefit could be related to the spatial cooperation between local and systemic treatment. In our opinion, the use of local treatment alone would be justified in a prospective trial conducted on patients with a more precise staging aimed to exclude subclinical disease outside the prostate bed. However, the majority of patients (74%) were affected by disease with ISUP scores ≤ 3, and the likelihood of subclinical microscopic disease is lower in a similar population if compared to Gleason 8 or higher prostate cancer. For this reason, escalation in terms of local treatment might have been effective even in the absence of concomitant ADT administration.

4.3. Current Status of PET-Directed sRT

Tailoring the treatment volume on the basis of PET/CT and MRI allowed a reduction of the overall treatment volume and the profitably spare organs at risk. Interestingly, no data about regional, distant or local relapse detection rate with PSMA or Choline imaging are available from this series, because patients with regional or metastatic disease were excluded from the trial and screening failure procedures were not recorded. Insights about these issues may be related to early PSMA detection results reported within a parallel project running in our center (PSICHE trial, NCT05022914). Of note, further reduction in terms of acute toxicity may be related to the use of the Cyberknife[R] robotic stereotactic technique, as suggested by a post hoc analysis of a PACE-B trial [15]. Thus, SSRT may have the potential to increase the benefit-to-risk ratio in the complex scenario of postoperative recurrence. Nevertheless, salvage radiotherapy is currently a debated issue, especially regarding correct prognostic stratification and the addition of concomitant ADT [14,16]. However, many of the pivotal trials published in this scenario were conducted on conventional imaging only, while recent evidence confirmed the significant impact that sensitive imaging methods may have on postoperative management. The availability of modern imaging and RT techniques allows the precise identification of the site and extension of disease, prompting the development of treatment strategies aimed at maximizing clinical outcomes. The EMPIRE-1 trial was a single center phase 2/3 trial including patients with a detectable PSA after RP, randomized to receive conventional imaging alone or with 18F-fluciclovine-PET/CT. In the experimental group, radiotherapy management and target delineation were determined by PET findings. The trial enrolled 165 patients, and results showed a significant advantage for patients undergoing next generation imaging in terms of three-year event free survival (75.5% vs. 63%, $p = 0.002$), and a similar toxicity in both study groups. Authors concluded that next generation imaging significantly improved survival free from biochemical recurrence or persistence, and that a novel PET radiotracer should be integrated into radiotherapy decisions [17]. Of note, the EMPIRE-1 trial did not included stereotactic radiotherapy within a pre-determined management algorithm, while other ongoing trials (e.g., PSICHE trial, NCT05022914) are currently implementing such treatment strategy within a PSMA guided framework. Despite the emerging role of next generation imaging and stereotactic RT, no standardized approach for patients with pelvic macroscopic evidence of disease detected after a postoperative PSA rise currently exists, and various strategies have been proposed.

4.4. Dose-Escalated Radiotherapy in Salvage Setting and Comparison with Other SSRT Series

Dose-escalated conventional radiotherapy was proposed within various retrospective studies, reporting biochemical progression free survival ranging between 44 and 89% and late G3 GU or GI toxicity ranging between 2 and 7.3% [4,6,18–22]. SSRT has been proposed as an alternative in this scenario in one previous retrospective series of 90 patients, reporting an overall biochemical free survival rate of 72% after an average follow up of 21.2 months and no G > 2 adverse events reported [11]. However, that series included both patients treated with Cyberknife[R] robotic technique and with intensity modulated RT (IMRT) using the VERO[R] system, while the present analysis is based only on Cyberknife[R] treated patients. This makes a direct comparison difficult; still, it suggests that SSRT may be feasible as well with various RT techniques, expanding this treatment possibility to different facilities experienced in stereotactic radiotherapy. Of note, this approach was compared within a propensity score matched analysis with conventional salvage radiotherapy. In brief, data from 185 patients treated in seven Italian centers for macroscopic prostate bed recurrence were retrospectively collected. After propensity matching, 90 patients in the conventional and SSRT group were selected and compared (45 in each group). Results did not show any significant difference in terms of biochemical relapse free and progression free survival.

However, a lower rate of toxicity was evidenced for patients treated with SSRT, with acute GI and GU adverse events reported in 4.4 versus 44.4% ($p < 0.001$) and 28.9 versus 46.7% ($p = 0.08$) of patients, and late GI and GU adverse events reported in 0 versus 13.3% ($p = 0.04$) and 6.7 versus 22.2% ($p = 0.03$) of patients, respectively [8]. SSRT to prostate bed was tested, as well, in two prospective phase I trials [23,24]. These demonstrated the feasibility of dose escalation up to 35–45 Gy without dose limiting toxicity, confirming the good safety profile of ultrahypofractionated treatment for postoperative RT. Ballas et al. published a phase I dose escalation trial aiming to evaluate the maximum tolerated dose after increasing hypofractionation to the prostate bed. Authors tested three dose levels (3.6 Gy $\times$ 15 fractions, 4.7 Gy $\times$ 10 fractions and 7.1 Gy $\times$ 5 fractions) on a twenty-four patient cohort with at least 6 months of follow-up. Results showed that no G $\geq$ 3 GI or GU toxicity was seen at any dose level. Seven of twelve patients enrolled in the 7.1 Gy $\times$ 5 fractions cohort experienced a G2 GI toxicity during treatment, and one out of twelve patients of the same group had an increase to G1 and G2 GU toxicity in the two weeks after RT. Moreover, 71% of patients had a minimally important difference in terms of Expanded Prostate Cancer Index Composite score bowel domain at week 2 after treatment, while International Prostate Symptom Scores worsened two weeks after treatment but improved by six to ten weeks. Authors concluded that long-term follow up was needed after SBRT due to the transient G2 increase in rectal toxicity occurring during and immediately after radiotherapy [23]. Sampath et al. published another dose escalation trial including patients with organ-confined, node-negative prostate cancer who had biochemical failure after prostatectomy with a PSA $\leq$ 2 ng/mL. In their cohort, the dose escalation protocol provided treatment with 35 Gy, 40 Gy and 45 Gy in five fractions administered on alternate days. After the enrollment of 26 patients, the median follow up was 60, 48 and 33 months in the 35, 40 and 45 Gy cohort, respectively. Results reported that no acute dose limiting toxicity events were observed, while late G $\geq$ 2 and $\geq$ 3 GI toxicity was reported in 11% and 0%, respectively, and 38% and 15% of patients suffered late grade $\geq$ 2 and $\geq$ 3 GU toxicity, respectively. Interestingly, no increase in terms of late GU toxicity was reported when comparing the 45 Gy to the 40 Gy cohort, and the crude rate of complete biochemical response was 42% [24]. Authors concluded that the recommended dose for a phase 2 study should have been 40 Gy in five fractions, which is slightly higher than the dose proposed within the STARR trial. However, a comparison between these two studies and the STARR trial is difficult because both of them included all the prostate bed within treatment volume, and included patients affected by biochemical recurrence only. From a safety reporting view, only patients with prostate bed relapse were enrolled in the STARR trial, with the target including only macroscopic evidence of disease and a lower extent of treatment volumes. Thus, the rate of adverse events in those Phase I trials may be negatively affected by larger target volumes, and the prognosis of patients enrolled within the STARR trial could be considered different due to the presence of macroscopic recurrence within the prostate bed. Despite the extreme heterogeneity of treatment approaches proposed, some sort of treatment intensification for these patients appears to be beneficial, as evidenced by a multicentric retrospective experience published in 2022, the SPIDER 01 study [25]. In this series, authors collected data about 363 patients treated in 16 European centers for biochemical recurrence and prostate bed macroscopic relapse within the prostate bed proven by functional imaging. Patients were treated between January 2000 and December 2019 and divided into four groups according to the delivered treatment (dose escalation on macroscopic recurrence, dose escalation on prostate bed, dose escalation on prostate bed and macroscopic recurrence, no dose escalation). After a median follow-up of 53.6 months, five-year progression free survival and metastasis free survival were 70% and 83.7%, respectively, with rate of G $\geq$ 2 GU and GI late toxicity of 12 and 3%, respectively. Of note, results showed a five-year progression free survival benefit for all groups with any dose escalation > 72 Gy (72.8% vs. 60.3%, $p = 0.03$). Authors concluded that the integration of functional imaging in the salvage treatment approach is effective when macroscopic relapse is detected inside the prostate bed, and that dose escalation had a significant impact on progression free survival. Thus, treatment intensification for patients with macroscopic prostate bed recurrence appears justified. Another ongoing prospective trial (SHORTER, NCT04422132) is currently enrolling patients randomized to receive either moderate hypofractionation (55 Gy in 20 fractions) or SSRT (32.5 Gy in 5 fractions) to the prostate bed +/− pelvic nodes, aiming to compare the rate of GI and GU symptoms after the two treatment approaches. Of course, the inclusion of prophylactic pelvic volumes in a five-fractions salvage treatment strategy would be an interesting field of debate, given the necessity to correctly assess the risk-to-benefit ratio in this particular scenario.

4.5. Potential Advantages of SSRT

SSRT on macroscopic appears an attractive approach due to the limited number of fractions and the potential favorable risk-to-benefit ratio. Altered fractionation (e.g., moderate hypofractionation) is already shown to be effective and feasible within this setting [26], but prospective evidence about more extreme fractionations (e.g., >5 Gy per fraction) is eagerly awaited. Of course, the postoperative management of prostate cancer in the era of next generation imaging is a complex issue, especially when pelvic disease has been detected. Different approaches exploiting the current advances in radiation therapy have been proposed [27], and real-world data confirmed that no increased or unexpected toxicity were detected after the use of hypofractionated regimens in this scenario [28]. Stereotactic radiotherapy constitutes a tailored approach aimed to treat macroscopic evidence of disease, avoiding wide prophylactic treatment volumes, and many prospective trials are currently testing this treatment strategy in different settings of prostate cancer treatment [29]. Furthermore, salvage radiotherapy guided by imaging has been shown to be effective in clinical practice [30]. The STARR trial (NCT05455736) is focused on implementing stereotactic radiotherapy in a well-selected cohort of patients affected by macroscopic prostate bed relapse. If the promising data reported in this early work are confirmed in a complete cohort, SSRT may represent an interesting treatment option allowing the performance of an effective salvage treatment in a low number of fractions. This could be particularly beneficial for patients' quality of life (one of the secondary endpoints of the STARR trial) and facilities' waiting lists. Moreover, longer treatments may be unhelpful in special situations, when hospital admittance is problematic (e.g., pandemics) [31]. Of note, concomitant ADT was not provided within the STARR trial, and biochemical outcomes in this early cohort are exclusively related to SSRT effect. This allows a reliance on clinical benefit from the curative local treatment, but spatial cooperation with ADT may improve the benefit in selected patients with adverse prognostic factors. The attitude of clinicians towards ADT is often heterogeneous [32], especially in a postoperative setting, and its benefit when SSRT is provided will be an interesting matter of debate.

5. Conclusions

Early results from the first cohort of patients enrolled within the STARR trial (NCT05455736) show promising biochemical outcomes and a favorable toxicity profile. Once completed, the STARR trial could constitute one of the first prospective pieces of evidence about treatment tailoring and intensification for patients affected by postsurgical relapse and macroscopic evidence of disease within the prostate bed. After the advent of modern RT techniques, and supported by the literature data, hypofractionation in the postoperative scenario is currently the mainstay approach for different pathologies (e.g., breast cancer) [33,34], and we advocate for the implementation of similar treatment strategies in prostate cancer. SSRT may represent a paradigm for the integration of novel imaging methods and modern RT techniques in routine clinical practice.

Author Contributions: Conceptualization, G.F. (Giulio Francolini) and P.G.; tables and figures preparation, V.D.C., B.D. and M.L.; manuscript drafting, S.S., C.M., I.D. and L.L.; medical writing, D.G. and G.S.; data collecting, I.M., I.B., A.G.A., G.F. (Giulio Frosini), M.G., M.G.C., V.S., E.O., L.V., C.B., M.V., C.M. and M.R. All authors have read and agreed to the published version of the manuscript.

Funding: This research received no external funding.

Institutional Review Board Statement: The study was conducted in accordance with the Declaration of Helsinki and approved by the Institutional Review Board (or Ethics Committee) of Area Vasta centro (protocol code 17086_oss and date of approval 9 March 2021).

Informed Consent Statement: Informed consent was obtained from all subjects involved in the study.

Data Availability Statement: The data presented in this study are available on request from the corresponding author. The data are not publicly available due to privacy policy.

Conflicts of Interest: The authors declare no conflict of interest.

References

1. Stensland, K.D.; Caram, M.V.; Burns, J.A.; Sparks, J.B.; Shin, C.; Zaslavsky, A.; Hollenbeck, B.K.; Tsodikov, A.; Skolarus, T.A. Recurrence, metastasis, and survival after radical prostatectomy in the era of advanced treatments. *J. Clin. Oncol.* **2022**, *40*, 5090. [CrossRef]
2. Vale, C.L.; Fisher, D.; Kneebone, A.; Parker, C.; Pearse, M.; Richaud, P.; Sargos, P.; Sydes, M.R.; Brawley, C.; Brihoum, M.; et al. Adjuvant or early salvage radiotherapy for the treatment of localised and locally advanced prostate cancer: A prospectively planned systematic review and meta-analysis of aggregate data. *Lancet* **2020**, *396*, 1422–1431. [CrossRef] [PubMed]
3. Emmett, L.; van Leeuwen, P.J.; Nandurkar, R.; Scheltema, M.J.; Cusick, T.; Hruby, G.; Kneebone, A.; Eade, T.; Fogarty, G.; Jagavkar, R. Treatment outcomesfrom 68Ga-PSMA PET/CT–informed salvage radiation treatment in menwith rising PSA after radical prostatectomy: Prognostic value of a negativePSMA PET. *J. Nucl. Med.* **2017**, *58*, 1972–1976. [CrossRef] [PubMed]
4. Shelan, M.; Odermatt, S.; Bojaxhiu, B.; Nguyen, D.P.; Thalmann, G.N.; Aebersold, D.M.; Pra, A.D. Disease Control with Delayed Salvage Radiotherapy for Macroscopic Local Recurrence Following Radical Prostatectomy. *Front. Oncol.* **2019**, *9*, 12. [CrossRef] [PubMed]
5. Tamihardja, J.; Zehner, L.; Hartrampf, P.E.; Cirsi, S.; Wegener, S.; Buck, A.K.; Flentje, M.; Polat, B. Dose-Escalated Salvage Radiotherapy for Macroscopic Local Recurrence of Prostate Cancer in the Prostate-Specific Membrane Antigen Positron Emission Tomography Era. *Cancers* **2022**, *14*, 4956. [CrossRef]
6. Mottet, N.; van den Bergh, R.C.N.; Briers, E.; Van den Broeck, T.; Cumberbatch, M.G.; De Santis, M.; Fanti, S.; Fossati, N.; Gandaglia, G.; Gillessen, S.; et al. EAU-EANM-ESTRO-ESUR-SIOG Guidelines on Prostate Cancer-2020 Update. Part 1: Screening, Diagnosis, and Local Treatment with Curative Intent. *Eur. Urol.* **2021**, *79*, 243–262. [CrossRef]
7. Schröder, C.; Tang, H.; Windisch, P.; Zwahlen, D.R.; Buchali, A.; Vu, E.; Bostel, T.; Sprave, T.; Zilli, T.; Murthy, V.; et al. Stereotactic Radiotherapy after Radical Prostatectomy in Patients with Prostate Cancer in the Adjuvant or Salvage Setting: A Systematic Review. *Cancers* **2022**, *14*, 696. [CrossRef]
8. Francolini, G.; Jereczek-Fossa, B.A.; Di Cataldo, V.; Simontacchi, G.; Marvaso, G.; Gandini, S.; Corso, F.; Ciccone, L.P.; Zerella, M.A.; Gentile, P.; et al. Stereotactic or conventional radiotherapy for macroscopic prostate bed recurrence: A propensity score analysis. *La Radiol. Medica* **2022**, *127*, 449–457. [CrossRef]
9. Scher, H.I.; Morris, M.J.; Stadler, W.M.; Higano, C.; Basch, E.; Fizazi, K.; Antonarakis, E.S.; Beer, T.M.; Carducci, M.A.; Chi, K.N.; et al. Trial Design and Objectives for Castration-Resistant Prostate Cancer: Updated Recommendations from the Prostate Cancer Clinical Trials Working Group 3. *J. Clin. Oncol.* **2016**, *34*, 1402–1418. [CrossRef]
10. U.S. Department of Health and Human Services NIH, National Cancer Institute. Common Terminology Criteria for Adverse Events (CTCAE) Version 4.0. Available online: http://evs.nci.nih.gov/ftp1/CTCAE/CTCAE_4.03_2010-0614_QuickReference_5x7.pdf (accessed on 21 December 2022).
11. Francolini, G.; Jereczek-Fossa, B.A.; Di Cataldo, V.; Simontacchi, G.; Marvaso, G.; Zerella, M.A.; Gentile, P.; Bianciardi, F.; Allegretta, S.; Detti, B.; et al. Stereotactic radiotherapy for prostate bed recurrence after prostatectomy, a multicentric series. *BJU Int.* **2020**, *125*, 417–425. [CrossRef]
12. Hoskin, P.J.; Rojas, A.M.; Bownes, P.J.; Lowe, G.J.; Ostler, P.J.; Bryant, L. Randomised trial of external beam radiotherapy alone or combined with high-dose-rate brachytherapy boost for localised prostate cancer. *Radiother. Oncol.* **2012**, *103*, 217–222. [CrossRef] [PubMed]
13. Carrie, C.; Magné, N.; Burban-Provost, P.; Sargos, P.; Latorzeff, I.; Lagrange, J.-L.; Supiot, S.; Belkacemi, Y.; Peiffert, D.; Allouache, N.; et al. Short-term androgen deprivation therapy combined with radiotherapy as salvage treatment after radical prostatectomy for prostate cancer (GETUG-AFU 16): A 112-month follow-up of a phase 3, randomised trial. *Lancet Oncol.* **2019**, *20*, 1740–1749. [CrossRef]
14. Shipley, W.U.; Seiferheld, W.; Lukka, H.R.; Major, P.P.; Heney, N.M.; Grignon, D.J.; Sartor, O.; Patel, M.P.; Bahary, J.-P.; Zietman, A.L.; et al. Radiation with or without Antiandrogen Therapy in Recurrent Prostate Cancer. *N. Engl. J. Med.* **2017**, *376*, 417–428. [CrossRef]
15. Tree, A.C.; Ostler, P.; van der Voet, H.; Chu, W.; Loblaw, A.; Ford, D.; Tolan, S.; Jain, S.; Martin, A.; Staffurth, J.; et al. Intensity-modulated radiotherapy versus stereotactic body radiotherapy for prostate cancer (PACE-B): 2-year toxicity results from an open-label, randomised, phase 3, non-inferiority trial. *Lancet Oncol.* **2022**, *23*, 1308–1320. [CrossRef]

16. Spratt, D.E. Evidence-based Risk Stratification to Guide Hormone Therapy Use with Salvage Radiation Therapy for Prostate Cancer. *Int. J. Radiat. Oncol.* **2018**, *102*, 556–560. [CrossRef]
17. Jani, A.B.; Schreibmann, E.; Goyal, S.; Halkar, R.; Hershatter, B.; Rossi, P.J.; Shelton, J.W.; Patel, P.R.; Xu, K.M.; Goodman, M.; et al. 18F-fluciclovine-PET/CT imaging versus conventional imaging alone to guide postprostatectomy salvage radiotherapy for prostate cancer (EMPIRE-1): A single centre, open-label, phase 2/3 randomised controlled trial. *Lancet* **2021**, *397*, 1895–1904. [CrossRef]
18. Bruni, A.; Ingrosso, G.; Trippa, F.; Di Staso, M.; Lanfranchi, B.; Rubino, L.; Parente, S.; Frassinelli, L.; Maranzano, E.; Santoni, R.; et al. Macroscopic locoregional relapse from prostate cancer: Which role for salvage radiotherapy? *Clin. Transl. Oncol.* **2019**, *21*, 1532–1537. [CrossRef]
19. Zaine, H.; Vandendorpe, B.; Bataille, B.; Lacornerie, T.; Wallet, J.; Mirabel, X.; Lartigau, E.; Pasquier, D. Salvage Radiotherapy for Macroscopic Local Recurrence Following Radical Prostatectomy. *Front. Oncol.* **2021**, *11*, 669261. [CrossRef]
20. Zilli, T.; Jorcano, S.; Peguret, N.; Caparrotti, F.; Hidalgo, A.; Khan, H.G.; Vees, H.; Miralbell, R. Results of Dose-adapted Salvage Radiotherapy After Radical Prostatectomy Based on an Endorectal MRI Target Definition Model. *Am. J. Clin. Oncol.* **2017**, *40*, 194–199. [CrossRef]
21. Lee, S.U.; Cho, K.H.; Kim, J.H.; Kim, Y.S.; Nam, T.-K.; Kim, J.-S.; Cho, J.; Choi, S.H.; Shim, S.J.; Chang, A.R. Clinical Outcome of Salvage Radiotherapy for Locoregional Clinical Recurrence After Radical Prostatectomy. *Technol. Cancer Res. Treat.* **2021**, *20*, 15330338211041212. [CrossRef]
22. Schmidt-Hegemann, N.S.; Stief, C.; Kim, T.H.; Eze, C.; Kirste, S.; Strouthos, I.; Li, M.; Schultze-Seemann, W.; Ilhan, H.; Fendler, W.P.; et al. Outcome after PSMA PET/CT based salvage radiotherapy in patients with biochemical recurrence after radical prostatectomy: A bi-institutional retrospective analysis. *J. Nucl. Med.* **2019**, *60*, 227–233. [CrossRef]
23. Ballas, L.K.; Luo, C.; Chung, E.; Kishan, A.U.; Shuryak, I.; Quinn, D.I.; Dorff, T.; Jhimlee, S.; Chiu, R.; Abreu, A.; et al. Phase 1 Trial of SBRT to the Prostate Fossa After Prostatectomy. *Int. J. Radiat. Oncol.* **2018**, *104*, 50–60. [CrossRef] [PubMed]
24. Sampath, S.; Frankel, P.; del Vecchio, B.; Ruel, N.; Yuh, B.; Liu, A.; Tsai, T.; Wong, J. Stereotactic Body Radiation Therapy to the Prostate Bed: Results of a Phase 1 Dose-Escalation Trial. *Int. J. Radiat. Oncol.* **2019**, *106*, 537–545. [CrossRef] [PubMed]
25. Benziane-Ouaritini, N.; Zilli, T.; Ingrosso, G.; di Staso, M.; Trippa, F.; Francolini, G.; Meyer, E.; Achard, V.; Schick, U.; Cosset, J.; et al. Salvage Radiotherapy Guided by Functional Imaging for Macroscopic Local Recurrence Following Radical Prostatectomy: A Multicentric Retrospective Study. *Int. J. Radiat. Oncol.* **2022**, *114*, S131–S132. [CrossRef]
26. Buyyounouski, M.; Pugh, S.; Chen, R.; Mann, M.; Kudchadker, R.; Konski, A.; Mian, O.; Michalski, J.; Vigneault, E.; Valicenti, R.; et al. Primary Endpoint Analysis of a Randomized Phase III Trial of Hypofractionated vs. Conventional Post-Prostatectomy Radiotherapy: NRG Oncology GU003. *Int. J. Radiat. Oncol.* **2021**, *111*, S2–S3. [CrossRef]
27. Francolini, G.; Stocchi, G.; Detti, B.; Di Cataldo, V.; Bruni, A.; Triggiani, L.; Guerini, A.E.; Mazzola, R.; Cuccia, F.; Mariotti, M.; et al. Dose-escalated pelvic radiotherapy for prostate cancer in definitive or postoperative setting. *La Radiol. Medica* **2021**, *127*, 206–213. [CrossRef]
28. Nicosia, L.; Mazzola, R.; Vitale, C.; Cuccia, F.; Figlia, V.; Giaj-Levra, N.; Ricchetti, F.; Rigo, M.; Ruggeri, R.; Cavalleri, S.; et al. Postoperative moderately hypofractionated radiotherapy in prostate cancer: A mono-institutional propensity-score-matching analysis between adjuvant and early-salvage radiotherapy. *La Radiol. Medica* **2022**, *127*, 560–570. [CrossRef]
29. Francolini, G.; Detti, B.; Di Cataldo, V.; Garlatti, P.; Aquilano, M.; Allegra, A.; Lucidi, S.; Cerbai, C.; Ciccone, L.P.; Salvestrini, V.; et al. Study protocol and preliminary results from a mono-centric cohort within a trial testing stereotactic body radiotherapy and abiraterone (ARTO-NCT03449719). *La Radiol. Medica* **2022**, *127*, 912–918. [CrossRef]
30. D'Angelillo, R.M.; Fiore, M.; Trodella, L.E.; Sciuto, R.; Ippolito, E.; Carnevale, A.; Iurato, A.; Miele, M.; Trecca, P.; Trodella, L.; et al. 18F-choline PET/CT driven salvage radiotherapy in prostate cancer patients: Up-date analysis with 5-year median follow-up. *La Radiol. Medica* **2020**, *125*, 668–673. [CrossRef]
31. Barra, S.; Guarnieri, A.; di Monale EBastia, M.B.; Marcenaro, M.; Tornari, E.; Belgioia, L.; Magrini, S.M.; Ricardi, U.; Corvò, R. Short fractionation radiotherapy for early prostate cancer in the time of COVID-19: Long-term excellent outcomes from a multicenter Italian trial suggest a larger adoption in clinical practice. *Radiol. Med.* **2021**, *126*, 142–146. [CrossRef]
32. Fersino, S.; Borghesi, S.; Jereczek-Fossa, B.A.; Arcangeli, S.; Mortellaro, G.; Magrini, S.M.; Alongi, F. Uro-Oncology study group of Italian association of Radiotherapy and Clinical Oncology (AIRO) PROACTA: A survey on the actual attitude of the Italian radiation oncologists in the management and prescription of hormonal therapy in prostate cancer patients. *La Radiol. Medica* **2020**, *126*, 460–465. [CrossRef]
33. Meattini, I.; Palumbo, I.; Becherini, C.; Borghesi, S.; Cucciarelli, F.; Dicuonzo, S.; Fiorentino, A.; Spoto, R.; Poortmans, P.; Aristei, C.; et al. The Italian Association for Radiotherapy and Clinical Oncology (AIRO) position statements for postoperative breast cancer radiation therapy volume, dose, and fractionation. *La Radiol. Medica* **2022**, *127*, 1407–1411. [CrossRef]
34. Gregucci, F.; Fozza, A.; Falivene, S.; Smaniotto, D.; Morra, A.; Daidone, A.; Barbara, R.; Ciabattoni, A. Present clinical practice of breast cancer radiotherapy in Italy: A nationwide survey by the Italian Society of Radiotherapy and Clinical Oncology (AIRO) Breast Group. *La Radiol. Medica* **2020**, *125*, 674–682. [CrossRef]

cancers

MDPI

Article

Disruption of CCL2 in Mesenchymal Stem Cells as an Anti-Tumor Approach against Prostate Cancer

Quoc Thang Bui [1], Kuan-Der Lee [1,2], Yu-Ching Fan [3], Branwen S. Lewis [4], Lih-Wen Deng [5,6,7] and Yuan-Chin Tsai [4,8,*]

1 International Ph.D. Program for Cell Therapy and Regeneration Medicine (IPCTRM), College of Medicine, Taipei Medical University, Taipei 110301, Taiwan
2 Department of Medical Research, Taichung Veterans General Hospital, Taichung 407219, Taiwan
3 Ph.D. Program for Cancer Molecular Biology and Drug Discovery, College of Medical Science and Technology, Taipei Medical University and Academia Sinica, Taipei 110301, Taiwan
4 Graduate Institute of Cancer Biology and Drug Discovery, College of Medical Science and Technology, Taipei Medical University, Taipei 110301, Taiwan
5 Department of Biochemistry, Yong Loo Lin School of Medicine, National University of Singapore, MD 7, 8 Medical Drive, Singapore 117596, Singapore
6 NUS Center for Cancer Research, Yong Loo Lin School of Medicine, National University of Singapore, 14 Medical Drive, Singapore 117599, Singapore
7 National University Cancer Institute, National University Health System, 5 Lower Kent Ridge Road, Singapore 119074, Singapore
8 Ph.D. Program for Cancer Molecular Biology and Drug Discovery, College of Medical Science and Technology, Taipei Medical University, Taipei 110301, Taiwan
* Correspondence: yuanchin@tmu.edu.tw

Simple Summary: Cancer cells and mesenchymal stem cells (MSCs) secrete C-C motif chemokine ligand 2 (CCL2), a small protein that attracts tumor-associated macrophages (TAMs), which promotes malignant progression, such as drug resistance and metastasis. In addition, MSCs can also be recruited by CCL2; thus, a local milieu consisting of tumor cells, MSCs, and TAMs can promote tumor progression via a CCL2-dependent paracrine. The aim of the current study was to examine the functions of endogenous CCL2 of MSCs in cancer biology. Using a genetic engineering technique, we blocked the CCL2 expression in murine bone marrow-derived MSCs (CCL2 KO MSCs) and analyzed the effects on cancer progression. We found that CCL2 KO MSCs showed anti-tumor function when injected with murine prostate cancer cells into mice. The inhibitory effect was associated with an increase of $CD45^+CD11b^+$ mononuclear myeloid cells in tumors.

Abstract: Background: MSCs are known to secrete abundant CCL2, which plays a crucial role in recruiting TAMs, promoting tumor progression. It is important to know whether disrupting MSC-derived CCL2 affects tumor growth. Methods: Murine bone marrow-derived MSCs were characterized by their surface markers and differentiation abilities. Proliferation and migration assays were performed in order to evaluate the functions of MSCs on cancer cells. CCL2 expression in MSCs was reduced by small interfering RNA (siRNA) or completely disrupted by CRISPR/Cas9 knockout (KO) approaches. An immune-competent syngeneic murine model of prostate cancer was applied in order to assess the role of tumor cell- and MSC-derived CCL2. The tumor microenvironment was analyzed to monitor the immune profile. Results: We confirmed that tumor cell-derived CCL2 was crucial for tumor growth and MSCs migration. CCL2 KO MSCs inhibited the migration of the monocyte/macrophage but not the proliferation of tumor cells in vitro. However, the mice co-injected with tumor cells and CCL2 KO MSCs exhibited anti-tumor effects when compared with those given tumor cell alone and with control MSCs, partly due to increased infiltration of $CD45^+CD11b^+Ly6G^-$ mononuclear myeloid cells. Conclusions: Disruption of MSC-derived CCL2 enhances anti-tumor functions in an immune-competent syngeneic mouse model for prostate cancer.

Keywords: CCL2; mesenchymal stem cells; tumor associated macrophages; tumor microenvironment; $CD11b^+Ly6G^-$

Citation: Bui, Q.T.; Lee, K.-D.; Fan, Y.-C.; Lewis, B.S.; Deng, L.-W.; Tsai, Y.-C. Disruption of CCL2 in Mesenchymal Stem Cells as an Anti-Tumor Approach against Prostate Cancer. *Cancers* **2023**, *15*, 441. https://doi.org/10.3390/cancers15020441

Academic Editor: Kouji Izumi

Received: 8 December 2022
Revised: 4 January 2023
Accepted: 6 January 2023
Published: 10 January 2023

1. Introduction

The androgen receptor (AR) plays a key role in the progression of prostate cancer, and androgen-deprivation therapy (ADT) is the first line of treatment against advanced metastatic prostate cancer after surgery of the primary site [1]. While ADT exhibits high efficacy against androgen-sensitive tumor cells at the beginning, patients eventually develop metastatic castration-resistant prostate cancer (CRPC) [2]. At this stage, many tumors have acquired mutations that overcome the castrated level of testosterone (e.g., amplification of AR gene or autogenic induction of androgen) [3,4]. Therefore, targeting AR function remains the mainstay of therapeutic approaches to CRPC [5].

Many molecular mechanisms underlying castration resistance or androgen independence have been identified in CRPC cells [6]; however, other factors in the complex tumor microenvironment (TME) also contribute to malignant progression. TAMs are capable of switching the functions of some AR antagonists from suppression to activation [7], and M2-polarized macrophages are associated with immunosuppression and poor survival rate [8]. Although several chemokines are capable of recruiting TAMs to the TME [9], the chemoattractant C-C motif ligand 2 (CCL2), alias MCP1, is the key factor and is known to be induced in prostate cancer in response to AR inhibition [10,11]. In addition to TAMs, MSCs can promote CRPC progression and metastasis by converting to cancer-associated fibroblasts [12,13]. Importantly, MSCs also secrete CCL2 [14,15]. MSC-derived CCL2 contributes to cancer progression not only by attracting TAMs but also by facilitating their M2-polarization [16]. Since tumor-derived CCL2 also recruits MSCs to the TME [17], an established CCL2 paracrine among tumor cells, MSCs, and TAMs in TME can support malignant progression.

Increased serum CCL2 has been demonstrated as a promising biomarker in diagnosis and prognosis [18–20]. Targeting CCL2 using its neutralizing antibody has been successful in mouse xenograft models in preventing prostate cancer metastasis [21,22]; however, it was reported that accelerated relapse and metastasis may occur once the antibody administration is interrupted [23]. Since CCL2-neutralizing antibodies inhibit not only TAMs but also all the normal monocyte/macrophages in the body (e.g., bone marrow), which contributes to systemic side effects, we thought to utilize the tumor-homing ability of MSCs [13] and to develop a genetically-engineered cellular therapy. We confirmed that tumor cell-derived CCL2 was crucial in regulating the migration activities of MSCs and in tumor growth using a syngeneic mouse prostate cancer model. The expression of endogenous CCL2 in MSCs was transiently inhibited by small interfering RNA (siRNA) or permanently by CRISPR/Cas9 KO. The role of CCL2-suppressed MSCs in cancer growth was examined by proliferation assays in vitro and a syngeneic mouse tumor model.

2. Materials and Methods

2.1. Cells and Conditioned Media Preparation

Mouse prostate cancer cell lines (TRAMP-C1, TRAMP-C2 and TRAMP-C3), mouse macrophages (RAW 264.7), and human monocytes (THP-1) were obtained from the American Type Culture Collection (ATCC, Manassas, VA, USA). Cells were maintained in the suggested culture medium according to the ATCC. Commercial mouse bone marrow-derived mesenchymal stem cells (BM/MSCs) were purchased from Cyagen (Santa Clara, CA, USA), and the cells were maintained following the manufacturer's guidelines. The preparation of primary BM/MSCs was modified from an established procedure [24]. In brief, the bone marrow cells of 8-week-old C57BL/6 mice were flushed out with Dulbecco's Modified Eagle's Medium supplemented with 100 U/mL penicillin/streptomycin and 10% fetal bovine serum (GIBCO, Grand Island, NY, USA). By washing with phosphate buffer saline (PBS) and filtering with 70 μm nylon mesh filter (Falcon Cell Strainers, Thermo Fisher Scientific, Waltham, MA, USA), cells were cultured in a 5% CO_2 incubator. Unbound cells were removed every 24 h for three consecutive days to enrich MSCs utilizing their plastic adherence property. The MSCs were further enriched from the flow through cells using an EasySep™ Mouse Mesenchymal Stem/Progenitor Cell Enrichment Kit (STEMCELL technologies, Vancouver, BC, Canada). An established procedure was modified in order to isolate MSCs in the TME [25]. In brief, MSCs in the TRAMP-C1-derived tumor-infiltrating leukocytes were isolated by the same Mouse Mesenchymal Stem/Progenitor Cell Enrichment Kit (STEMCELL Technologies). Culture media from the MSCs (ca. 80% confluence) were collected as conditioned media and stored at −80 °C.

Similar to the isolation of MSCs in the TME, an established procedure was modified in order to prepare the CD11b-positive ($CD11b^+$) cells [25]. In brief, $CD11b^+$ TRAMP-C1-derived tumor-infiltrating leukocytes were enriched by magnetic beads using the EasySep™ mouse CD11b-positive selection kit II (STEMCELL Technologies).

2.2. *In Vitro Cell Proliferation Analysis*

Colony assay was performed with 500 cells seeded into each well in 12-well plates which were incubated with either the conditioned media or complete media. After seven days of incubation, cells were fixed and stained with 0.2% crystal violet. The images of colonies were taken and analyzed by Image J using the ColonyArea plugin [26].

A colorimetric cell viability kit was used to determine cell proliferation in vitro. In brief, the cells were seeded in 96-well plates for 24 h followed by treatment with either the conditioned media, mouse IL-28α, or IL-28β (ProSpec, Rehovot, Israel) for 1–3 days. A CCK-8 solution (Sigma-Aldrich) was applied to each well and incubated for 1 h. The measurement was done by reading the absorbance at 450 nm on an Epoch Microplate Spectrophotometer (BioTek Instruments, Winooski, VT, USA).

2.3. *Western Blot Analysis*

Cell lysates were processed with 6× Laemmli sample buffer, followed by sodium dodecyl sulfate-polyacrylamide gel electrophoresis (SDS-PAGE). Samples were transferred onto the polyvinylidene difluoride (PVDF) membranes and blocked with 5% milk in TBST (Sigma-Aldrich, St. Louis, MO, USA). Western blotting was performed with specific antibodies at 4 °C overnight: anti-CD11b antibody (ABclonal, Woburn, MA, USA) and anti-GAPDH antibody (GeneTex, Irvne, CA, USA) (Supplementary Table S1). Membranes were washed with TBST twice and incubated with an HRP-labeled antibody at room temperature for 1 h. After incubation with an HRP substrate (Western Bright ECL HRP Substrate, Advansta, San Jose, CA, USA), images were taken with an Amersham™ Imager 600 (GE Healthcare, Chicago, IL, USA).

2.4. *Enzyme-Linked Immunosorbent Assay (ELISA)*

Mouse CCL2 (Quantikine ELISA Kit; R&D Systems, Minneapolis, MN, USA), and mouse Interleukin 1 Receptor Antagonist (IL1RA) ELISA Kit (MyBioSource, CA, USA) were used to detect specific cytokine secretion. The procedure was performed following the manufacturer's protocol. In brief, conditioned media (C.M.) were collected and stored at −80 °C until being measured. After incubation for 2 h at room temperature in 96-well ELISA plates, each well was washed and incubated with 100 μL of conjugate solution for 2 h. After washing, each well was incubated with 100 μL of substrate solution for 30 min, followed by the addition of 100 μL of stop solution. Measurements were made by reading the absorbance at 450 nm on an Epoch Microplate Spectrophotometer (BioTek Instruments, Winooski, VT, USA).

In order to analyze the cytokine/chemokine profile, the conditioned media of MSCs were collected and analyzed using a Proteome Profiler™ Array kit (R&D Systems) following the manufacturer's guidelines.

2.5. *Differentiation of MSCs and Staining Assays*

Osteoblast differentiation was assayed with 10,000 cells/cm^2 in a basal culture medium. At 80% cell confluence, cultured media were changed to an osteogenic induction medium consisting of DMEM (GIBCO, Grand Island, NY, USA) containing 10% FBS, 100 U/mL of penicillin, 100 mg/mL of streptomycin, 50 μg/mL of vitamin C, 10 nM dexamethasone, and

10 mM β-glycerol-phosphate (Sigma-Aldrich). The media were changed every 3–4 days during the culture. Cells were induced to osteoblast differentiation for 28 days. After fixing, cells were stained with 40mM Alizarin red S (Sigma-Aldrich), pH 4.2 at room temperature (RT) for 30 min, followed by washing with water. The images of calcium acceleration were taken and analyzed.

Adipocyte differentiation was assayed with 10,000 cells/cm^2 in a basal culture medium. At 80% cell confluence, cultured media were changed to an adipogenic induction medium consisting of DMEM supplemented with 10% FBS, 100 U/mL of penicillin, 100 mg/mL of streptomycin, 1 μM dexamethasone, 500 μM 1-methyl-3-isobutyl-xanthine (IBMX), 1 μM rosiglitazone, 100 μM indomethacin, and 5 μg/mL insulin (Sigma-Aldrich). The media were changed every 3–4 days during the culture. Cells were induced to adipocyte differentiation for 21 days. After fixing, cells were stained with 0.5% Oil red O solution (Sigma-Aldrich) for 60 min at RT, followed by washing with water. The images of lipid droplets were taken and analyzed.

2.6. Flow Cytometry Analysis

Monitoring of bone marrow-derived MSCs was performed by a Mouse Mesenchymal Stem Cell Multi-Color Flow Kit (R&D Systems, Minneapolis, MN, USA). Briefly, cells were stained with specific antibodies (anti CD29-PE, anti-Sca-1-APC, anti-CD45-PerCP) or isotype controls (anti-IgG2A-APC, anti-IgG2A-PE, anti-IgG2A-PerCP) in the dark at 4 °C for 45 min.

In order to investigate the profile of the tumor microenvironment, the tumors were isolated into single cells, blocked with FcR Blocking Reagent (Miltenyi Biotec, Gaithersburg, MD, USA), followed by staining with fluorescent dye–conjugated anti-CD45, anti-CD11b, and anti-Ly6G (Supplementary Table S2) in the dark at 4 °C for 30 min. The profiles were analyzed by Attune NxT Cytofluorimeter (Invitrogen, Carlsbad, CA, USA).

2.7. Generation of CCL2-KO Cell Lines and Conditioned Media Preparation

Guide (g)RNA targeting mouse CCL2 exons 1 (NM_011333.3) was generated based on the CRISPR/CRISPR-associated protein 9 (Cas9) editing technique. Mouse CCL2 gRNA sequences were selected from a CRISPR-designed website (https://chopchop.cbu.uib.no, accessed on 16 October 2018) and cloned into pSpCas9(BB)-2A-Puro (PX459) V2.0, a gift from Feng Zhang (Addgene plasmid # 62988) (Supplementary Table S3). Following transient transfection, MSCs or TRAMP-C2 cells were treated with puromycin (2.5 μg/mL) to select puromycin-resistant clones. CCL2-KO clones were confirmed by several approaches: ELISA for CCL2 secretion, DNA sequencing for mutation profiles, and a cytokine/chemokine analysis (Proteome Profiler Mouse Cytokine Array, R&D Systems). Genomic DNA isolated from KO clones was amplified by a polymerase chain reaction (PCR) using specific primers (Supplementary Table S4) to identify mutation sequence.

2.8. siRNA Knockdown of the il1rn & ccl2 Expression

MSCs were seeded into six-well plates at a density of 2 × 10^5 cells/well. When the cell reached ~80% confluence, small interfering RNA targeting CCL2 (Supplementary Table S5) or IL1RN (Sigma-Aldrich) was transfected into MSCs using RNAiMAX (Invitrogen). After 20 h, the medium was replaced with complete media. After two days of cultivation, the supernatants were collected and stored at −80 °C until use.

2.9. Migration Assay

Migration assays were performed in a Transwell Chamber with 8 μm pore size filters (BD Biosciences, Corning, NY, USA). A total of 2.5 × 10^4 cells were seeded in 1% FBS medium into the upper chamber and allowed to migrate/invade toward the bottom section containing either the conditioned or complete media for 24 h. Migrated cells were fixed, stained with 0.2% Crystal violet, and counted in 2–3 randomly chosen fields. For each condition, two replicate chambers were assayed. For THP-1, 2.5 × 10^4 cells were seeded into the upper chamber with 1% FBS and allowed to migrate through the bottom section for 6 h. The average number of migrated cells per field was calculated for each group.

2.10. Syngeneic Prostate Cancer Mouse Model

An animal experiment was performed in accordance with a protocol approved by the Taipei Medical University Animal Care and Use Committee (approval no.: LAC-2017-0274, Taipei, Taiwan). For tumor growth analysis, 10^6 TRAMP-C2 cells with or without 10^6 MSCs cells were subcutaneously injected into 8-week-old male C57BL/6 mice (NLAC, Taipei, Taiwan). Tumor sizes were quantified according to the formula: length (mm) $\times$ width $(mm)^2/2$, and mice were sacrificed to collect tumors at size ~900 (mm^3).

2.11. In Vitro Cytotoxicity Assay

In vitro cytotoxicity assay was performed with a cytotoxicity assay kit (CFSE, 7AAD) (Abcam, Cambridge, UK). Briefly, TRAMP-C2 was stained with CSFE at RT for 20 min before co-culturing with parental or CCL2 KO MSCs with a tumor-to-MSC ratio from 3:1 to 1:1. After two days of incubation, the staining dye 7AAD was added to stain all necrotic cells red by binding to the DNA of membrane-compromised cells. A positive control (dead cells) was performed by incubating the cells at 56 °C for 15 min, followed by staining with 7-AAD. The percentage of dead TRAMP-C2 cells (CSFE$^+$ 7AAD$^+$ population) was analyzed by Attune NxT Cytofluorimeter (Invitrogen, Carlsbad CA, USA).

2.12. Statistical Analysis

All data were presented as the mean $\pm$ standard deviation (SD). Differences between groups were analyzed by Student's *t*-test. Statistical calculations were performed with Prism analytical tools (GraphPad Software). A *p*-value of < 0.05 was considered significant.

3. Results

3.1. Inhibition of Tumor Growth by CCL2 Knockout (KO) in a Syngeneic Prostate Cancer Model

In order to study the role of CCL2 in a network consisting of tumor cells, MSCs, and TAMs in the TME, we disrupted the CCL2 gene in the transgenic adenocarcinoma of the mouse prostate (TRAMP)-C2 cell line [27]. We isolated three CCL2 knockout (KO) clones (KOA-KOC, Figure 1a) and confirmed the absence of CCL2 (Figure 1b). We also compared the cytokines/chemokines secreted into the conditioned media and confirmed again the loss of CCL2 expression (red box, Figure 1c). When we monitored the in vitro proliferation, all of the CCL2 KO clones showed increased rates compared to the control (Figure 1d). Many studies have shown the positive regulatory role of CCL2 in tumor growth; indeed, we also observed reduced proliferation in TRAMP-C1 following CCL2 knockdown by siRNA (Supplementary Figure S1). Therefore, the selected CCL2 KO clones may already bypass the CCL2-CCR2 signaling and even acquire mutations involved in mitogenic pathway, leading to enhanced proliferation in vitro. However, all of the KO clones failed to form tumors when subcutaneously injected into immune competent, syngeneic mice (Figure 1e). It was shown that mice deficient in CCL2 exhibited inhibitory effects to skin carcinogenesis [28], showing its role in maintaining the TME. Our results confirmed that tumor cell-derived CCL2 plays an essential role in the syngeneic prostate cancer model, possibly due to the recruitment of many immunosuppressive cells (e.g., TAMs).

3.2. Tumor Cell-Derived CCL2 Is Crucial in Recruiting Mesenchymal Stem Cells (MSCs)

By analyzing the cytokine/chemokine profiles of the tumor cell-derived TME using mouse Lewis lung cancer and transgenic adenocarcinoma of the mouse prostate cell lines, we demonstrated that a population deficient in cluster differentiation 11b (CD11b) contributed to the anti-inflammatory environment in the TME, partly via secretion of a natural anti-inflammatory cytokine, IL1RN, and promoted tumor cell proliferation [29]. Indeed, we observed again the promotional effect of the CD11b$^-$ population in the TME (Figure 2a,b). It was shown that MSCs were deficient in CD11b [30]; therefore, we analyzed the CD11b expression in primary MSCs derived from either the TME or bone marrow (BM) (Figure 2c). We confirmed that the ratio between CD11b and GAPDH drastically decreased in MSC-enriched populations (MSCs^{h} vs MSCs^{L}) both in the TME (0.5 vs. 2.0) and BM (0.4 vs. 1.5) (Figure 2c; Supplementary Figure S2). It was shown that the MSC-derived IL1RN plays an important role [31,32]. By monitoring the MSCs-derived C.M. collected on different days (D6, D12), we confirmed the secretion of IL1RN by MSCs (Figure 2d). In summary, our results suggest the recruitment of MSCs in the TME.

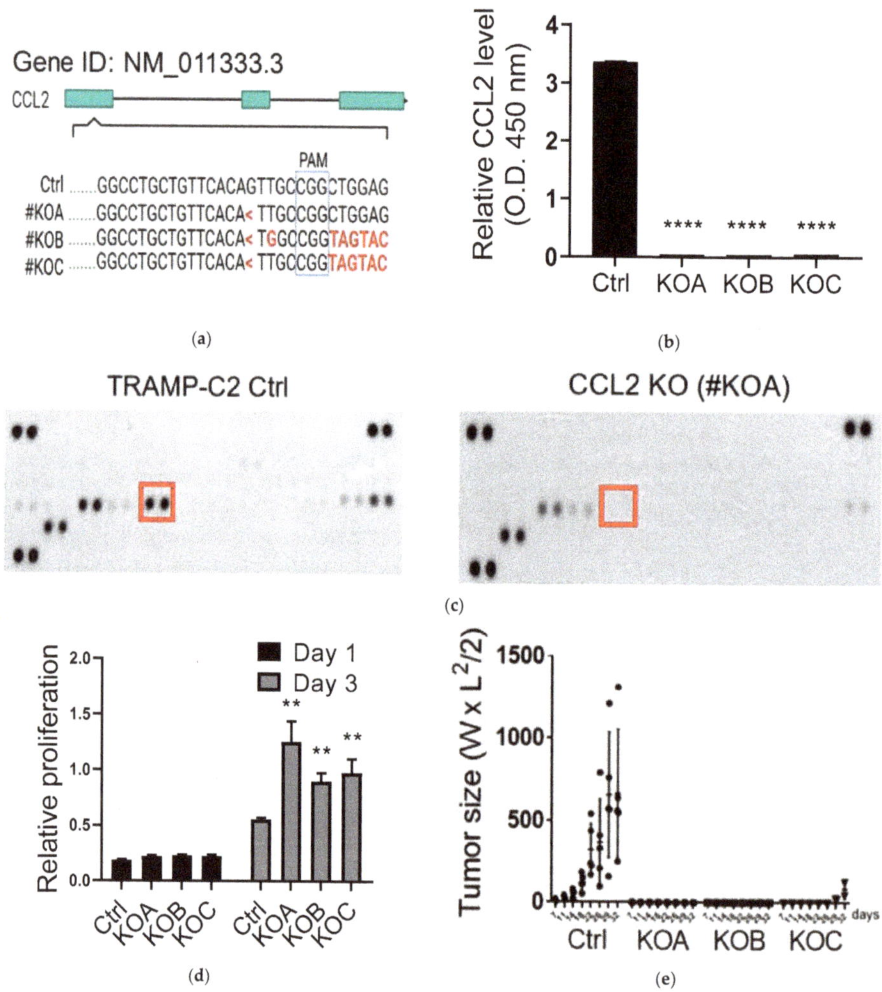

Figure 1. The requirement of tumor-derived CCL2 in tumor growth. (**a**) Establishment of CCL2 knockout (KO) in TRAMP-C2 cell line (Ctrl vs. KOA-KOC). PAM: the protospacer-adjacent motif. <: deletion; Red: mutation. (**b**) Comparison of CCL2 protein secretion in cell media (Ctrl vs. KOA-KOC) by ELISA. (**c**) Comparison of cytokine/chemokine profiles of TRAMP-C2 (Ctrl) and its CCL2 KO derivative (KOA); Red box: CCL2. (**d**) Comparison of cell proliferation rates in vitro among TRAMP-C2-derived clones (Ctrl vs. KOA-KOC); n = 6. (**e**) Comparison of tumor growth rates in vivo. Immune competent syngeneic mice (C57BL/6) were injected with different TRAMP-C2-derived clones (Ctrl/n = 5 vs. KOA-KOC/n = 3 each). Student's *t*-test. ** $p < 0.01$. **** $p < 0.0001$.

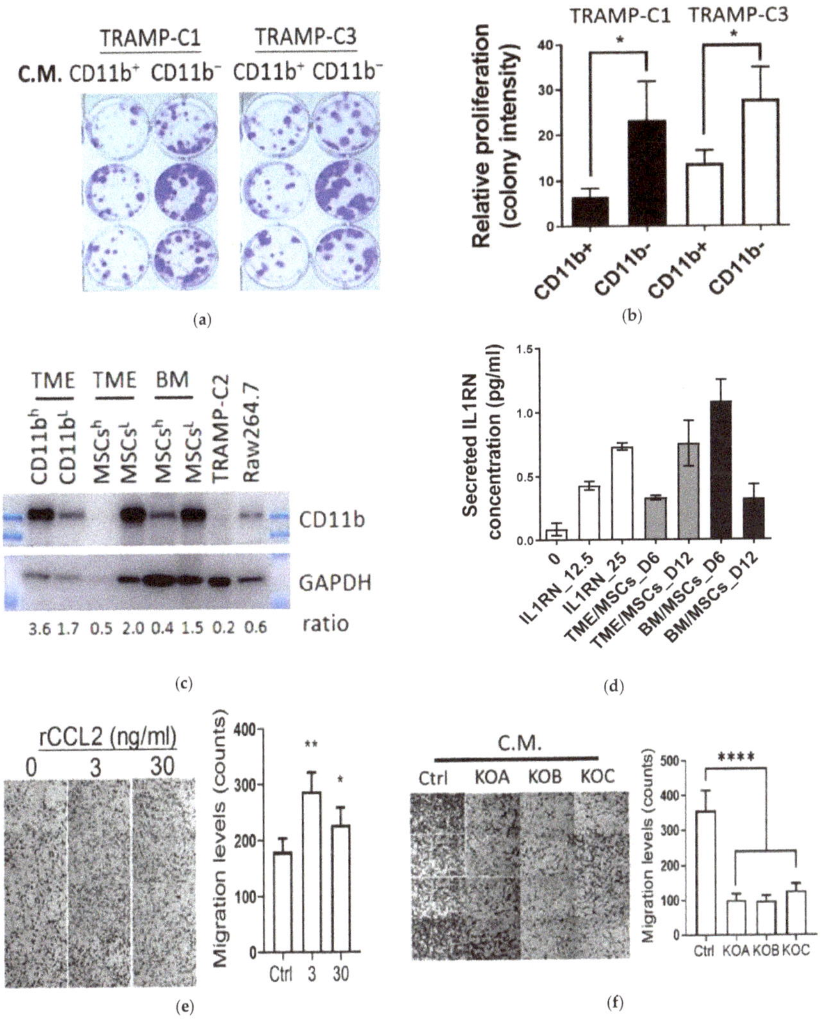

Figure 2. Tumor cell-derived CCL2 is involved in regulation of the migration activities of MSCs (**a**) Colony-formation assays using conditioned media (C.M.) collected from the CD11b$^+$ and CD11b$^-$ leukocytes in the TRAMP-C1-derived tumors. C.M. was applied to two mouse prostate cancer cells (TRAMP-C1 and TRAMP-C3). (**b**) Colony numbers were quantified and compared (right). n = 3. (**c**) Comparison of the CD11b expression of different cell populations by Western blotting assay. Single cell suspension collected from the TME or bone marrow (BM) was treated with either a CD11b or MSCs enrichment kit. CD11b^h and MSC^h: enriched populations. CD11b^L and MSC^L: non-enriched populations. Ratio: images were quantified and presented as CD11b/GAPDH. (**d**) Detection of IL1RN secretion in the conditioned media of MSC^h populations from the TME (TME/MSCs) and bone marrow (BM/MSCs). D6 and D12: condition media collected on day 6 (D6) and day 12 (D12). (**e**) Transwell analyses of BM/MSCs in response to different concentrations of recombinant CCL2 (rCCL2); n = 4. (**f**) Transwell analyses of BM/MSCs in response to different C.M. collected from TRAMP-C2-derived CCL2 KO clones (Ctrl vs. KOA–KOC); n = 4. Student's t-test. * $p < 0.05$. ** $p < 0.01$. **** $p < 0.0001$.

We hypothesized that the CCL2 paracrine in the TME establishes a network consisting of tumor cells, MSCs, and TAMs; consistently, it was suggested that breast cancer-derived CCL2 is involved in the homing effect of human MSCs [17]. Thus, we examined the role of tumor-derived CCL2 in regulating the migration activities of the MSCs. In order to secure the abundance and consistency of MSCs for further investigation, we used commercially available mouse bone marrow-derived MSCs and confirmed again their low expression of CD11b (Supplementary Figure S3). Consistently, using recombinant CCL2 protein enhanced the migration activities of MSCs (Figure 2e). Furthermore, the conditioned media collected from all the CCL2 KO TRAMP-C2 cell lines (KOA-KOC) showed significantly reduced migration activities of MSCs (Figure 2f). In summary, our results suggest that tumor cell-derived CCL2 is involved in the recruitment of MSCs to TME.

3.3. Inhibitory Effects of Condition Media Collected from the Bone Marrow-Enriched Mesenchymal Stem Cells (MSCs) with CCL2 Knockdown by Specific Small Interfering RNA (siRNA)

Although MSCs exhibit a tumor promotion function [12,13], it was shown that MSCs also exerted anti-proliferation effects on bone metastatic prostate cancer via an IL-28-mediated signaling pathway and contributed to the development of drug-resistant clones [33]. Thus, we asked whether endogenous IL1RN and CCL2 expressed in MSCs were involved in growth regulation. We utilized the MSCs from bone marrow and confirmed their properties in differentiation (Figure 3a) and surface marker expression (CD45^{-}Sca-1^{+}CD29^{+}, Figure 3b). After confirmation of the source of MSCs, the expression of endogenous IL1RN and CCL2 was reduced by the siRNA approach (Figure 3c), and the C.M. was collected for further analysis. We performed a colony assay in order to monitor the effects of C.M. in both TRAMP-C1 (Figure 3d) and TRAMP-C2 (Figure 3e). While we did not observe a significant reduction of proliferation using the C.M. from parental MSCs (med. vs. scr., Figure 3d,e), downregulation of IL1RN (siIL1RN) and CCL2 (siCCL2) showed enhanced anti-proliferation effects on both cell lines (Figure 3f). However, the inhibitory effects were not dependent on IL-28 as previously reported [33], since the cell line was not sensitive to either IL-28α or IL-28β recombinant protein (Figure 3g,h). In summary, our results suggest that disrupting MSC-derived IL1RN and CCL2 can enhance anti-proliferation effects.

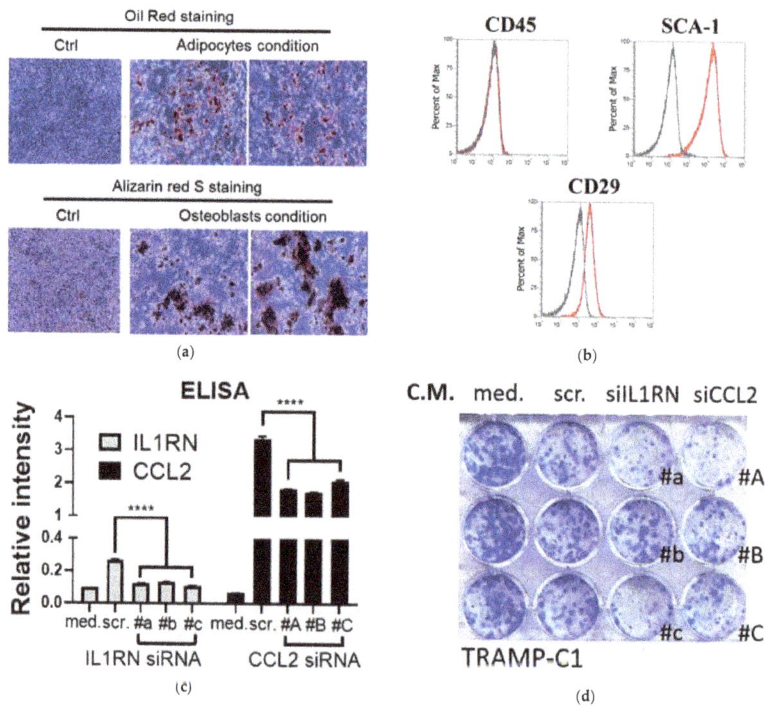

Figure 3. *Cont.*

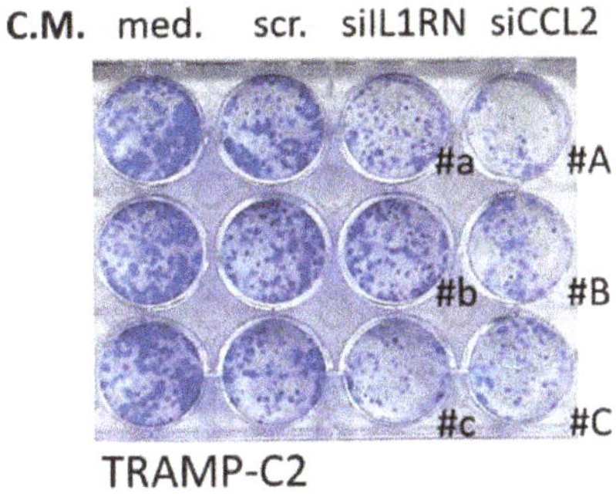

(e)

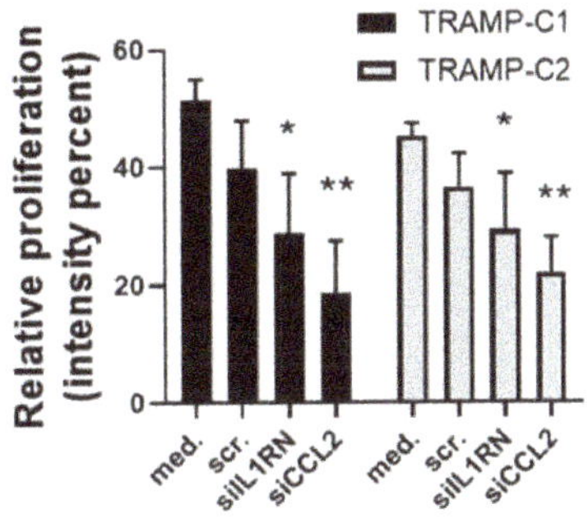

(f)

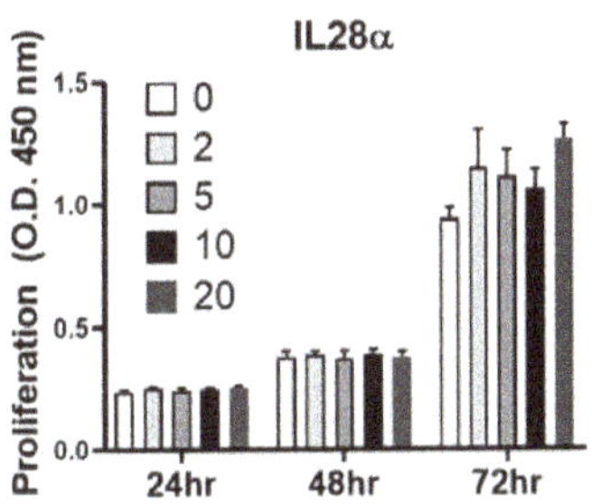

(g)

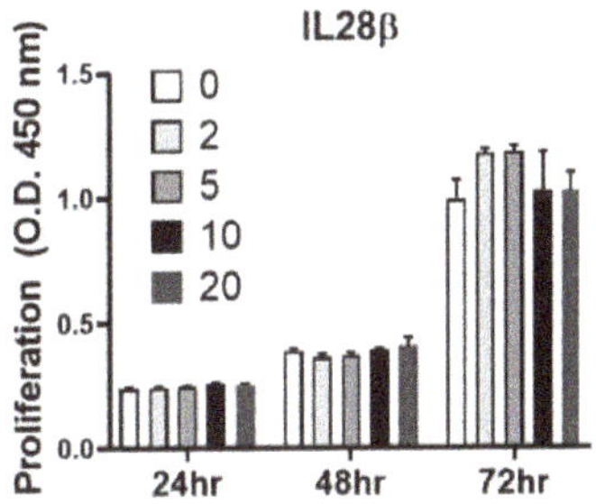

(h)

Figure 3. Anti-proliferation function of the conditioned media (C.M.) derived from the MSCs with knockdown of IL1RN and CCL2. (**a**) Differentiation of MSCs to adipocytes (oil red) and osteoblasts (Alizarin red S). MSCs without differentiation treatment serve as control (Ctrl). (**b**) Characterization of MSC markers using flow cytometry to detect several surface markers. Black: isotype antibody control. Red: specific antibody. (**c**) Confirmation of knockdown efficiency by measuring IL1RN and CCL2 protein secretion in the MSCs treated with respective siRNAs: siIL1RN (#a–#c) and siCCL2 (#A–#C). Protein secretion was measured by ELISA. (Ctrl vs. KOA-KOC) by ELISA; n = 3; med: fresh medium, scr: siRNA control. (**d**,**e**) Colony-formation assays using C.M. collected from the siRNA-treated MSCs in panel (**a**). C.M. was applied to TRAMP-C1 [panel (**d**)] and TRAMP-C2 [panel (**e**)]. (**f**) Colony numbers and staining intensities were quantified and compared; n = 3. (**g**,**h**) Proliferation analysis using TRAMP-C2 cell line in response to IL-28α [panel (**g**)] and IL-28β [panel (**h**)] recombinant proteins (ng/mL); n = 4. Student's *t*-test. * $p < 0.05$. ** $p < 0.01$. **** $p < 0.0001$.

3.4. Establishment of CCL2 Knockout (KO) in Mesenchymal Stem Cells (MSCs)

Many studies have aimed to apply MSCs as a therapeutic approach in clinics [34]; we hypothesized that genetically engineered MSCs with CCL2 KO can enhance the anti-proliferation activities against tumors. To test this idea, we utilized CRISPR/Cas9 system to disrupt the CCL2 gene in mouse bone marrow-enriched MSCs (#1-#2, Figure 4a). We confirmed the mutations of these KO clones (#1-#2, Figure 4a) and their lack of CCL2 expression by ELISA (Figure 4b). In addition, we collected the C.M. and tested their abilities to recruit monocytes using the THP-1 cell line. As shown in Figure 4c, the transwell activities were lost using the C.M. collected from the CCL2 KO clones. When we performed a differentiation assay, CCL2 KO in the MSCs did not affect their abilities to differentiate into either adipocytes or osteoblasts (Figure 4d).

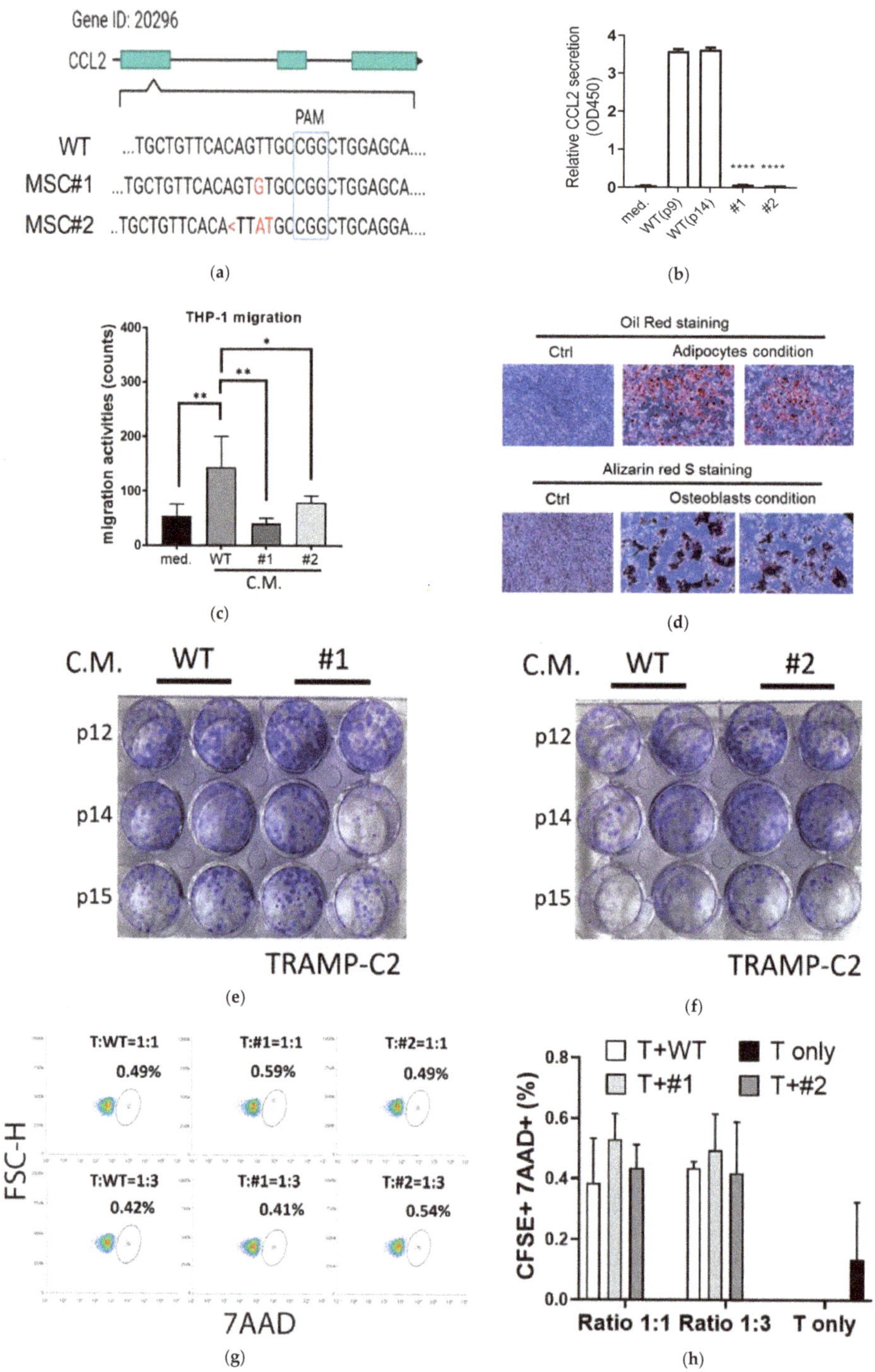

Figure 4. Lack of anti-proliferation function of MSCs in vitro. (**a**) Establishment of CCL2 knockout (KO) in bone marrow-derived MSCs. (WT vs. MSC#1-#2). PAM: the protospacer adjacent motif. <: deletion.

Red: mutation. (**b**) Comparison of CCL2 protein secretion in cell media by ELISA. Different passage numbers of MSCs (p9 and p14) were compared with CCL2-KO MSCs (#1 and #2). med: negative control of the fresh medium. (**c**) Transwell analyses of THP-1 cells in response to different conditioned media (C.M.) collected from MSCs (WT vs. #1-#2). n = 3. (**d**) Differentiation of CCL2-KO MSCs to adipocytes (oil red) and osteoblasts (Alizarin red S). MSCs without differentiation treatment serve as control (Ctrl). (**e**,**f**) Colony-formation assays using C.M. collected from the MSCs [panel (**e**): WT vs. #1; panel (**f**): WT vs. #2]. C.M. collected from different passage numbers (p12, p14, p15) was applied to TRAMP-C2; n = 2. (**g**) Co-culture assay using TRAMP-C2 cells (T) labeled with CFSE and then mixed with different MSCs (WT, #1, #2). After 48 h, the mixture was stained with 7AAD, and the CFSE$^+$7AAD$^+$ population was analyzed by flow cytometry. (**h**) Quantification of CFSE$^+$7AAD$^+$ population in TRAMP-C2 (T) collected from panel (**g**); n = 3. Student's *t*-test. * $p < 0.05$. ** $p < 0.01$. **** $p < 0.0001$.

Since the C.M. from CCL2 siRNA-treated MSCs showed enhanced anti-proliferation effects (Figure 3f), we further examined the functions of the CCL2 KO clones in proliferation. However, compared with parental MSCs (WT), we did not observe inhibitory effects using C.M. collected from several passages of the CCL2 KO clones (Figure 4e,f). This discrepancy may be due to adaption (e.g., crosstalk from other signaling pathways) or acquired mutations, replacing the need of CCL2 for CCR2 signaling in the CCL2 KO MSCs. Thus, we asked whether MSCs may trigger cytotoxic effects in tumor cells via direct cell-to-cell interaction. In order to address this issue, we performed a co-culture assay using TRAMP-C2 and the MSCs. The TRAMP-C2 cell line was labeled with a protein-conjugating dye (carboxyfluorescein diacetate succinimidyl ester, CFSE) and then mixed with MSCs. After incubation for 2 days, the percentage of dead cells in the CFSE$^+$ population was measured by using a DNA intercalating dye (7-aminoactinomycin D, 7AAD) (Figure 4g). Although we tested two different tumor-to-MSC ratios (1:1 and 1:3), the CFSE$^+$ 7AAD$^+$ percentages were very low and not statistically different from TRAMP-C2 (T) only in all the experimental settings (Figure 4h). In summary, our results show that the CCL2 KO MSCs do not induce anti-proliferation effects against TRAMP-C2 cells in vitro.

3.5. Enhanced Anti-Tumor Effects of the CCL2 KO MSCs in a Syngeneic Prostate Cancer Model

MSC-derived CCL2 is involved in the tumor-promoting functions of macrophages [16], and targeting CCL2 has been a therapeutic approach [21,22]. Although we did not observe the anti-proliferation effects of the CCL2 KO MSCs in vitro, we sought to examine their roles in the TME developed in an immune-competent syngeneic mouse prostate cancer model. We analyzed the profiles of secreted cytokine and confirmed again the lack of CCL2 in CCL2 KO MSCs clones (#1-#2, Figure 5a). Using a TRAMP-C2 cell line (TRAMP-C2/Luc-eGFP), expressing a fusion protein containing both an enhanced green fluorescent protein (EGFP) and luciferase (Luc), we found that the tumors co-injected with both CCL2 KO MSCs showed reduced growth rates compared with parental MSCs (T+WT vs. T+ #1/or #2, Supplementary Figure S4). However, mice injected with TRAMP-C2/Luc-eGFP cells only, without MSCs, did not show tumor formation either (tumor only, Supplementary Figure S4), which could be due to the anti-tumor immunogenic effects of the neo-antigens derived from both the EGFP and Luc genes. Therefore, we performed the animal study again using a parental TRAMP-C2 cell line without EGFP and Luc expression.

Surprisingly, compared with mice injected with parental TRAMP-C2 cells only, co-injection with either WT or CCL2 KO MSCs significantly reduced the tumor growth rates; however, the CCL2 KO (#1) exhibited enhanced inhibitory effects (Figure 5b). After we collected the tumors and measured their weights, only the tumor co-injected with CCL2 KO MSCs showed a reduction with statistical significance (T vs. T+#1, Figure 5c,d). Therefore, these results support that CCL2 KO MSCs exhibited enhanced anti-tumor functions. The distinct effects between in vitro (Figure 4) and in vivo (Figure 5) suggest that the MSCs established an anti-tumor microenvironment in the syngeneic tumor model. In order to address this issue, we analyzed the immune profile in the tumors and found a significant increase (~20%) of CD45$^+$CD11b$^+$Ly6G$^-$ populations (Figure 5e). Since CD45$^+$CD11b$^+$Ly6G$^-$

populations primarily contain monocytes and macrophages, our results suggest that the CCL2 KO MSCs promote anti-tumor responses via mononuclear myeloid cell-mediated pathways in the TME.

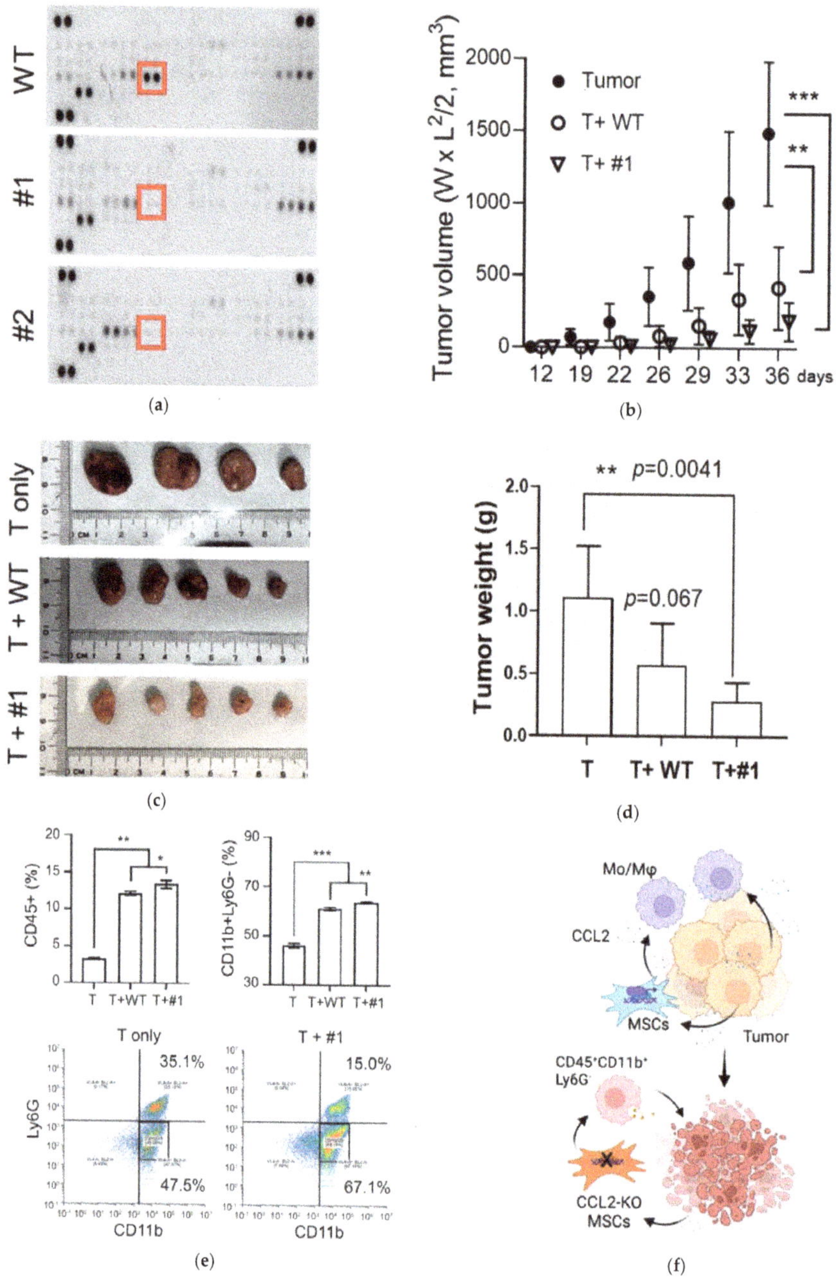

Figure 5. Enhanced anti-tumor effects of the CCL2 knockout (KO) MSCs in vivo. (**a**) Monitoring cytokine/chemokine profiles in C.M. collected from the MSCs (WT) and CCL2-KO MSCs (#1–#2). Red box: CCL2. (**b–d**) Comparison of tumor growth rates in vivo. Immune competent, syngeneic mi-

ce (C57BL/6) were co-injected with TRAMP-C2 (T) and MSCs (WT vs. #1). Time course of tumor size [panel (**b**)]. Images of the collected tumors from each group [panel (**c**)] and final tumor weights [panel (**d**)]. (**e**) Immune profile analysis of $CD11b^+LyG6^-$ populations in the tumor microenvironment. n = 3. (**f**) A working model. Prostate cancer and MSCs secret CCL2 to recruit monocyte/macrophage (Mo/Mφ). Using CCL2-KO MSCs to suppress tumor growth indireclty via $CD45^+CD11b^+Ly6G^-$ mediated functions. Student's *t*-test. * $p < 0.05$. ** $p < 0.01$. *** $p < 0.001$.

4. Discussion

The role of MSCs in prostate cancer remains unclear. While the malignant progression of prostate cancer was shown to be promoted by MSCs [12,13], it was also reported that MSCs can suppress growth via IL-28 mediated apoptosis [33]. Using C.M. collected from MSCs treated with siRNA targeting either IL1RN or CCL2, we also observed the inhibition of proliferation; however, the mechanism was not likely due to the IL-28 related pathway, since the tumor cells were not sensitive to exogenous IL-28 at high concentrations (Figure 3). Surprisingly, we did not observe a significant anti-proliferation effect when either the parental or CCL2 KO MSCs were co-cultured with tumor cells in vitro (Figure 4). It is possible that tumor cells are capable of compromising the anti-tumor functions of MSCs either by secreted cytokines or direct interactions; therefore, under the in vitro experimental setting as the co-culture assay, we only focused on the signaling between tumor cells and MSCs, recapitulating part of the communications in the tumor microenvironment. On the contrary, when the MSCs were co-injected with tumor cells in the immune competent syngeneic mice, the CCL2 KO MSCs indeed showed increased anti-tumor effects compared to wildtype MSCs (Figure 5d). Since MSCs do not express the CD45 marker, marked increase of $CD45^+$ and $CD45^+CD11b^+Ly6G^-$ mononuclear populations in the tumor microenvironment confirmed the immune modulating functions of MSCs.

Although both WT and CCL2 KO MSCs reduced tumor growth in mice injected with the parental TRAMP-C2, we suspected that the WT MSCs can be tumor-promoting in certain situations. In mice injected with the TRAMP-C2/Luc-eGFP cells, only co-injection of WT MSCs (T+WT) showed significant tumor growth, compared with those with CCL2 KO MSCs (T+#1 and T+#2) or no MSCs (Tumor only) (Supplementary Figure S4). Therefore, the anti-tumor mechanism against the TRAMP-C2/Luc-eGFP is different from that against the parental TRAMP-C2 in a syngeneic model. The anti-tumor immunity against TRAMP-C2/Luc-eGFP cells in the TME may be induced by the neo-antigens derived from Luc and EGFP foreign proteins, and only the WT MSCs can suppress this immunogenic environment leading to tumor growth. On the other hand, the parental TRAMP-C2 cell line is a selected clone from the TRAMP model [27], the anti-tumor effect observed in both WT and CCL2 KO MSCs was less likely to be due to immunogenic neo-antigens but rather to the elevated $CD45^+CD11b^+Ly6G^-$ mononuclear population (Figure 5d). Our earlier studies demonstrated tumor type-specific TME in syngeneic mice in that parental TRAMP-C1 cells established an anti-inflammatory TME while a lung cancer cell line resulted in an inflammatory one [25,29]. Similar to TRAMP-C1, the parental TRAMP-C2 may exhibit an anti-inflammatory TME that influences the functions of the MSCs (WT and CCL2 KO), supporting mononuclear population and anti-tumor effects. Since the CCL2 KO MSCs showed enhanced anti-tumor effects compared to WT MSCs in mice injected with either TRAMP-C2 or its derived TRAMP-C2/Luc-eGFP cells, we proposed a working model depicting the potential therapeutic benefit of this genetically engineered cell therapy (Figure 5f). Further investigation is required to address whether tumor cells exhibiting inflammatory TME exhibit distinct immune responses to WT and CCL2 MSCs.

Neutrophils ($CD45^+CD11b^+Ly6G^+$) occupy a high percentage of leukocytes in the TME; however, using the Ly6G marker, we showed that co-injection with MSCs reduced the neutrophil-to-mononuclear ratio in $CD11b^+$ myeloid cells. Thus, although neutrophils can exhibit anti-tumor function, our results suggested that the mononuclear $CD45^+CD11b^+Ly6G^-$ cells play an important role. The role of $CD11b^+$ myeloid cells in tumor biology is controversial. It was reported that using CD11b neutralizing antibodies can sensitize the therapeutic effect of radiation by reducing infiltration of myeloid cells [35]; however, using a CD11b-activating molecule was shown to suppress tumor growth via pro-inflammatory macrophages, likely M1-polarized macrophages [36]. Consistently, a negative association between CD11b signaling and M2-polarized macrophages was shown in that CD11b deletion in macrophages induced anti-inflammatory cytokines, and immune suppressive signals inhibited CD11b expression [36]. Since MSCs were shown to increase CD11b expression in dendritic cells [37], it is possible that MSCs can maintain and activate CD11b signaling in the $CD45^{+}CD11b^{+}Ly6G^{-}$ myeloid cells, promoting their anti-inflammatory functions. Furthermore, MSC-derived CCL2 and CXCL12 form a complex to induce M2-polarized macrophages, and disrupting CCL2 evidently obstructs this process [16]. Thus, delivering CCL2 KO MSCs into the TME may prevent immunosuppressing TAMs and facilitate the M1-polarized macrophages, promoting anti-tumor function. However, it is not clear how the mice co-injected with both tumor cells and MSCs exhibited a drastic increase (~20%) in $CD45^{+}CD11b^{+}Ly6^{-}$ population (Figure 5e). It is possible that abundant MSCs in the TME perturb the balance of different chemokines; consequently, it provides a unique niche favoring the recruitment or proliferation of $CD45^{+}CD11b^{+}Ly6^{-}$ population. It would be interesting to study the underlying mechanism in the future.

In addition to CCL2, the C.M. collected from MSCs with the downregulation of IL1RN by the siRNA approach exhibited anti-proliferation activity against the prostate cancer cells (Figure 3). Although we do not know the effect in vivo on the TME, it was reported that MSC-derived IL1RN promoted differentiation of M2 macrophages, similar to the role of CCL2 [32,38]. Additionally, IL1RN is known to be the key anti-inflammatory factor of both human and murine M2 macrophages, suppressing the IL-1-related pro-inflammatory functions [39]. Based on our previous studies, using the TRAMP-C1-derived tumors collected from immune-competent mice indeed exhibited an anti-inflammatory TME partly due to IL1RN induction [25]. The source of IL1RN in the TRAMP-C1-derived tumors was likely from both the MSCs and M2-macrophages, but not tumor cells per se [29]. Based on these results, it would be interesting to know whether delivering IL1RN KO MSCs also enhances anti-tumor effects. Further investigation is required to address this issue.

5. Conclusions

Genetically engineered MSCs with CCL2 knockout can enhance the anti-tumor effect in an immune-competent syngeneic mouse model of prostate cancer.

Supplementary Materials: The following supporting information can be downloaded at: https://www.mdpi.com/article/10.3390/cancers15020441/s1, Figure S1: Monitor CD11b expression. Figure S2: CD11b expression in MSCs. Figure S3: tumor growth rate using TRAMP-C2 expressing a luciferase-eGFP fusion protein. Figure S4: Comparison of tumor growth rates using TRAMP-C2/Luc-eGFP cell line. Table S1: Antibodies for Western blotting; Table S2: Antibodies for Flow cytometry; Table S3: Guide RNA (gRNA) sequences targeting the CCL2 genes; Table S4: Primers for sequencing CCL2 KO; Table S5: siRNA sequences targeting the CCL2.

Author Contributions: Conceptualization, Y.-C.T.; data curation, Q.T.B., K.-D.L. and Y.-C.F.; formal analysis, Q.T.B., K.-D.L., Y.-C.F., B.S.L. and L.-W.D.; investigation, Q.T.B., Y.-C.F. and Y.-C.T.; methodology, Y.-C.T.; project administration, Y.-C.T.; resources, K.-D.L.; supervision, Y.-C.T.; validation, Q.T.B. and Y.-C.F.; writing—original draft, Y.-C.T.; writing—review and editing, B.S.L., L.-W.D. and Y.-C.T. All authors have read and agreed to the published version of the manuscript.

Funding: This research was funded by the Ministry of Science and Technology of Taiwan, grant number 110-2314-B-038-135-MY3.

Institutional Review Board Statement: The study was conducted according to the guidelines of the Declaration of Helsinki and approved by the Institutional Animal Care and Use Committee or Panel (IACUC/IACUP) of Taipei Medical University (approval no.: LAC-2017-0274, Taipei, Taiwan).

Data Availability Statement: Data is contained within the article or supplementary material.

Acknowledgments: We appreciate the technical support of Yu-Cin Fong (BioGate Precision Medicine Corp, Taipei, Taiwan).

Conflicts of Interest: The authors declare no conflict of interest.

References

1. Leuprolide Study Group. Leuprolide versus diethylstilbestrol for metastatic prostate cancer. *N. Engl. J. Med.* **1984**, *311*, 1281–1286. [CrossRef]
2. Eisenberger, M.A.; Blumenstein, B.A.; Crawford, E.D.; Miller, G.; McLeod, D.G.; Loehrer, P.J.; Wilding, G.; Sears, K.; Culkin, D.J.; Thompson, I.M., Jr.; et al. Bilateral orchiectomy with or without flutamide for metastatic prostate cancer. *N. Engl. J. Med.* **1998**, *339*, 1036–1042. [CrossRef] [PubMed]
3. Linja, M.J.; Savinainen, K.J.; Saramaki, O.R.; Tammela, T.L.; Vessella, R.L.; Visakorpi, T. Amplification and overexpression of androgen receptor gene in hormone-refractory prostate cancer. *Cancer Res.* **2001**, *61*, 3550–3555. [PubMed]
4. Chang, K.H.; Li, R.; Papari-Zareei, M.; Watumull, L.; Zhao, Y.D.; Auchus, R.J.; Sharifi, N. Dihydrotestosterone synthesis bypasses testosterone to drive castration-resistant prostate cancer. *Proc. Natl. Acad. Sci. USA* **2011**, *108*, 13728–13733. [CrossRef] [PubMed]
5. Schrader, A.J.; Boegemann, M.; Ohlmann, C.H.; Schnoeller, T.J.; Krabbe, L.M.; Hajili, T.; Jentzmik, F.; Stoeckle, M.; Schrader, M.; Herrmann, E.; et al. Enzalutamide in castration-resistant prostate cancer patients progressing after docetaxel and abiraterone. *Eur. Urol.* **2014**, *65*, 30–36. [CrossRef]
6. Karantanos, T.; Corn, P.G.; Thompson, T.C. Prostate cancer progression after androgen deprivation therapy: Mechanisms of castrate resistance and novel therapeutic approaches. *Oncogene* **2013**, *32*, 5501–5511. [CrossRef]
7. Zhu, P.; Baek, S.H.; Bourk, E.M.; Ohgi, K.A.; Garcia-Bassets, I.; Sanjo, H.; Akira, S.; Kotol, P.F.; Glass, C.K.; Rosenfeld, M.G.; et al. Macrophage/cancer cell interactions mediate hormone resistance by a nuclear receptor derepression pathway. *Cell* **2006**, *124*, 615–629. [CrossRef]
8. Erlandsson, A.; Carlsson, J.; Lundholm, M.; Falt, A.; Andersson, S.O.; Andren, O.; Davidsson, S. M2 macrophages and regulatory T cells in lethal prostate cancer. *Prostate* **2019**, *79*, 363–369. [CrossRef]
9. Argyle, D.; Kitamura, T. Targeting Macrophage-Recruiting Chemokines as a Novel Therapeutic Strategy to Prevent the Progression of Solid Tumors. *Front. Immunol.* **2018**, *9*, 2629. [CrossRef]
10. Izumi, K.; Fang, L.Y.; Mizokami, A.; Namiki, M.; Li, L.; Lin, W.J.; Chang, C. Targeting the androgen receptor with siRNA promotes prostate cancer metastasis through enhanced macrophage recruitment via CCL2/CCR2-induced STAT3 activation. *EMBO Mol. Med.* **2013**, *5*, 1383–1401. [CrossRef]
11. Tsai, Y.C.; Chen, W.Y.; Abou-Kheir, W.; Zeng, T.; Yin, J.J.; Bahmad, H.; Lee, Y.C.; Liu, Y.N. Androgen deprivation therapy-induced epithelial-mesenchymal transition of prostate cancer through downregulating SPDEF and activating CCL2. *Biochim. Et Biophys. Acta* **2018**, *1864*, 1717–1727. [CrossRef] [PubMed]
12. Cheng, J.; Yang, K.; Zhang, Q.; Yu, Y.; Meng, Q.; Mo, N.; Zhou, Y.; Yi, X.; Ma, C.; Lei, A.; et al. The role of mesenchymal stem cells in promoting the transformation of androgen-dependent human prostate cancer cells into androgen-independent manner. *Sci. Rep.* **2016**, *6*, 16993. [CrossRef]
13. Jung, Y.; Kim, J.K.; Shiozawa, Y.; Wang, J.; Mishra, A.; Joseph, J.; Berry, J.E.; McGee, S.; Lee, E.; Sun, H.; et al. Recruitment of mesenchymal stem cells into prostate tumours promotes metastasis. *Nat. Commun.* **2013**, *4*, 1795. [CrossRef] [PubMed]
14. Whelan, D.S.; Caplice, N.M.; Clover, A.J.P. Mesenchymal stromal cell derived CCL2 is required for accelerated wound healing. *Sci. Rep.* **2020**, *10*, 2642. [CrossRef] [PubMed]
15. Boomsma, R.A.; Geenen, D.L. Mesenchymal stem cells secrete multiple cytokines that promote angiogenesis and have contrasting effects on chemotaxis and apoptosis. *PLoS ONE* **2012**, *7*, e35685. [CrossRef]
16. Giri, J.; Das, R.; Nylen, E.; Chinnadurai, R.; Galipeau, J. CCL2 and CXCL12 Derived from Mesenchymal Stromal Cells Cooperatively Polarize IL-10+ Tissue Macrophages to Mitigate Gut Injury. *Cell Rep.* **2020**, *30*, 1923–1934.e4. [CrossRef]
17. Dwyer, R.M.; Potter-Beirne, S.M.; Harrington, K.A.; Lowery, A.J.; Hennessy, E.; Murphy, J.M.; Barry, F.P.; O'Brien, T.; Kerin, M.J. Monocyte chemotactic protein-1 secreted by primary breast tumors stimulates migration of mesenchymal stem cells. *Clin. Cancer Res. Off. J. Am. Assoc. Cancer Res.* **2007**, *13*, 5020–5027. [CrossRef]
18. Izumi, K.; Mizokami, A.; Lin, H.P.; Ho, H.M.; Iwamoto, H.; Maolake, A.; Natsagdorj, A.; Kitagawa, Y.; Kadono, Y.; Miyamoto, H.; et al. Serum chemokine (CC motif) ligand 2 level as a diagnostic, predictive, and prognostic biomarker for prostate cancer. *Oncotarget* **2016**, *7*, 8389–8398. [CrossRef]
19. Iwamoto, H.; Izumi, K.; Nakagawa, R.; Toriumi, R.; Aoyama, S.; Shimada, T.; Kano, H.; Makino, T.; Kadomoto, S.; Yaegashi, H.; et al. Usefulness of serum CCL2 as prognostic biomarker in prostate cancer: A long-term follow-up study. *Jpn. J. Clin. Oncol.* **2022**, *52*, 1337–1344. [CrossRef]
20. Iwamoto, H.; Izumi, K.; Nakagawa, R.; Toriumi, R.; Aoyama, S.; Kamijima, T.; Shimada, T.; Kano, H.; Makino, T.; Naito, R.; et al. Serum CCL2 Is a Prognostic Biomarker for Non-Metastatic Castration-Sensitive Prostate Cancer. *Biomedicines* **2022**, *10*, 2369. [CrossRef]
21. Kirk, P.S.; Koreckij, T.; Nguyen, H.M.; Brown, L.G.; Snyder, L.A.; Vessella, R.L.; Corey, E. Inhibition of CCL2 signaling in combination with docetaxel treatment has profound inhibitory effects on prostate cancer growth in bone. *Int. J. Mol. Sci.* **2013**, *14*, 10483–10496. [CrossRef]
22. Loberg, R.D.; Ying, C.; Craig, M.; Day, L.L.; Sargent, E.; Neeley, C.; Wojno, K.; Snyder, L.A.; Yan, L.; Pienta, K.J. Targeting CCL2 with systemic delivery of neutralizing antibodies induces prostate cancer tumor regression in vivo. *Cancer Res.* **2007**, *67*, 9417–9424. [CrossRef] [PubMed]
23. Bonapace, L.; Coissieux, M.M.; Wyckoff, J.; Mertz, K.D.; Varga, Z.; Junt, T.; Bentires-Alj, M. Cessation of CCL2 inhibition accelerates breast cancer metastasis by promoting angiogenesis. *Nature* **2014**, *515*, 130–133. [CrossRef] [PubMed]

24. Abdallah, B.M.; Alzahrani, A.M.; Abdel-Moneim, A.M.; Ditzel, N.; Kassem, M. A simple and reliable protocol for long-term culture of murine bone marrow stromal (mesenchymal) stem cells that retained their in vitro and in vivo stemness in long-term culture. *Biol. Proced. Online* **2019**, *21*, 3. [CrossRef] [PubMed]
25. Fan, Y.C.; Chen, W.Y.; Lee, K.D.; Tsai, Y.C. Tumor-infiltrating Leukocytes Suppress Local Inflammation Via Interleukin-1 Receptor Antagonist in a Syngeneic Prostate Cancer Model. *Biology* **2020**, *9*, 67. [CrossRef] [PubMed]
26. Guzman, C.; Bagga, M.; Kaur, A.; Westermarck, J.; Abankwa, D. ColonyArea: An ImageJ plugin to automatically quantify colony formation in clonogenic assays. *PLoS ONE* **2014**, *9*, e92444. [CrossRef] [PubMed]
27. Foster, B.A.; Gingrich, J.R.; Kwon, E.D.; Madias, C.; Greenberg, N.M. Characterization of prostatic epithelial cell lines derived from transgenic adenocarcinoma of the mouse prostate (TRAMP) model. *Cancer Res.* **1997**, *57*, 3325–3330.
28. Moore, R.J.; Owens, D.M.; Stamp, G.; Arnott, C.; Burke, F.; East, N.; Holdsworth, H.; Turner, L.; Rollins, B.; Pasparakis, M.; et al. Mice deficient in tumor necrosis factor-alpha are resistant to skin carcinogenesis. *Nat. Med.* **1999**, *5*, 828–831. [CrossRef] [PubMed]
29. Fan, Y.C.; Lee, K.D.; Tsai, Y.C. Roles of Interleukin-1 Receptor Antagonist in Prostate Cancer Progression. *Biomedicines* **2020**, *8*, 602. [CrossRef]
30. Cheng, C.C.; Lian, W.S.; Hsiao, F.S.; Liu, I.H.; Lin, S.P.; Lee, Y.H.; Chang, C.C.; Xiao, G.Y.; Huang, H.Y.; Cheng, C.F.; et al. Isolation and characterization of novel murine epiphysis derived mesenchymal stem cells. *PLoS ONE* **2012**, *7*, e36085. [CrossRef]
31. Ortiz, L.A.; Dutreil, M.; Fattman, C.; Pandey, A.C.; Torres, G.; Go, K.; Phinney, D.G. Interleukin 1 receptor antagonist mediates the antiinflammatory and antifibrotic effect of mesenchymal stem cells during lung injury. *Proc. Natl. Acad. Sci. USA* **2007**, *104*, 11002–11007. [CrossRef] [PubMed]
32. Luz-Crawford, P.; Djouad, F.; Toupet, K.; Bony, C.; Franquesa, M.; Hoogduijn, M.J.; Jorgensen, C.; Noel, D. Mesenchymal Stem Cell-Derived Interleukin 1 Receptor Antagonist Promotes Macrophage Polarization and Inhibits B Cell Differentiation. *Stem. Cells* **2016**, *34*, 483–492. [CrossRef] [PubMed]
33. McGuire, J.J.; Frieling, J.S.; Lo, C.H.; Li, T.; Muhammad, A.; Lawrence, H.R.; Lawrence, N.J.; Cook, L.M.; Lynch, C.C. Mesenchymal stem cell-derived interleukin-28 drives the selection of apoptosis resistant bone metastatic prostate cancer. *Nat. Commun.* **2021**, *12*, 723. [CrossRef] [PubMed]
34. Pittenger, M.F.; Discher, D.E.; Peault, B.M.; Phinney, D.G.; Hare, J.M.; Caplan, A.I. Mesenchymal stem cell perspective: Cell biology to clinical progress. *NPJ Regen. Med.* **2019**, *4*, 22. [CrossRef]
35. Ahn, G.O.; Tseng, D.; Liao, C.H.; Dorie, M.J.; Czechowicz, A.; Brown, J.M. Inhibition of Mac-1 (CD11b/CD18) enhances tumor response to radiation by reducing myeloid cell recruitment. *Proc. Natl. Acad. Sci. USA* **2010**, *107*, 8363–8368. [CrossRef]
36. Schmid, M.C.; Khan, S.Q.; Kaneda, M.M.; Pathria, P.; Shepard, R.; Louis, T.L.; Anand, S.; Woo, G.; Leem, C.; Faridi, M.H.; et al. Integrin CD11b activation drives anti-tumor innate immunity. *Nat. Commun.* **2018**, *9*, 5379. [CrossRef]
37. Jo, H.; Eom, Y.W.; Kim, H.S.; Park, H.J.; Kim, H.M.; Cho, M.Y. Regulatory Dendritic Cells Induced by Mesenchymal Stem Cells Ameliorate Dextran Sodium Sulfate-Induced Chronic Colitis in Mice. *Gut Liver* **2018**, *12*, 664–673. [CrossRef]
38. Oh, S.H.; Choi, C.; Noh, J.E.; Lee, N.; Jeong, Y.W.; Jeon, I.; Shin, J.M.; Kim, J.H.; Kim, H.J.; Lee, J.M.; et al. Interleukin-1 receptor antagonist-mediated neuroprotection by umbilical cord-derived mesenchymal stromal cells following transplantation into a rodent stroke model. *Exp. Mol. Med.* **2018**, *50*, 1–12. [CrossRef]
39. Abdelaziz, M.H.; Abdelwahab, S.F.; Wan, J.; Cai, W.; Huixuan, W.; Jianjun, C.; Kumar, K.D.; Vasudevan, A.; Sadek, A.; Su, Z.; et al. Alternatively activated macrophages; a double-edged sword in allergic asthma. *J. Transl. Med.* **2020**, *18*, 58. [CrossRef]

cancers

MDPI

Article

Tumor Location and a Tumor Volume over 2.8 cc Predict the Prognosis for Japanese Localized Prostate Cancer

Haruki Baba [1,†], Shinichi Sakamoto [1,*,†], Xue Zhao [1,†], Yasutaka Yamada [1], Junryo Rii [1], Ayumi Fujimoto [1], Manato Kanesaka [1], Nobuyoshi Takeuchi [1], Tomokazu Sazuka [1], Yusuke Imamura [1], Koichiro Akakura [2] and Tomohiko Ichikawa [1]

1 Department of Urology, Chiba University Graduate School of Medicine, Chiba 260-8670, Japan
2 Department of Urology, Japan Community Health-Care Organization Tokyo Shinjuku Medical Center, Tokyo 162-8543, Japan
* Correspondence: rbatbat1@chiba-u.jp; Tel.: +81-43-226-2134; Fax: +81-43-226-2136
† These authors contributed equally to this work.

Simple Summary: About 40% of men with localized prostate cancer experience biochemical recurrence after radical prostatectomy. The early detection of disease progression is important for optimal post-operative treatment and follow-up. Our study reviewed 557 patients with prostate cancer who underwent radical prostatectomy and found that a tumor volume over 2.8 cc was a novel independent predictive factor for biochemical recurrence. We further established a novel risk assessment model based on tumor volume and location (posterior and peripheral zone). We confirmed that the risk model could stratify patients' prognoses. In addition to the previously reported biomarkers, these novel factors obtained from the surgical specimen may provide better prognostic information in patients with prostate cancer.

Abstract: (1) Objective: Our study investigated the prognostic value of tumor volume and location in prostate cancer patients who received radical prostatectomy (RP). (2) Methods: The prognostic significance of tumor volume and location, together with other clinical factors, was studied using 557 patients who received RP. (3) Results: The receiver operating characteristic (ROC) curve identified the optimal cutoff value of tumor volume as 2.8 cc for predicting biochemical recurrence (BCR). Cox regression analysis revealed that a tumor in the posterior area ($p = 0.031$), peripheral zone ($p = 0.0472$), and tumor volume $\geq$ 2.8 cc ($p < 0.0001$) were predictive factors in univariate analysis. After multivariate analysis, tumor volume $\geq$ 2.8 cc ($p = 0.0225$) was an independent predictive factor for BCR. Among them, a novel risk model was established using tumor volume and location in the posterior area and peripheral zone. The progression-free survival (PFS) of patients who met the three criteria (unfavorable group) was significantly worse than other groups ($p \leq 0.001$). Furthermore, multivariate analysis showed that the unfavorable risk was an independent prognostic factor for BCR. The prognostic significance of our risk model was observed in low- to intermediate-risk patients, although it was not observed in high-risk patients. (4) Conclusion: Tumor volume ($\geq$2.8 cc) and localization (posterior/peripheral zone) may be a novel prognostic factor in patients undergoing RP.

Keywords: tumor volume; tumor location; prostate cancer; biochemical recurrence; prognostic factor

Citation: Baba, H.; Sakamoto, S.; Zhao, X.; Yamada, Y.; Rii, J.; Fujimoto, A.; Kanesaka, M.; Takeuchi, N.; Sazuka, T.; Imamura, Y.; et al. Tumor Location and a Tumor Volume over 2.8 cc Predict the Prognosis for Japanese Localized Prostate Cancer. *Cancers* **2022**, *14*, 5823. https://doi.org/10.3390/cancers14235823

Academic Editor: Grace Lu-Yao

Received: 5 November 2022
Accepted: 24 November 2022
Published: 25 November 2022

1. Introduction

Prostate cancer (Pca) is the most common malignant tumor in men. About 2.6 million cases are newly diagnosed and 34,500 deaths of Pca are estimated per year in the United States [1]. Radical prostatectomy (RP) for the treatment of prostate cancer has made remarkable progress since it widely emerged around 1900. At present, RP is still the standard treatment option for localized Pca [2]. However, the frequency of biochemical recurrence (BCR) has been reported to be about 40% within 10 years after RP [3]. Once BCR occurs, about 3.5% of patients will inevitably develop resistance to androgen deprivation therapy, also known as castration-resistant prostate cancer (CRPC) [4]. CRPC has been reported to cause death within 2 to 4 years [5]. Therefore, BCR is the major clinical issue to be detected and addressed in patients who received RP.

A lot of clinical studies have evaluated predictive factors and/or risk models for BCR after RP. Serum prostate-specific antigen (PSA) is the mainstay to detect the BCR of patients after surgery [6], and it has been recommended to keep close monitoring until PSA reaches 0.2 ng/mL [7]. In addition to PSA kinetics, Gleason score, PSA density, pathological and clinical stages, surgical margin, and other clinical factors have been studied for their prognostic significance, however, these factors could not predict BCR independently [8]. To better distinguish the recurrence risk and evaluate the prognosis after RP, more innovative predictors or models are unmet clinical needs. The individualized management after treatment requires effective recurrence risk prediction to implement timely intervention and avoid overtreatment. Previous studies showed that the tumor volume was related to the clinical manifestations of prostate cancer [9]. A tumor with a volume of less than 0.5 cc is considered as insignificant prostate cancer, and aggressive treatment may not be needed [10,11]. Recently, several studies proposed the novel definition of insignificant prostate cancer as a tumor volume of less than 2.5 cc [11–17], or less than 2.0 cc [18]. However, it was found that the BCR risk increased with tumor volume over 2.49 cc, indicating that the tumor volume was deeply involved in the progression of Pca [19]. Furthermore, little is known about the relationship between different prostate areas and tumor volumes, and their impact on BCR. Herein, we examined the prognostic role of tumor volume and location in patients with localized Pca for a better treatment strategy and postoperative follow-up.

2. Methods

2.1. Study Design and Setting

Clinical data of 557 patients who received RP at Chiba University Hospital and affiliated hospitals between 2006 and 2020 were retrospectively reviewed. The study was approved by the clinical review committee of our institution (#1768) and the written informed consent of all patients participating in the study was obtained. All participants or designated agents accepted a standardized data collection protocol, including personal postoperative follow-up information and medical record. The study is in accordance with the Japanese ethical document.

2.2. Patients

The inclusion criteria were RP for biopsy-proven prostate cancer performed at Chiba University Hospital and affiliated hospitals; whole-mount step-section pathologic maps available for tumor volume-calculation and localization. The exclusion criteria were neoadjuvant hormone therapy; radiation therapy; poor pathologic map quality; short follow-up term (<12 months).

2.3. Variables

Baseline clinical data included age, BMI, serum PSA, PSA F/T ratio, serum testosterone, biopsy positive rate, Gleason score (GS), clinical TNM staging, surgical prostate specimen, tumor volume, tumor location, surgical resect margin, and pathological TNM staging. Each patient came to our institution every 3 months after RP and had blood samples taken for PSA measurement until the occurrence of BCR or death was confirmed.

After RP, an elevated serum PSA level (>0.2 ng/mL) was defined as BCR [6].

2.4. Tumor Volume and Location Estimation Method

2.4.1. Measurement of Tumor Volume

The prostatectomy specimens were step-sectioned transversely at 5-mm intervals. All the specimens were mounted on slides. Tumor volume was calculated by scanning the sliced specimen, and the area of the tumor was analyzed using ImageJ software. Total tumor volume = tumor area × thickness of specimen × 1.2 (correction for shrinkage).

2.4.2. Tumor Localization

All specimens were serially sectioned from the tip to the base at 5 mm intervals, and the bladder neck and vertex edges were submitted as vertical sections. According to the anatomical structure, the specimen was divided into the following regions: the peripheral zone (PZ), the transition zone (TZ), and the central zone (CZ). The region within 1.0 cm or 1.5 cm from the tip of the prostate was identified as the Apex region. The prostatic urethra is an anatomic marker for a tumor to be classified as anterior or posterior (Figure 1). If a tumor showed a slight extension to another site, >80% volume in the main area was the criterion for defining the origin of the tumor in this area. Each RP sample was reviewed by two pathologists.

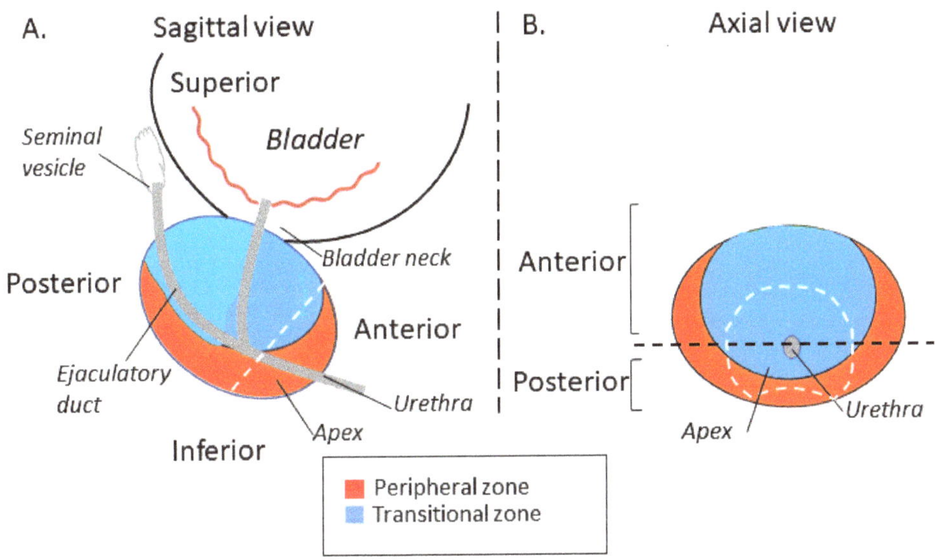

Figure 1. Schematic diagram of an anatomical division of the prostate. The location of the Anterior/Posterior and Peripheral/Transitional Zones are described. (**A**) Sagittal view. (**B**) Axial view.

2.5. Statistical Methods

JMP Pro (Version 16.0; SAS Institute Inc., Cary, NC, USA) was used for statistical analysis. Univariate cox proportional hazards model analysis was performed on the baseline data classified by the median value of the outcome measurement to determine the predictive factors of the BCR. The significant variables ($p < 0.05$) were further analyzed by multivariable cox proportional hazards model regression. The optimal cutoff value of tumor volume was obtained by calculating Area Under the Curve (AUC) from the Receiver Operating Characteristic (ROC) curve analysis. To evaluate the interaction between tumor volume and location, 3 risk factors related to volume and location obtained from univariate and multivariate cox regression analysis were combined into a risk classification model. This model was grouped according to the number of risk factors displayed: favorable; 0 risk factor, moderate; 1 or 2 risk factors, unfavorable; all 3 risk factors. Kaplan–Meier method was used to evaluate progression-free survival (PFS). Statistical significance was set at $p < 0.05$.

3. Results

3.1. Participants

In total, 557 patients were enrolled in the study. Follow-up terms ranged from 12 to 161.5 months, with a median follow-up time of 45.3 months. As of the end of the study, 66 (11.8%) patients had BCR, and 9 (1.6%) patients died (not due to prostate cancer). The median age of all patients was 67 years old. The median preoperative PSA level was 7.71 ng/mL. The biopsy GS was 7 or less in 79.7%, 8 in 8.6%, and 9 or more in 11%. Overall, 64.8% of patients were pathological TNM stage 2c or above, and 1.4% were positive for lymph node metastasis. According to the risk grouping of Pca by the American Cancer Society (ACS), 77 (13.8%) patients were classified into the low-risk group, 279 (50.1%) were classified into the intermediate-risk group, and 201 (36.1%) were classified into the high-risk group. The median tumor volume was 2.12 cc. Seminal vesicle invasion was observed in 8.6%, the extracapsular invasion was seen in 24.8%, and 30.3% had positive margins. The tumor distributions were in the apex area (63.7%), middle area (63.4%), and bladder neck (21.4%). Regarding the anterior or posterior area of the prostate, 48.1% of the tumors were in the anterior, and 52.4% were in the posterior. Overall, 67.1% were located in the PZ and 37.3% were in the TZ (Table 1).

Table 1. Characteristics of patients.

Characteristics	
Number of patients	557
Median age at operation (range), years	67 (46–77)
Median follow-up time (range), months	45.3 (12–161.5)
Median initial PSA (range) (ng/mL)	7.71 (2.15–87.16)
Gleason score sum, n (%)	
≤7	444 (79.7)
8	48 (8.6)
≥9	61 (11.0)
T stage, n (%)	
≤2b	195 (35.0)
≥2c	361 (64.8)
Risk Group; Low/Intermediate/High, n (%)	77 (13.8)/279 (50.1)/201 (36.1)
Tumor Volume (range), cc	2.12 (0.02–57)
Tumor Location, n (%)	
apex	355 (63.7)
middle	353 (63.4)
bladder neck	119 (21.4)
Tumor Location, n (%)	
anterior	268 (48.1)
posterior	292 (52.4)
Tumor Location, n (%)	
PZ	374 (67.1)
TZ	208 (37.3)
N stage, n (%)	
positive	8 (1.4)
Seminal Vesicle Invasion, n, (%)	48 (8.6)
Extracapsular Extension, n, (%)	138 (24.8)
Resection Margins, n, (%)	169 (30.3)
PSA Recurrence, n, (%)	66 (11.8)

PSA = prostate-specific antigen; T stage = tumor stage; N stage = lymph node stage; PZ = peripheral zone; TZ = transition zone.

3.2. Predictive Factors for Progression-Free Survival (PFS)

The ROC curve was used to calculate the relationship between BCR and tumor volume, and the optimal cutoff value was identified as 2.8 cc (AUC = 0.69) (Supplementary Figure S1A). We analyzed different tumor volume cutoff values (0.5 cc, 1.0 cc, 2.0 cc, 2.8 cc, 3.0 cc, 3.5 cc) and compared HR and p-values. The results confirmed that 2.8 cc is the optimal cut-off value as a predictive factor for BCR (Table 2). (The cutoff values of two tumor volumes with $p < 0.0001$ that were not selected (3.0 cc and 3.5 cc) were also verified by corresponding models, as shown in Supplementary Figures S2 and S3).

Table 2. Univariable and multivariable cox proportional hazard regression models in predictive factors for PFS in localized Pca (overall risk).

	Univariable				Multivariable		
	Cut Off	**HR**	**95% CI**	***p* Value**	**HR**	**95% CI**	***p* Value**
Age	≥67	0.96	0.59–1.57	0.8842			
initial PSA	≥7.71 ng/mL	1.65	1.00–2.73	0.0505			
PSAD	≥0.26	2.06	1.21–3.53	0.0082	1.51	0.73–3.09	0.2643
GS	≥7	1.15	0.46–2.88	0.7593			
T stage	≥T3	4.66	2.81–7.73	<0.0001	1.69	0.77–3.71	0.1894
RM	positive	4.18	2.46–7.10	<0.0001	1.99	0.94–4.20	0.0712
Tumor location							
	Apex	1.45	0.70–3.02	0.3166			
	PZ	3.28	1.01–10.60	0.0472	2.21	0.49–10.05	0.3030
	posterior	2.24	1.07–4.65	0.0314	1.72	0.72–4.12	0.2193
TV							
	≥0.5 cc	1.61	0.73–3.53	0.2344			
	≥1.0 cc	2.18	1.11–4.27	0.0240			
	≥2.0 cc	2.74	1.55–4.82	0.0005			
	≥2.8 cc **	3.10	1.86–5.17	<0.0001	2.47	1.14–5.36	0.0225 *
	≥3.0 cc	2.96	1.80–4.88	<0.0001			
	≥3.5 cc	2.80	1.72–4.58	<0.0001			

PSA = prostate-specific antigen; PSAD = prostate-specific antigen density; GS = Gleason score; T stage = tumor stage; RM = resection margins; HR = hazard ratio; CI = confidence interval; * *p*-value < 0.05, ** tumor volume cutoff value based on the ROC curve.

Univariate and multivariate predictors for BCR obtained from cox proportional hazard analysis are shown in Table 2. The predictors for BCR were pathological stage $T \geq 3$ (HR = 4.66 [95% CI: 2.81–7.73], $p < 0.0001$), positive surgical margin (HR = 4.18 [95% CI: 2.46–7.10], $p < 0.0001$), tumor volume ≥ 2.8 cc (HR = 3.10 [95% CI: 1.86–5.17], $p < 0.0001$), followed by PSA density ≥0.26 (HR = 2.06 [95% CI: 1.21–3.53], $p = 0.0082$), tumor located in the Posterior region (HR = 2.24 [95% CI: 1.07–4.65], $p = 0.0314$), tumor located in the PZ (HR = 3.28 [95% CI: 1.01–10.6], $p = 0.0472$). The multivariate analysis showed that the independent predictor of BCR was only tumor volume ≥ 2.8 cc (HR = 2.47 [95% CI: 1.14–5.36], $p = 0.0225$) (Table 2).

The Kaplan–Meier method was used to evaluate the PFS curve. The PFS of patients with tumors located in the PZ was inferior to those in the TZ (Figure 2A $p = 0.0354$). Furthermore, patients harboring tumors located in the posterior had shorter PFS than those in the anterior area (Figure 2B $p = 0.027$). Consistent with cox analysis, there was no significant difference between the PFS of the patients with tumors in the apex and not-apex area (Figure 2C $p = 0.3135$). PFS in the patients with tumor volume ≥ 2.8 cc was significantly inferior to those with less than 2.8 cc (Figure 2D $p < 0.0001$).

3.3. Model for Predicting PFS by Tumor Volume at Specific Location

Based on the analysis of clinical factors related to BCR in Table 2 and Figure 2, tumor volume and tumor location (PZ and Posterior location) were statistically significant predictive factors. Therefore, we established a risk classification model using tumor volume and location to stratify patients on the basis of risk of progression. The three risk factors that predict BCR in the model are tumor volume ≥ 2.8 cc, tumor located in PZ, and tumor located in the posterior area. The capability of the unfavorable risk to predict BCR was shown in Table 3 and only these risk factors predicted BCR on multivariable analysis (HR 3.16 [95% CI: 1.52–6.56], $p = 0.002$).

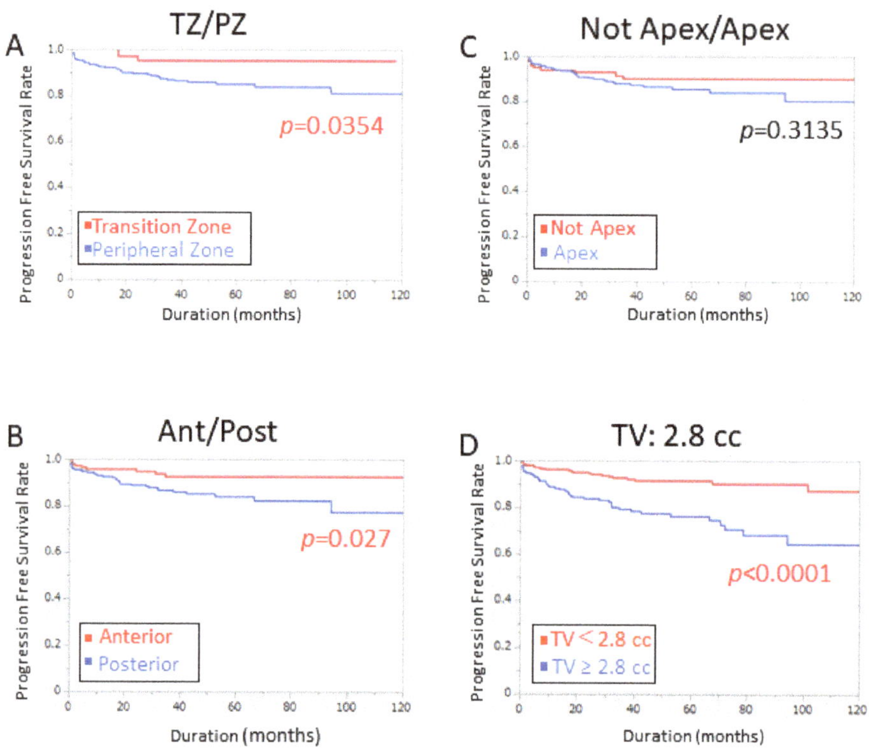

Figure 2. Prognostic significance of tumor location and tumor volume. (**A**) Patients with tumor in the PZ had significantly worse PFS than those in the TZ ($p = 0.0354$). (**B**) Patients with tumor in the posterior region had significantly worse PFS than those in the anterior region ($p = 0.027$). (**C**) There was no difference in PFS between apex and non-apex regions. (**D**) Patients with tumor volume $\geq$ 2.8 cc had significantly worse PFS than those <2.8 cc ($p < 0.0001$).

Table 3. Univariable and multivariable cox proportional hazard regression models in predictive factors for PFS in localized Pca (overall risk) with unfavorable risk.

	Univariable				Multivariable		
	Cut Off	HR	95% CI	*p* Value	HR	95% CI	*p* Value
Age	≥67	0.96	0.59–1.57	0.8842	-	-	-
initial PSA	≥7.71 ng/mL	1.65	1.00–2.73	0.0505	-	-	-
PSAD	≥0.26	2.06	1.21–3.53	0.0082	1.55	0.76–3.15	0.2307
GS	≥7	1.15	0.46–2.88	0.7593	-	-	-
T stage	≥T3	4.66	2.81–7.73	<0.0001	1.64	0.74–3.65	0.2261
RM	positive	4.18	2.46–7.10	<0.0001	2.09	0.99–4.42	0.0548
Unfavorable Risk	PZ + Post + TV2.8 cc	4.74	2.60–8.65	<0.0001	3.16	1.52–6.56	0.0020 *

PSA = prostate-specific antigen; PSAD = prostate-specific antigen density; GS = Gleason score; T stage = tumor stage; RM = resection margins; PZ + Post + TV2.8 cc = tumor volume $\geq$ 2.8 cc in posterior location of peripheral zone; HR = hazard ratio; CI = confidence interval; * *p*-value < 0.05.

To further explore the predictive ability of the novel risk model, we divided the patients into the low-risk group, intermediate-risk group, and high-risk group according to the risk grouping of Pca by the American Cancer Society (ACS) [20] and validated the predictive value of the risk models among different ACS risk groups. In the analysis of the high-risk group, our unfavorable risk model could not predict disease progression independently (Table 4). However, the risk factors were the only independent predictor for PFS among patients with low to intermediate-risk groups (HR 4.43 [95% CI: 1.51–13.01], $p = 0.0068$) (Table 5).

Table 4. Univariable and multivariable cox proportional hazard regression models in predictive factors for PFS in localized Pca (high risk).

		Univariable			Multivariable		
	Cut Off	HR	95% CI	*p* Value	HR	95% CI	*p* Value
Age	≥67	0.76	0.40–1.47	0.4167	-	-	-
initial PSA	≥7.71 ng/mL	1.04	0.52–2.08	0.9097	-	-	-
PSAD	≥0.26	1.9	0.82–4.40	0.1326	-	-	-
GS	≥7	1.29	0.18–9.46	0.7991	-	-	-
T stage	≥T3	4.38	2.11–9.10	<0.0001	1.98	0.75–5.25	0.1701
RM	positive	4.65	2.16–10.02	<0.0001	2.37	0.95–5.91	0.0649
Unfavorable Risk	PZ + Post + TV2.8 cc	3.5	1.64–7.47	0.0012	1.87	0.77–4.53	0.1653

PSA = Prostate Specific Antigen; PSAD = Prostate Specific Antigen Density; GS = Gleason Score; T stage = Tumor Stage; RM = Resection Margins; HR = Hazard Ratio; CI = Confidence Interval.

Table 5. Univariable and multivariable cox proportional hazard regression models in predictive factors for PFS in localized Pca (low to intermediate risk).

		Univariable			Multivariable		
	Cut Off	HR	95% CI	*p* Value	HR	95% CI	*p* Value
Age	≥67	1.07	0.51–2.25	0.8546	-	-	-
initial PSA	≥7.71 ng/mL	1.56	0.74–3.28	0.2458	-	-	-
PSAD	≥0.26	1.52	0.72–3.19	0.2716	-	-	-
GS	≥7	0.74	0.26–2.15	0.5855	-	-	-
T stage	≥T3	3.34	1.59–7.01	0.0015	0.97	0.28–3.38	0.961
RM	positive	3.03	1.42–6.47	0.0043	1.38	0.43–4.41	0.5904
Unfavorable Risk	PZ + Post + TV2.8 cc	4.71	1.75–12.69	0.0022	4.43	1.51–13.01	0.0068 *

PSA = prostate-specific antigen; PSAD = prostate-specific antigen density; GS = Gleason score; T stage = tumor stage; RM = resection margins; HR = hazard ratio; CI = confidence interval; PZ + Post + TV2.8 cc = tumor volume ≥ 2.8 cc in posterior location of the peripheral zone. * *p*-value < 0.05.

3.4. Risk Model to Stratify Patient Prognosis

According to our established risk model, we divided the patients into three groups (favorable; displayed zero risk factors, moderate; displayed one or two risk factors, unfavorable; displayed all three risk factors). Overall, 61, 343, and 104 patients were classified as belonging to the favorable, moderate, and unfavorable group, respectively (Figure 3A).

The PFS curves of the three groups of patients (Figure 3B) showed that the PFS of the unfavorable group was significantly worse than that of the moderate group ($p < 0.0001$) and the favorable group ($p = 0.001$), while there was no significant difference between the moderate group and the favorable group ($p = 0.1150$).

The median tumor volume of the three groups was 1.33 cc, 1.81 cc, and 4.92 cc, respectively and there were significant differences between the three groups (Figure 3C).

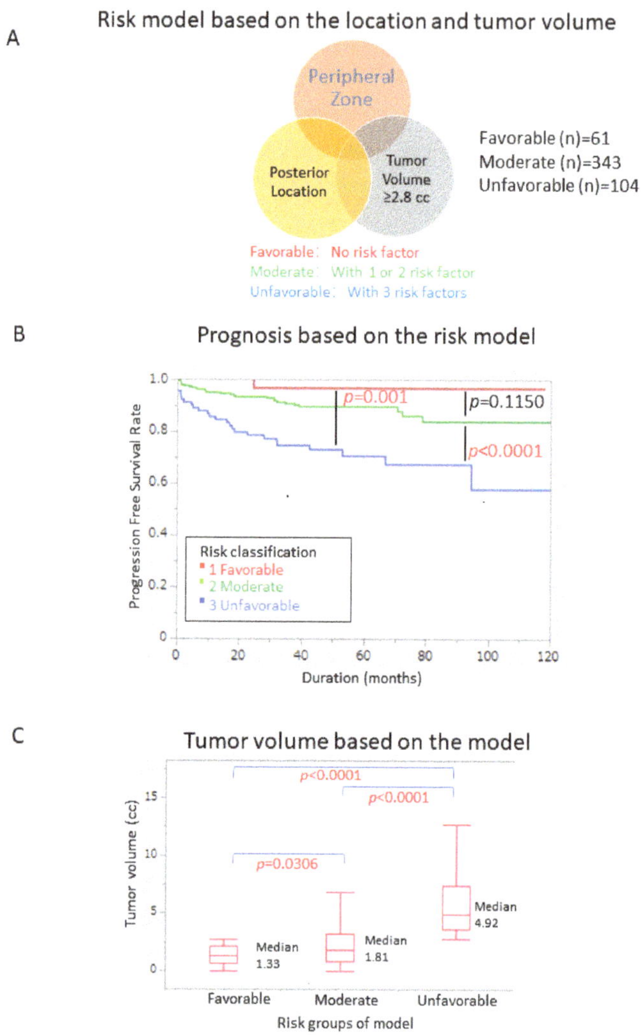

Figure 3. Prognostic model based on the location and tumor volume (**A**) Venn diagram of risk model based on the location and tumor volume. (**B**) Risk classification significantly differentiated the PFS between the Favorable and Unfavorable group ($p = 0.001$) and the Moderate and Unfavorable group ($p < 0.0001$). (**C**) The tumor volume showed significant differences among different risk groups.

In addition, we analyzed the impact of tumor volume on PFS in different prostate regions with the tumor volume of 2.8 cc as the threshold (Figure 4). The results suggested that the PFS of tumor $\geq$ 2.8 cc in the PZ is significantly worse than that of less than 2.8 cc (Figure 4A $p < 0.0001$). Similar results were observed for tumors $\geq$ 2.8 cc in the posterior location (Figure 4C $p < 0.0001$). Of note, the 2.8 cc cutoff value in TZ also showed a significant difference in PFS between the two groups (Figure 4B $p = 0.0345$). On the other hand, the significant difference was not seen in the anterior area (Figure 4D $p = 0.0873$).

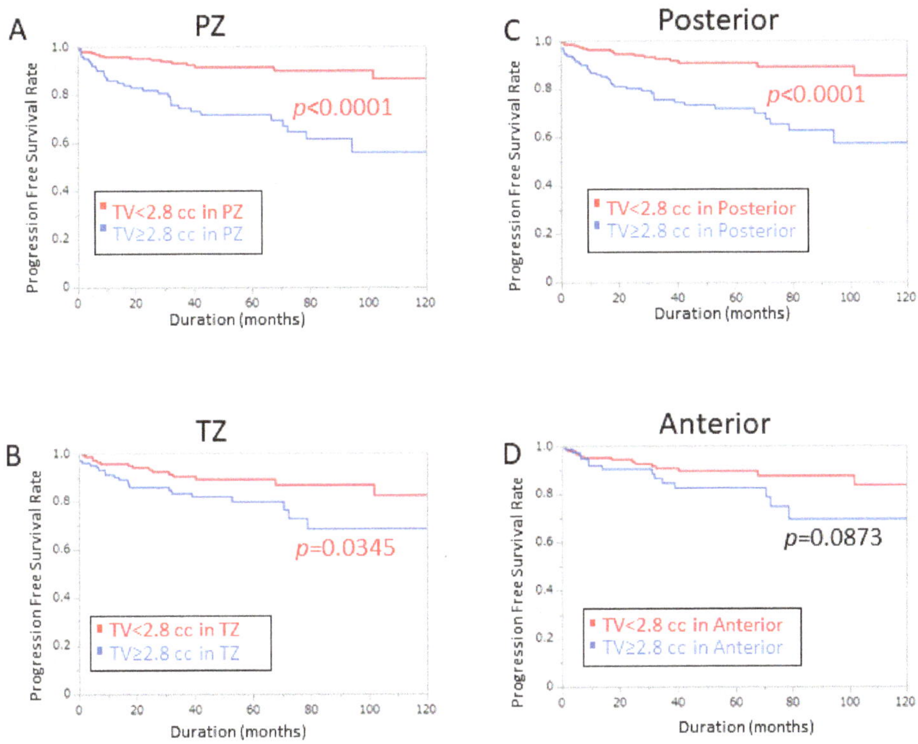

Figure 4. Prognostic significance of Tumor volume 2.8 cc based on the location. (**A**) Patients with tumor volume $\geq$ 2.8 cc had significantly worse PFS in the PZ ($p < 0.0001$). (**B**) Patients with tumor volume $\geq$ 2.8 cc had significantly worse PFS in the TZ ($p = 0.0345$). (**C**) Patients with tumor volume $\geq$ 2.8 cc had significantly worse PFS in the posterior region ($p < 0.0001$). (**D**) In the anterior region, there was no difference in PFS by tumor volume cutoff of 2.8 cc.

4. Discussion

In our study, a tumor with a volume $\geq$ 2.8 cc was identified as an independent predictive factor for BCR ($p = 0.0225$). Furthermore, we established novel risk classification together with PZ and posterior location, which distinguished PFS between different risk groups. We believe this risk model will provide novel prognostic significance in patients who received RP.

Previous studies showed the positive surgical margin after RP is a potential predictive factor for BCR [21–29]. It is difficult to completely avoid the incidence of positive surgical margins through objective methods. Several studies found that positive surgical margins with limited length [30,31], locations [32], or quantity [33] decreased the correlation with BCR. Another study showed that tumor volume was associated with BCR in patients who underwent RP with negative surgical margins [34]. In addition, tumor volume and GS were even more significant predictors for BCR than positive margins [35] and the location of the tumor could predict the incidence of positive surgical margins [36–39]. Multivariate analysis showed that the predictive value of our risk model was superior to the positive surgical margin. These findings suggested that focusing on tumor volume and location, not only resection margins will give us better prognostic information in the treatment of localized Pca.

Regarding the prognostic significance of tumor localization, tumors originating in the TZ have been reported to be associated with a better prognosis in comparison with those in the PZ [39–41]. Augustin et al. found that the location of prostate cancer in the TZ was associated with better progression-free survival after RP (p = 0.0402) [40]. However, the zonal location offers no advantage over the well-established prognostic factors in predicting recurrence. Some more detailed anatomical differentiation (anterior, posterior, the apex of prostate, bladder neck) also revealed the difference in tumor location on prognosis [42,43]. Magheli et al. found that tumors in the anterior prostate were associated with favorable pathological features and improved biochemical-free survival, although it was not an independent predictor of BCR [42]. There are also some studies that have concluded that tumor location is not related to prognosis [44,45].

Tumor volume has been reported to show a significant correlation with BCR after RP [46–50]. Generally, tumor volume < 0.5 cc has been considered as an insignificant Pca, which has a low potential of recurrence [51]. The predictive factors for BCR in patients with low-volume prostate cancer (≤0.5 cc) have not been well studied [52]. Several reports proposed to increase the thresholds of volume for insignificant cancer to avoid over-treatment [14], however, other studies showed that the modified criteria had a higher risk of BCR in Gleason 4/5 cancer [53]. The tumor volume was superior to the percentage of cancer (tumor volume/prostate volume ratio) for predicting the prognosis after RP [54]. Different tumor volume cut-off values were proposed to determine the prognosis of Pca. Friedersdorff et al. suggested that tumor volume ≥ 5 cc (AUC = 0.79) was a significant prognostic factor for BCR [55]. Another study set the cut-off values as: minimal (≤1.0 cc), middle (1.1–5.0 cc), or extended (>5.0 cc) [47]. Shin et al. divided the tumor volume into three groups according to 2 cc and 5 cc, in multivariate analysis, recurrence-free survival could be independently predicted [56]. The tumor volume in the surgical specimen after neoadjuvant therapy was investigated and the study showed that patients with residual tumors ≥ 1.0 cc in the specimen had a higher risk of BCR [57]. Raison et al. studied 685 British patients who underwent laparoscopic and robot-assisted RP and revealed that 2.5 cc (AUC = 0.71) was the best cutoff value for predicting BCR [58]. Of note, some studies showed that the tumor volume alone may not be able to evaluate the prognosis of recurrence and prognosis after RP [13,59]. O'Neil et al. suggested that tumors in some locations are larger and more likely to invade the sites that are prone to recurrence [37]. However, there have been no studies that have analyzed the prognostic value of tumor volume combined with tumor localization.

In our study, we attempted to evaluate the potential interaction between tumor volume and location, the tumor volume cutoff value obtained by the ROC curve was 2.8 cc (AUC = 0.69). Therefore, we used the tumor volume threshold (≥2.8 cc) of the specific location to improve the capability of our risk model. We hypothesized that the larger tumor volume in the PZ and/or posterior of the prostate may be associated with BCR. Our findings demonstrated that the prognostic significance of tumor volume over 2.8 cc varied by tumor localization (Figure 4). In our model, the interaction between prostate tumor location and volume was a promising predictor of prostate BCR. Interestingly, our risk model was an independent predictor in patients with low and intermediate risk while it was not in patients with high risk. Extended dissection during surgery and close follow-up after surgery may enhance clinical benefit in patients who met our criteria.

The limitations of this study are as follows. First, our study included a single Asian race. Compared with the western population, the Asian population has a lower incidence and mortality of prostate cancer [60]. The tumor volume of African American men with prostate cancer is larger than that of white men [61]. The risk of BCR in black Americans has been reported to be 1.6 times higher than that in white Americans [62]. These results suggested that there may be differences in clinical and pathological features between races. Further validation of our risk model will be warranted in other patients' cohorts. Second, our study may need to be further investigated using genomic analysis. The previous study has revealed that prostate cancer risk alleles are associated with prostate cancer volume and prostate size [63]. Downregulation of PAH and AOC1 and upregulation of DDC, LIN01436, and ORM1 were associated with the development of prostate cancer [8,64].

Molecular and cellular biological studies are also closely related to the site of prostate tumorigenesis [41]. Studying the specific genes behind it could improve understanding of the region or cell-type characteristics of prostate cancer. These features account for differences in tumor progression and invasion between different regions of the prostate [41]. The unique biological characteristics of tumor types in different prostate regions can help guide individualized treatment and patient risk stratification. Finally, further validation of our clinical parameters using the latest imaging system PSMA/PET [65] or artificial intelligence system (deep learning) [66] may enhance the clinical importance of this study.

5. Conclusions

Tumor volume $\geq$ 2.8 cc was an independent predictive factor for BCR in patients who received RP. Furthermore, we established a novel risk model using tumor volume over 2.8 cc and tumor location (PZ and/or posterior). Our risk classification could predict patient prognosis and will help us to optimize peri-operative and post-operative treatment strategies.

Supplementary Materials: The following supporting information can be downloaded at: https://www.mdpi.com/article/10.3390/cancers14235823/s1, Figure S1: (A) Tumor volume cut off based on the ROC curve. (B) Tumor volume based on the location; Figure S2: (A) A supplemental model that included the 3.0 cc tumor volume as one of the factors in the risk model. (B) Risk classification significantly differentiated the PFS between the Favorable and Unfavorable group (p = 0.0008) and the Moderate and Unfavorable group (p < 0.0001); Figure S3: (A) A supplemental model that included the 3.5 cc tumor volume as one of the factors in the risk model. (B) Risk classification significantly differentiated the PFS between the Favorable and Unfavorable group (p = 0.0001) and the Moderate and Unfavorable group (p < 0.0001).

Author Contributions: H.B. contributed to collecting data, preparing figures, and writing; S.S. and X.Z. contributed to analyzing data, collecting bibliography, drawing tables, and writing; Y.Y. and J.R. contributed to analyzing data; A.F., M.K., N.T., T.S., Y.I. and K.A. contributed to collecting data; S.S. and T.I. contributed to the supervision of all the activities; The first draft of the manuscript was prepared by H.B. and X.Z. performed subsequent amendments. S.S. revised the manuscript. All authors have read and agreed to the published version of the manuscript.

Funding: The present study was supported by grants from Grant-in-Aid for Scientific Research (C) (20K09555 to S.S.), Grant-in-Aid for Scientific Research (B) (20H03813 to T.I.), and the Japan China Sasakawa Medical Fellowship (to X.Z.).

Institutional Review Board Statement: The study was conducted in accordance with the Declaration of Helsinki, and approved by the Institutional Review Board (or Ethics Committee) of Chiba University of Graduate School of Medicine and School of Medicine (protocol code 1768 and date of approval 1 March 2018).

Informed Consent Statement: Informed consent was obtained from all subjects involved in the study.

Data Availability Statement: The data presented in this study are available on request from the corresponding author.

Conflicts of Interest: The authors declare no conflict of interest. The funders had no role in the design of the study; in the collection, analyses, or interpretation of data; in the writing of the manuscript, or in the decision to publish the results.

Abbreviations

Pca	prostate cancer
RP	radical prostatectomy
BCR	biochemical recurrence
CRPC	castration-resistant prostate cancer
PSA	prostate-specific antigen
PZ	peripheral zone

TZ	transition zone
CZ	central zone
TV	tumor volume
GS	Gleason score
ROC	Receiver Operating Characteristic
AUC	Area Under the Curve
PFS	Progression-Free Survival
ACS	American Cancer Society

References

1. Siegel, R.L.; Miller, K.D.; Fuchs, H.E.; Jemal, A. Cancer statistics, 2022. *CA Cancer J. Clin.* **2022**, *72*, 7–33. [CrossRef]
2. Costello, A.J. Considering the role of radical prostatectomy in 21st century prostate cancer care. *Nat. Rev. Urol.* **2020**, *17*, 177–188. [CrossRef] [PubMed]
3. Han, M.; Partin, A.W.; Pound, C.R.; Epstein, J.I.; Walsh, P.C. Long-term biochemical disease-free and cancer-specific survival following anatomic radical retropubic prostatectomy. The 15-year Johns Hopkins experience. *Urol. Clin. N. Am.* **2001**, *28*, 555–565. [CrossRef]
4. Everist, M.M.; Howard, L.E.; Aronson, W.J.; Kane, C.J.; Amling, C.L.; Cooperberg, M.R.; Terris, M.K.; Freedland, S.J. Socioeconomic status, race, and long-term outcomes after radical prostatectomy in an equal access health system: Results from the SEARCH database. *Urol. Oncol.* **2019**, *37*, 289.e11–289.e17. [CrossRef] [PubMed]
5. Pagliarulo, V. Androgen Deprivation Therapy for Prostate Cancer. *Adv. Exp. Med. Biol.* **2018**, *1096*, 1–30. [CrossRef] [PubMed]
6. Cookson, M.S.; Aus, G.; Burnett, A.L.; Canby-Hagino, E.D.; D'Amico, A.V.; Dmochowski, R.R.; Eton, D.T.; Forman, J.D.; Goldenberg, S.L.; Hernandez, J. Variation in the definition of biochemical recurrence in patients treated for localized prostate cancer: The American Urological Association Prostate Guidelines for Localized Prostate Cancer Update Panel report and recommendations for a standard in the reporting of surgical outcomes. *J. Urol.* **2007**, *177*, 540–545. [PubMed]
7. Teeter, A.E.; Griffin, K.; Howard, L.E.; Aronson, W.J.; Terris, M.K.; Kane, C.J.; Amling, C.L.; Cooperberg, M.R.; Freedland, S.J. Does Early Prostate Specific Antigen Doubling Time after Radical Prostatectomy, Calculated Prior to Prostate Specific Antigen Recurrence, Correlate with Prostate Cancer Outcomes? A Report from the SEARCH Database Group. *J. Urol.* **2018**, *199*, 713–718. [CrossRef] [PubMed]
8. Wei, J.; Wu, X.; Li, Y.; Tao, X.; Wang, B.; Yin, G. Identification of Potential Predictor of Biochemical Recurrence in Prostate Cancer. *Int. J. Gen. Med.* **2022**, *15*, 4897–4905. [CrossRef]
9. Stamey, T.A.; Freiha, F.S.; McNeal, J.E.; Redwine, E.A.; Whittemore, A.S.; Schmid, H.P. Localized prostate cancer. Relationship of tumor volume to clinical significance for treatment of prostate cancer. *Cancer* **1993**, *71*, 933–938. [CrossRef] [PubMed]
10. Epstein, J.I.; Walsh, P.C.; Carmichael, M.; Brendler, C.B. Pathologic and clinical findings to predict tumor extent of nonpalpable (stage t1 c) prostate cancer. *JAMA* **1994**, *271*, 368–374. [CrossRef] [PubMed]
11. Wolters, T.; Roobol, M.J.; van Leeuwen, P.J.; van den Bergh, R.C.; Hoedemaeker, R.F.; van Leenders, G.J.; Schröder, F.H.; van der Kwast, T.H. A critical analysis of the tumor volume threshold for clinically insignificant prostate cancer using a data set of a randomized screening trial. *J. Urol.* **2011**, *185*, 121–125. [CrossRef]
12. Ploussard, G.; Epstein, J.I.; Montironi, R.; Carroll, P.R.; Wirth, M.; Grimm, M.-O.; Bjartell, A.S.; Montorsi, F.; Freedland, S.J.; Erbersdobler, A. The contemporary concept of significant versus insignificant prostate cancer. *Eur. Urol.* **2011**, *60*, 291–303. [CrossRef]
13. Ito, Y.; Udo, K.; Vertosick, E.A.; Sjoberg, D.D.; Vickers, A.J.; Al-Ahmadie, H.A.; Chen, Y.B.; Gopalan, A.; Sirintrapun, S.J.; Tickoo, S.K.; et al. Clinical Usefulness of Prostate and Tumor Volume Related Parameters following Radical Prostatectomy for Localized Prostate Cancer. *J. Urol.* **2019**, *201*, 535–540. [CrossRef] [PubMed]
14. Ting, F.; van Leeuwen, P.J.; Delprado, W.; Haynes, A.M.; Brenner, P.; Stricker, P.D. Tumor volume in insignificant prostate cancer: Increasing the threshold is a safe approach to reduce over-treatment. *Prostate* **2015**, *75*, 1768–1773. [CrossRef]
15. Fugini, A.V.; Antonelli, A.; Giovanessi, L.; Gardini, V.C.; Abuhilal, M.; Zambolin, T.; Tardanico, R.; Simeone, C.; Cunico, S.C. Insignificant Prostate Cancer: Charateristics and Predictive Factors. *Urol. J.* **2011**, *78*, 184–186. [CrossRef] [PubMed]
16. Antonelli, A.; Vismara Fugini, A.; Tardanico, R.; Giovanessi, L.; Zambolin, T.; Simeone, C. The percentage of core involved by cancer is the best predictor of insignificant prostate cancer, according to an updated definition (tumor volume up to 2.5 cm^3): Analysis of a cohort of 210 consecutive patients with low-risk disease. *Urology* **2014**, *83*, 28–32. [CrossRef]
17. Yamada, Y.; Sakamoto, S.; Sazuka, T.; Goto, Y.; Kawamura, K.; Imamoto, T.; Nihei, N.; Suzuki, H.; Akakura, K.; Ichikawa, T. Validation of active surveillance criteria for pathologically insignificant prostate cancer in Asian men. *Int. J. Urol.* **2016**, *23*, 49–54. [CrossRef] [PubMed]
18. Frankcombe, D.E.; Li, J.; Cohen, R.J. Redefining the Concept of Clinically Insignificant Prostate Cancer. *Urology* **2020**, *136*, 176–179. [CrossRef]
19. Schiffmann, J.; Connan, J.; Salomon, G.; Boehm, K.; Beyer, B.; Schlomm, T.; Tennstedt, P.; Sauter, G.; Karakiewicz, P.I.; Graefen, M.; et al. Tumor volume in insignificant prostate cancer: Increasing threshold gains increasing risk. *Prostate* **2015**, *75*, 45–49. [CrossRef] [PubMed]

20. Wolf, A.M.; Wender, R.C.; Etzioni, R.B.; Thompson, I.M.; D'Amico, A.V.; Volk, R.J.; Brooks, D.D.; Dash, C.; Guessous, I.; Andrews, K.; et al. American Cancer Society guideline for the early detection of prostate cancer: Update 2010. *CA Cancer J. Clin.* **2010**, *60*, 70–98. [CrossRef]
21. Sooriakumaran, P.; Dev, H.S.; Skarecky, D.; Ahlering, T. The importance of surgical margins in prostate cancer. *J. Surg. Oncol.* **2016**, *113*, 310–315. [CrossRef] [PubMed]
22. Matti, B.; Reeves, F.; Prouse, M.; Zargar-Shoshtari, K. The impact of the extent and location of positive surgical margins on the risk of biochemical recurrence following radical prostatectomy in men with Gleason 7 prostate cancers. *Prostate* **2021**, *81*, 1428–1434. [CrossRef]
23. Ploussard, G.; Drouin, S.J.; Rode, J.; Allory, Y.; Vordos, D.; Hoznek, A.; Abbou, C.C.; de la Taille, A.; Salomon, L. Location, extent, and multifocality of positive surgical margins for biochemical recurrence prediction after radical prostatectomy. *World J. Urol.* **2014**, *32*, 1393–1400. [CrossRef] [PubMed]
24. Meeks, J.J.; Eastham, J.A. Radical prostatectomy: Positive surgical margins matter. *Urol. Oncol.* **2013**, *31*, 974–979. [CrossRef] [PubMed]
25. Li, K.; Li, H.; Yang, Y.; Ian, L.H.; Pun, W.H.; Ho, S.F. Risk factors of positive surgical margin and biochemical recurrence of patients treated with radical prostatectomy: A single-center 10-year report. *Chin. Med. J.* **2011**, *124*, 1001–1005. [PubMed]
26. Sammon, J.D.; Trinh, Q.D.; Sukumar, S.; Ravi, P.; Friedman, A.; Sun, M.; Schmitges, J.; Jeldres, C.; Jeong, W.; Mander, N.; et al. Risk factors for biochemical recurrence following radical perineal prostatectomy in a large contemporary series: A detailed assessment of margin extent and location. *Urol. Oncol.* **2013**, *31*, 1470–1476. [CrossRef]
27. Wu, S.; Lin, S.X.; Wirth, G.J.; Lu, M.; Lu, J.; Subtelny, A.O.; Wang, Z.; Dahl, D.M.; Olumi, A.F.; Wu, C.L. Impact of Multifocality and Multilocation of Positive Surgical Margin After Radical Prostatectomy on Predicting Oncological Outcome. *Clin. Genitourin. Cancer* **2019**, *17*, e44–e52. [CrossRef] [PubMed]
28. Eastham, J.A.; Kuroiwa, K.; Ohori, M.; Serio, A.M.; Gorbonos, A.; Maru, N.; Vickers, A.J.; Slawin, K.M.; Wheeler, T.M.; Reuter, V.E.; et al. Prognostic significance of location of positive margins in radical prostatectomy specimens. *Urology* **2007**, *70*, 965–969. [CrossRef] [PubMed]
29. Aydin, H.; Tsuzuki, T.; Hernandez, D.; Walsh, P.C.; Partin, A.W.; Epstein, J.I. Positive proximal (bladder neck) margin at radical prostatectomy confers greater risk of biochemical progression. *Urology* **2004**, *64*, 551–555. [CrossRef] [PubMed]
30. Sooriakumaran, P.; Ploumidis, A.; Nyberg, T.; Olsson, M.; Akre, O.; Haendler, L.; Egevad, L.; Nilsson, A.; Carlsson, S.; Jonsson, M.; et al. The impact of length and location of positive margins in predicting biochemical recurrence after robot-assisted radical prostatectomy with a minimum follow-up of 5 years. *BJU Int.* **2015**, *115*, 106–113. [CrossRef] [PubMed]
31. Shikanov, S.; Song, J.; Royce, C.; Al-Ahmadie, H.; Zorn, K.; Steinberg, G.; Zagaja, G.; Shalhav, A.; Eggener, S. Length of positive surgical margin after radical prostatectomy as a predictor of biochemical recurrence. *J. Urol.* **2009**, *182*, 139–144. [CrossRef] [PubMed]
32. Kang, Y.J.; Abalajon, M.J.; Jang, W.S.; Kwon, J.K.; Yoon, C.Y.; Lee, J.Y.; Cho, K.S.; Ham, W.S.; Choi, Y.D. Association of Anterior and Lateral Extraprostatic Extensions with Base-Positive Resection Margins in Prostate Cancer. *PLoS ONE* **2016**, *11*, e0158922. [CrossRef] [PubMed]
33. Vrang, M.L.; Røder, M.A.; Vainer, B.; Christensen, I.J.; Gruschy, L.; Brasso, K.; Iversen, P. First Danish single-institution experience with radical prostatectomy: Impact of surgical margins on biochemical outcome. *Scand. J. Urol. Nephrol.* **2012**, *46*, 172–179. [CrossRef]
34. You, D.; Jeong, I.G.; Song, C.; Cho, Y.M.; Hong, J.H.; Kim, C.S.; Ahn, H. High percent tumor volume predicts biochemical recurrence after radical prostatectomy in pathological stage T3a prostate cancer with a negative surgical margin. *Int. J. Urol.* **2014**, *21*, 484–489. [CrossRef]
35. De La Roca, R.L.; Da Cunha, I.W.; Bezerra, S.M.; Da Fonseca, F.P. Radical prostatectomy and positive surgical margins: Relationship with prostate cancer outcome. *Int. Braz. J. Urol.* **2014**, *40*, 306–315. [CrossRef]
36. Hashine, K.; Ueno, Y.; Shinomori, K.; Ninomiya, I.; Teramoto, N.; Yamashita, N. Correlation between cancer location and oncological outcome after radical prostatectomy. *Int. J. Urol.* **2012**, *19*, 855–860. [CrossRef] [PubMed]
37. O'Neil, L.M.; Walsh, S.; Cohen, R.J.; Lee, S. Prostate carcinoma with positive margins at radical prostatectomy: Role of tumour zonal origin in biochemical recurrence. *BJU Int.* **2015**, *116* (Suppl. 3), 42–48. [CrossRef] [PubMed]
38. Song, C.; Kang, T.; Yoo, S.; Jeong, I.G.; Ro, J.Y.; Hong, J.H.; Kim, C.S.; Ahn, H. Tumor volume, surgical margin, and the risk of biochemical recurrence in men with organ-confined prostate cancer. *Urol. Oncol.* **2013**, *31*, 168–174. [CrossRef]
39. Shannon, B.A.; McNeal, J.E.; Cohen, R.J. Transition zone carcinoma of the prostate gland: A common indolent tumour type that occasionally manifests aggressive behaviour. *Pathology* **2003**, *35*, 467–471. [CrossRef]
40. Augustin, H.; Hammerer, P.G.; Blonski, J.; Graefen, M.; Palisaar, J.; Daghofer, F.; Huland, H.; Erbersdobler, A. Zonal location of prostate cancer: Significance for disease-free survival after radical prostatectomy? *Urology* **2003**, *62*, 79–85. [CrossRef]
41. Ali, A.; Du Feu, A.; Oliveira, P.; Choudhury, A.; Bristow, R.G.; Baena, E. Prostate zones and cancer: Lost in transition? *Nat. Rev. Urol.* **2022**, *19*, 101–115. [CrossRef] [PubMed]
42. Magheli, A.; Rais-Bahrami, S.; Peck, H.J.; Walsh, P.C.; Epstein, J.I.; Trock, B.J.; Gonzalgo, M.L. Importance of tumor location in patients with high preoperative prostate specific antigen levels (greater than 20 ng/ml) treated with radical prostatectomy. *J. Urol.* **2007**, *178*, 1311–1315. [CrossRef] [PubMed]

43. Hayee, A.; Lugo, I.; Iakymenko, O.A.; Kwon, D.; Briski, L.M.; Zhao, W.; Nemov, I.; Punnen, S.; Ritch, C.R.; Pollack, A.; et al. Anterior or Posterior Prostate Cancer Tumor Nodule Location Predicts Likelihood of Certain Adverse Outcomes at Radical Prostatectomy. *Arch. Pathol. Lab. Med.* **2022**, *146*, 833–839. [CrossRef]
44. Mygatt, J.G.; Cullen, J.; Streicher, S.A.; Kuo, H.C.; Chen, Y.; Young, D.; Gesztes, W.; Williams, G.; Conti, G.; Porter, C.; et al. Race, tumor location, and disease progression among low-risk prostate cancer patients. *Cancer Med.* **2020**, *9*, 2235–2242. [CrossRef]
45. Augustin, H.; Erbersdobler, A.; Graefen, M.; Fernandez, S.; Palisaar, J.; Huland, H.; Hammerer, P. Biochemical recurrence following radical prostatectomy: A comparison between prostate cancers located in different anatomical zones. *Prostate* **2003**, *55*, 48–54. [CrossRef]
46. Meng, Y.; Li, H.; Xu, P.; Wang, J. Do tumor volume, percent tumor volume predict biochemical recurrence after radical prostatectomy? A meta-analysis. *Int. J. Clin. Exp. Med.* **2015**, *8*, 22319–22327.
47. Kim, K.H.; Lim, S.K.; Shin, T.Y.; Kang, D.R.; Han, W.K.; Chung, B.H.; Rha, K.H.; Hong, S.J. Tumor volume adds prognostic value in patients with organ-confined prostate cancer. *Ann. Surg. Oncol.* **2013**, *20*, 3133–3139. [CrossRef] [PubMed]
48. Thompson, I.M., III; Salem, S.; Chang, S.S.; Clark, P.E.; Davis, R.; Herrell, S.D.; Kordan, Y.; Baumgartner, R.; Phillips, S.; Smith, J.A., Jr.; et al. Tumor volume as a predictor of adverse pathologic features and biochemical recurrence (BCR) in radical prostatectomy specimens: A tale of two methods. *World J. Urol.* **2011**, *29*, 15–20. [CrossRef]
49. Yuk, H.D.; Byun, S.S.; Hong, S.K.; Lee, H. The tumor volume after radical prostatectomy and its clinical impact on the prognosis of patients with localized prostate cancer. *Sci. Rep.* **2022**, *12*, 6003. [CrossRef]
50. Ates, M.; Teber, D.; Gözen, A.S.; Tefekli, A.; Sugiono, M.; Hruza, M.; Rassweiler, J. Do tumor volume, tumor volume ratio, type of nerve sparing and surgical experience affect prostate specific antigen recurrence after laparoscopic radical prostatectomy? A matched pair analysis. *J. Urol.* **2007**, *177*, 1771–1775; discussion 1775–1776. [CrossRef] [PubMed]
51. Hashimoto, Y.; Okamoto, A.; Imai, A.; Yoneyama, T.; Hatakeyama, S.; Yoneyama, T.; Koie, T.; Kaminura, N.; Ohyama, C. Biochemical outcome of small-volume or insignificant prostate cancer treated with radical prostatectomy in Japanese population. *Int. J. Clin. Oncol.* **2012**, *17*, 119–123. [CrossRef]
52. Furusato, B.; Rosner, I.L.; Osborn, D.; Ali, A.; Srivastava, S.; Davis, C.J.; Sesterhenn, I.A.; McLeod, D.G. Do patients with low volume prostate cancer have prostate specific antigen recurrence following radical prostatectomy? *J. Clin. Pathol.* **2008**, *61*, 1038–1040. [CrossRef]
53. Lee, D.H.; Koo, K.C.; Lee, S.H.; Rha, K.H.; Choi, Y.D.; Hong, S.J.; Chung, B.H. Analysis of different tumor volume thresholds of insignificant prostate cancer and their implications for active surveillance patient selection and monitoring. *Prostate Int.* **2014**, *2*, 76–81. [CrossRef] [PubMed]
54. Chung, B.I.; Tarin, T.V.; Ferrari, M.; Brooks, J.D. Comparison of prostate cancer tumor volume and percent cancer in prediction of biochemical recurrence and cancer specific survival. *Urol. Oncol.* **2011**, *29*, 314–318. [CrossRef]
55. Friedersdorff, F.; Groß, B.; Maxeiner, A.; Jung, K.; Miller, K.; Stephan, C.; Busch, J.; Kilic, E. Does the Prostate Health Index Depend on Tumor Volume?-A Study on 196 Patients after Radical Prostatectomy. *Int. J. Mol. Sci.* **2017**, *18*, 488. [CrossRef] [PubMed]
56. Shin, S.J.; Park, C.K.; Park, S.Y.; Jang, W.S.; Lee, J.Y.; Choi, Y.D.; Cho, N.H. Total intraglandular and index tumor volumes predict biochemical recurrence in prostate cancer. *Virchows Arch.* **2016**, *469*, 305–312. [CrossRef] [PubMed]
57. Miyake, H.; Sakai, I.; Harada, K.; Takechi, Y.; Hara, I.; Eto, H. Prognostic significance of the tumor volume in radical prostatectomy specimens after neoadjuvant hormonal therapy. *Urol. Int.* **2005**, *74*, 27–31. [CrossRef] [PubMed]
58. Raison, N.; Servian, P.; Patel, A.; Santhirasekaram, A.; Smith, A.; Yeung, M.; Lloyd, J.; Mannion, E.; Rockall, A.; Ahmed, H.; et al. Is tumour volume an independent predictor of outcome after radical prostatectomy for high-risk prostate cancer? *Prostate Cancer Prostatic Dis.* **2021**, 1–5. [CrossRef]
59. Salomon, L.; Levrel, O.; Anastasiadis, A.G.; Irani, J.; De La Taille, A.; Saint, F.; Vordos, D.; Cicco, A.; Hoznek, A.; Chopin, D.; et al. Prognostic significance of tumor volume after radical prostatectomy: A multivariate analysis of pathological prognostic factors. *Eur. Urol.* **2003**, *43*, 39–44. [CrossRef]
60. Akaza, H.; Onozawa, M.; Hinotsu, S. Prostate cancer trends in Asia. *World J. Urol.* **2017**, *35*, 859–865. [CrossRef] [PubMed]
61. Fuletra, J.G.; Kamenko, A.; Ramsey, F.; Eun, D.D.; Reese, A.C. African-American men with prostate cancer have larger tumor volume than Caucasian men despite no difference in serum prostate specific antigen. *Can. J. Urol.* **2018**, *25*, 9193–9198.
62. Gupta, K.; Mehrotra, V.; Fu, P.; Scarberry, K.; MacLennan, G.T.; Gupta, S. Racial disparities in biochemical recurrence of prostate cancer. *Am. J. Clin. Exp. Urol.* **2022**, *10*, 266–270. [PubMed]
63. Reinhardt, D.; Helfand, B.T.; Cooper, P.R.; Roehl, K.A.; Catalona, W.J.; Loeb, S. Prostate cancer risk alleles are associated with prostate cancer volume and prostate size. *J. Urol.* **2014**, *191*, 1733–1736. [CrossRef] [PubMed]
64. Helfand, B.T.; Paterakos, M.; Wang, C.H.; Talaty, P.; Abran, J.; Bennett, J.; Hall, D.W.; Lehman, A.; Aboushwareb, T. The 17-gene Genomic Prostate Score assay as a predictor of biochemical recurrence in men with intermediate and high-risk prostate cancer. *PLoS ONE* **2022**, *17*, e0273782. [CrossRef]
65. Santos, A.; Mattiolli, A.; Carvalheira, J.B.; Ferreira, U.; Camacho, M.; Silva, C.; Costa, F.; Matheus, W.; Lima, M.; Etchebehere, E. PSMA whole-body tumor burden in primary staging and biochemical recurrence of prostate cancer. *Eur. J. Nucl. Med. Mol. Imaging* **2021**, *48*, 493–500. [CrossRef]
66. Pinckaers, H.; van Ipenburg, J.; Melamed, J.; De Marzo, A.; Platz, E.A.; van Ginneken, B.; van der Laak, J.; Litjens, G. Predicting biochemical recurrence of prostate cancer with artificial intelligence. *Commun. Med.* **2022**, *2*, 64. [CrossRef] [PubMed]

cancers

MDPI

Article

Prognostic Impact of Lymphatic Invasion in Patients with High-Risk Prostate Cancer after Robot-Assisted Radical Prostatectomy and Extended Lymph Node Dissection: A Single-Institution Prospective Cohort Study

Shimpei Yamashita, Satoshi Muraoka, Takahito Wakamiya, Kazuro Kikkawa, Yasuo Kohjimoto * and Isao Hara

Department of Urology, Wakayama Medical University, 811-1 Kimiidera, Wakayama 641-0012, Japan; keito608@wakayama-med.ac.jp (S.Y.); muraoka@wakayama-med.ac.jp (S.M.); wakataka@wakayama-med.ac.jp (T.W.); kzro@wakayama-med.ac.jp (K.K.); hara@wakayama-med.ac.jp (I.H.)

* Correspondence: ykohji@wakayama-med.ac.jp

Simple Summary: The aim of our prospective cohort study was to assess the impact of lymphatic invasion on biochemical recurrence (BCR) in patients who underwent robot-assisted radical prostatectomy (RARP) and extended lymph node dissection (eLND) for high-risk prostate cancer (PC). Of 183 patients, lymphatic invasion and lymph node metastasis were observed in 47 (26%) and 17 patients (9%), respectively, whereas BCR was observed in 48 patients (26%). The BCR rate was significantly higher in patients with lymphatic invasion than in patients without lymphatic invasion. Moreover, according to multivariable analyses, lymphatic invasion was an independent significant predictor of BCR in the overall patient group and in patients without lymph node metastasis. Evaluation of lymphatic invasion could therefore be a useful predictor of BCR in patients who have undergone RARP and eLND for high-risk PC.

Abstract: The prognostic impact of lymphatic invasion in patients with high-risk prostate cancer (PC) remains unclear. The aim of our single-institution prospective cohort study was to examine the impact of lymphatic invasion on biochemical recurrence (BCR) in patients with high-risk PC according to National Comprehensive Cancer Network (NCCN) criteria who underwent robot-assisted radical prostatectomy (RARP) and extended lymph node dissection (eLND). A total of 183 patients were included who underwent RARP and eLND for NCCN high-risk PC between June 2014 and August 2019. Lymphatic invasion in resected specimens was observed in 47 patients (26%), whereas lymph node metastasis was observed in 17 patients (9%). During follow-up, BCR was observed in 48 patients (26%). The BCR rate in patients with lymphatic invasion was significantly higher than that in patients without lymphatic invasion ($p < 0.01$). According to multivariable Cox proportional hazards regression analyses, lymphatic invasion was a significant independent predictor of BCR in the overall patient group and was independently associated with BCR, even in patients without lymph node metastasis. In conclusion, evaluation of lymphatic invasion could be useful in predicting BCR in patients undergoing RARP and eLND for high-risk PC.

Keywords: prostate cancer; lymphatic invasion; biochemical recurrence; robot-assisted radical prostatectomy

Citation: Yamashita, S.; Muraoka, S.; Wakamiya, T.; Kikkawa, K.; Kohjimoto, Y.; Hara, I. Prognostic Impact of Lymphatic Invasion in Patients with High-Risk Prostate Cancer after Robot-Assisted Radical Prostatectomy and Extended Lymph Node Dissection: A Single-Institution Prospective Cohort Study. *Cancers* **2022**, *14*, 3466. https://doi.org/10.3390/cancers14143466

Academic Editor: Kouji Izumi

Received: 7 June 2022
Accepted: 15 July 2022
Published: 17 July 2022

1. Introduction

Prostate cancer is the second most common cause of tumors and the fifth leading cause of cancer mortality [1]. Radical prostatectomy is a standard treatment method for localized prostate cancer (PC) and has been shown to have cancer-specific survival benefits compared with watchful waiting [2]. Robot-assisted radical prostatectomy (RARP) has become a preferred treatment choice for localized PC as an alternative to open radical prostatectomy (ORP) or laparoscopic radical prostatectomy (LRP) [3]. Advantages of this treatment include shallow learning curves, low blood loss, low transfusion rate and short hospitalization duration [4,5]. Additionally, the oncological and functional outcomes of RARP are equivalent to those of ORP or LRP [4].

Despite the therapeutic efficacy of radical prostatectomy for localized PC, biochemical recurrence (BCR) has been reported in 10–25% of patients within five years after radical prostatectomy [6–11]. BCR could lead to the development of clinical metastases and cancer mortality with a median duration of 8 years from BCR to metastases and 5 years from metastases to death [12]. The National Comprehensive Cancer Network (NCCN) risk classification is a representative risk classification that is used clinically for decisions with respect to treatment policies [13]. In a recent study, five- and eight-year BCR-free rates in patients who underwent radical prostatectomy and pelvic lymph node dissection for NCCN high-risk PC were 47.8% and 39.6%, respectively [13].

Although attention should be paid to BCR after radical prostatectomy, especially in patients with high-risk PC, the risk of BCR may vary depending on histopathological findings of resected prostate specimens. Several risk factors, including extracapsular spread and positive surgical margin, are traditionally considered with respect to BCR after radical prostatectomy [14]. Moreover, lymph node metastasis has been reported to be a significant predictor of unfavorable postoperative progress, including BCR and cancer death [15–17]. Despite recent advances in imaging technologies, pelvic lymph node dissection remains the gold-standard technique for lymph node staging [18]. The direct therapeutic effect of lymph node dissection remains unclear, but it is generally accepted that extended lymph node dissection (eLND) provides appropriate prognostic information to assist with follow-up after surgery [19,20]. On the other hand, the presence of microlymphatic invasion in resected prostate specimens could be a useful predictor of BCR after surgery [14,21]. However, evidence of the prognostic impact of microlymphatic invasion is still limited, and, to the best of our knowledge, its predictive power for BCR in patients who have undergone radical prostatectomy and eLND for high-risk PC remains unclear. The aim of this prospective cohort study was to examine the association between microlymphatic invasion and postoperative BCR in patients who underwent RARP with eLND for NCCN high-risk PC.

2. Materials and Methods

This single-institutional prospective cohort study includes the 183 consecutive patients with NCCN high-risk PC who underwent RARP with eLND between June 2014 and August 2019. According to the NCCN guidelines, patients with high-risk PC are those with at least one of the following factors: clinical T stage 3a, maximum biopsy Gleason score of 8–10 and initial serum prostate serum antigen (PSA) >20 ng/mL [13]. The study was approved by the Wakayama Medical University Hospital Institutional Review Board (approval number 1670), and informed consent was preoperatively obtained from all subjects involved in the study.

We prospectively recorded preoperative patient backgrounds, including age, body mass index (BMI), smoking history, initial serum PSA, PSA density, maximum biopsy Gleason score, number of biopsy-positive cores and clinical stage. Initial serum PSA was defined as the PSA value just before prostate biopsy. PSA density was calculated by dividing the initial serum PSA by the prostate volume based on ultrasound examination. We also postoperatively recorded histopathological findings of resected specimens, including maximum Gleason score, pathological T stage, extraprostatic extension (EPE), seminal vesicle invasion (sv), lymphatic invasion (ly), venous invasion (v), resected margin (RM) and pathological N stage. Postoperative serum PSA value was evaluated and recorded every three months in the two years after surgery and every six months thereafter. BCR was defined as elevation of postoperative PSA > 0.20 ng/mL. If postoperative PSA was not reduced to <0.2 ng/mL, the operation date was taken as the recurrence date.

Three surgeons (I.H., Y.K. and K.K.), who are all experienced and skilled at ORP, LRP and RARP, performed RARP using a standard six-port, transperitoneal technique, employing the da Vinci Si system or da Vinci Xi system (Intuitive Surgical Inc., Sunnyvale, CA, USA) [22,23]. Our eLND template consisted of common iliac up to the ureteric crossing, external and internal iliac and obturator. eLND was performed, followed by cutting of the endopelvic fascia, transection of the bladder neck and dissection of the seminal vesicle and the prostate in an antegrade fashion. Nerve sparing was performed on the side, which met the following requirements according to the policies of our department: (1) non-detection of tumor by digital rectal examination, (2) no observation of disease lesion in the peripheral zone by magnetic resonance imaging and (3) two or fewer positive biopsy cores. After posterior musculofascial reconstruction and periurethral suspension stitching, vesicourethral anastomosis was performed with a running barbed suture. Resected specimens, including prostate and lymph nodes, were evaluated by two genitourinary pathologists, both of whom have more than 10 years of experience.

All statistical analyses were performed using JMP Pro 14, (SAS Institute Inc., Cary, NC, USA). Chi-square test and Mann-Whitney U test were used to compare patient demographics and histopathological findings of resected specimens between patients with ly0 and those with ly1. The Kaplan–Meier method and log-rank test were used to estimate the BCR rate and to compare the rates between groups. By using Cox proportional hazards regression analyses, univariable analyses and two models of multivariable analyses were performed to identify predictors of BCR. In model 1, Gleason-grade group of resected specimens, pathological T stage, RM, venous invasion (v) and pathological N stage were selected as predictors. In model 2, lymphatic invasion (ly) was used as a predictor in place of pathological N stage.

3. Results

3.1. Patient Demographics and Histopathological Findings of Resected Specimens

Preoperative patient demographics are summarized in Table 1. The median age was 69 years (quartile: 66–72 years). The median initial PSA was 10.9 ng/mL (quartile: 7.5–17.1 ng/mL). The biopsy Gleason-grade group was 4 in 110 patients (60%) and 5 in 42 patients (23%). Clinical T stage was T3 in 42 patients (23%).

Table 1. Summary of preoperative patient demographics.

Age, years	69 (66–72) [1]
BMI, kg/m^2	24.1 (22.0–26.2) [1]
Smoking history, *n* (%)	120 (66)
PSA, ng/mL	10.9 (7.5–17.1) [1]
PSA density	0.43 (0.26–0.67) [1]
Biopsy Gleason-grade group, *n* (%)	
1	4 (2)
2	10 (6)
3	17 (9)
4	110 (60)
5	42 (23)
Clinical T stage, *n* (%)	
T1c	16 (9)
T2	125 (68)
T3	42 (23)

[1] Continuous variables are shown in median (quartile) form.

Lymphatic invasion in the resected specimen was observed in 47 patients (26%). Table 2 shows a comparison of patient demographics and histopathological finding of resected specimens between patients with lymphatic invasion (ly1 group, *n* = 47) and without lymphatic invasion (ly0 group, *n* = 136). There was no significant difference in initial PSA, but the distribution of Gleason-grade group and pathological T stage was significantly different between the groups ($p < 0.01$ and $p < 0.01$, respectively), and the proportions of high Gleason grade and advanced pathological T stage in the ly1 group were higher than those in the ly0 group. Moreover, the percentages of EPE1, sv1,v1 and RM1 in the ly1 group were also higher than those in the ly0 group ($p < 0.01$, $p < 0.01$, $p < 0.01$ and $p < 0.01$, respectively). The median number of dissected lymph nodes was 21 (quartile: 14–28), and the percentage of nodal metastasis (pN1) in the ly1 group was higher than that in the ly0 group (26% vs. 4%, $p < 0.01$). Lymphatic invasion was observed in 35 patients (21%) in the pN0 group and 12 patients (71%) in the pN1 group ($p < 0.01$).

Table 2. Comparison of patient demographics and histopathological findings of resected specimens between the ly0 and ly1 groups.

	ly0 Group (*n* = 136)	ly1 Group (*n* = 47)	*p* Value
Age, years [1]	69 (65–72)	69 (66–72)	0.94
PSA, mg/dL [1]	10.3 (7.0–17.0)	11.9 (8.6–17.6)	0.22
PSA density [1]	0.42 (0.25–0.66)	0.47 (0.30–0.74)	0.28
Gleason-grade group, *n* (%)			<0.01
2	38 (28)	6 (13)	
3	59 (44)	17 (36)	
4	12 (9)	5 (11)	
5	26 (19)	19 (40)	
Pathological T stage, *n* (%)			<0.01
pT2	74 (54)	12 (26)	
pT3a	49 (36)	16 (34)	
pT3b	13 (10)	19 (40)	
EPE1, *n* (%)	58 (43)	31 (66)	<0.01
sv1, *n* (%)	13 (10)	19 (40)	<0.01
v1, *n* (%)	3 (2)	8 (17)	<0.01
RM1, *n* (%)	31 (23)	20 (43)	<0.01
pN1, *n* (%)	5 (4)	12 (26)	<0.01

[1] Continuous variables are shown in median (quartile) form.

3.2. BCR Rates

The median postoperative follow-up period was 20 months (quartile: 10–34 months). During the follow-up period, BCR was observed in 48 patients (26%), and 1-year, 2-year and 3-year BCR rates were 18.0%, 27.5% and 32.6%, respectively.

A comparison of BCR rates according to the presence of nodal metastasis (pathological N0 vs. N1) and lymphatic invasion (ly0 vs. ly1) is shown in Figure 1. The BCR rate in the pN1 group was significantly higher than that in the pN0 group ($p < 0.01$) (Figure 1A). Moreover, the BCR rate in the ly1 group was significantly higher than that in the ly0 group (Figure 1B) ($p < 0.01$).

A comparison of BCR rates according to the combination of nodal metastasis and lymphatic invasion is shown in Figure 2. The BCR rates were significantly different among the groups ($p < 0.01$). The BCR rate in the pN1/ly0 and pN1/ly1 groups was higher than that in the pN0/ly0 group. The BCR rate in the pN0/ly1 group was also higher than that in the pN0/ly0 group.

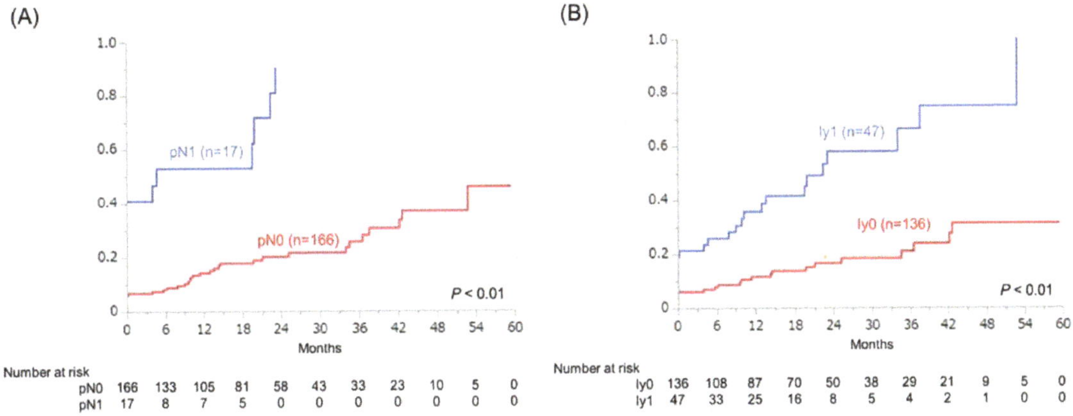

Figure 1. Kaplan–Meier analyses of BCR rates according to the presence of (**A**) nodal metastasis and (**B**) lymphatic invasion.

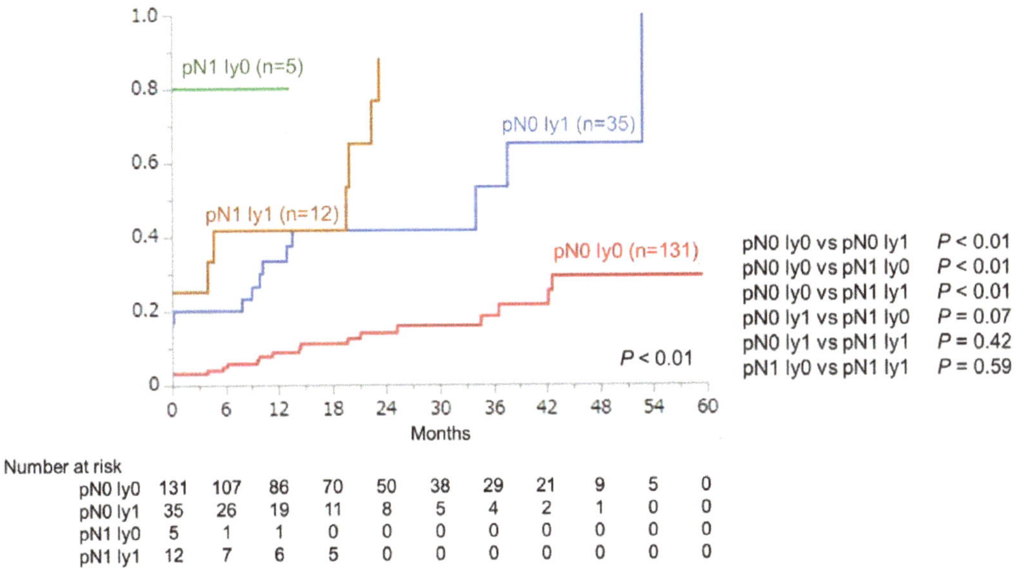

Figure 2. Kaplan–Meier analyses of BCR rates according to the combination of nodal metastasis and lymphatic invasion.

3.3. Predictive Value of Lymphatic Invasion for BCR

The results of univariable analyses and two models of multivariable analyses of associations between predictive factors and BCR in overall patients are shown in Table 3. In model 1, significant independent predictors of BCR were venous invasion (v1), resected margin-positive (RM1) and nodal metastasis (pN1). In model 2, venous invasion (v1) and lymphatic invasion (ly1) were significant independent predictors of BCR.

Table 3. Univariable and multivariable analyses of associations between various parameters and BCR in the overall patient group.

Univariable Analyses				Multivariable Analyses					
				Model 1			Model 2		
	HR	95% CI	*p* Value	HR	95% CI	*p* Value	HR	95% CI	*p* Value
Age, years	0.98	0.93–1.03	0.41						
PSA, ng/mL	1.02	0.98–1.05	0.18						
PSA density	1.22	0.57–2.36	0.57						
Gleason-grade groups 4–5 (vs. 2–3)	2.48	1.40–4.39	<0.01	1.70	0.90–3.18	0.09	1.81	0.97–3.38	0.06
pT3 (vs. pT2)	3.13	1.62–6.02	<0.01	1.95	0.96–3.96	0.06	1.94	0.96–3.89	0.06
v1 (vs. v0)	5.57	2.67–11.61	<0.01	2.73	1.19–6.24	0.01	2.58	1.13–5.84	0.02
RM1 (vs. RM0)	2.17	1.22–3.86	<0.01	1.92	1.06–3.48	0.03	1.70	0.93–3.10	0.08
pN1 (vs. pN0)	6.34	3.24–12.36	<0.01	2.73	1.29–5.75	<0.01			
ly1 (vs. ly0)	4.11	2.67–11.61	<0.01				2.33	1.22–4.42	0.01

The results of multivariable Cox proportional regression analyses of associations between predictive factors and BCR in only patients with pN0 are shown in Table 4. For patients without nodal metastasis, lymphatic invasion (ly1) was a significant independent predictor of BCR, as well as venous invasion (v1).

Table 4. Multivariable analyses of associations between various parameters and BCR only in patients with pN0.

	HR	95% CI	*p* Value
Gleason-grade groups 4–5 (vs. 2–3)	2.03	0.99–4.11	0.05
pT3 (vs. pT2)	1.75	0.82–3.67	0.14
RM1 (vs. RM0)	1.93	0.95–3.91	0.06
v1 (vs. v0)	4.10	1.50–11.19	<0.01
ly1 (vs. ly0)	2.59	1.25–5.32	0.01

4. Discussion

In this prospective cohort study, we evaluated the association between microlymphatic invasion and postoperative BCR in patients who underwent RARP with eLND for NCCN high-risk PC. Lymphatic invasion was shown to be independently associated with BCR both in the overall patient group and in patients without lymph node metastasis. Although several previous studies have focused on the prognostic impact of microlymphatic invasion in patients who underwent radical prostatectomy, to the best of our knowledge, there has been no investigation into the impact in patients who underwent eLND and radical prostatectomy [14,21]. Moreover, the prognostic impact of microlymphatic invasion has not been properly evaluated in a prospective study. Therefore, this is the first study to prospectively examine the association between microlymphatic invasion and postoperative BCR in patients who underwent RARP with eLND.

Lymph node metastasis is known to be one of the most important prognostic factors and is associated with a high BCR rate and high risk of death from PC [15–17]. The direct therapeutic effect of lymph node dissection remains controversial. eLND may reduce the BCR rate and improve survival [11,16,24,25]. However, a recent systematic review showed that there was inadequate evidence of a direct therapeutic effect of eLND [19]. Moreover, in two recent randomized, controlled trials, no significant difference was observed in oncological outcomes, including BCR rate, between the limited lymph dissection group and the eLND group [20,26]. eLND could still have a therapeutic effect in certain patients with high-risk PC, and large-scale studies are expected [20,27,28]. On the other hand, another role of lymph node dissection is to provide exact pathological information about lymph node metastasis. The pathological diagnosis of lymph node metastasis offers appropriate prognostic information and assists with follow-up after surgery. eLND for high-risk PC could improve pathological staging and remove more metastatic lymph nodes compared to limited lymph node dissection [29]. Moreover, a recent randomized, controlled trial showed that eLND for intermediate and high-risk PC achieved improved pathological staging [20]. Performance of eLND for optimal staging in patients who require lymph node dissection has therefore been widely accepted. Although selection criteria for patients who require eLND have not yet been established, it is often practically performed in patients who are strongly suspected to have lymph node metastasis according to various nomograms or intermediate- and/or high-risk patients as classified by D'Amico risk stratification or NCCN risk stratification [30–34]. In the present study, we performed eLND, as well as RARP, in patients with NCCN high-risk PC.

In addition to traditional risk factors, including lymph node metastases, lymphovascular invasion (LVI) in prostate specimens has been widely reported to have a prognostic impact in patients who underwent radical prostatectomy. LVI is recommended as part of the standard examination of radical prostatectomy specimens by the International Society of Urological Pathology and defined as the presence of tumor cells in the endothelium-lined space [35]. In previous systematic reviews, LVI was suggested to be associated with a higher risk of BCR in patients who have undergone radical prostatectomy [35,36]. On the other hand, several recent studies evaluated lymphatic invasion separately from vascular invasion and investigated the prognostic impact of microlymphatic invasion. In a study that included 299 radical prostatectomy cases, Okubo et al. showed that lymphatic invasion was independently associated with lymph node metastasis, whereas venous invasion was not. They recommended that lymphatic and venous invasion should be evaluated separately rather than being combined into the category of LVI [37]. Wilczak et al. retrospectively analyzed pathological and clinical data from 14,528 consecutive patients who underwent radical prostatectomy and examined of the prognostic value of lymphatic invasion [21]. They concluded that evaluation of lymphatic invasion could provide comparable prognostic information to that of lymph node analysis. However, the study included a combination of patients who did and did not undergo lymph node dissection. Hashimoto et al. retrospectively reviewed 1096 patients with pT2 PC and RM negativity and investigated predictors for BCR after RARP [14]. Microlymphatic invasion was found to be an independent predictor of BCR, whereas microvascular invasion was not. However, their study also included patients who both did and did not undergo lymph node dissection.

In the present study, we prospectively evaluated the prognostic impact of microlymphatic invasion in patients who underwent RARP and eLND for high-risk PC. In our cohort, venous invasion and lymphatic invasion were observed in 11 and 47 patients, respectively. As shown in Tables 3 and 4, whereas venous invasion was also related to BCR, lymphatic invasion was significantly associated with BCR independently of venous invasion. The association between lymph node metastasis and lymphatic invasion is summarized in Table 5. Lymph node metastasis (pN1) was observed in 17 patients in our cohort (9%) and was significantly associated with BCR after RARP. Moreover, lymph node metastasis was found to be an independent predictor of BCR. These results are consistent with those of previous studies. On the other hand, microlymphatic invasion (ly1) was observed in 12 patients with pN1 and 35 patients with pN0. Five patients with ly0 (5/136, 3.7%) had lymph node metastasis. Wilczan et al. reported that 4.3% of patients with ly0 had lymph node metastasis [21]. These discrepancies are considered to be due to microlymphatic invasion being overlooked. Complete detection of microlymphatic invasion is difficult, even with immunohistochemical staining by endothelial markers. eLND is therefore considered to have a diagnostic role in patients with high-risk PC. However, microlymphatic invasion was also found to be an independent predictor of BCR both in the overall patient group and in patients without lymph node metastasis. Thirty-five patients with pN0 (35/166, 21%) had microlymphatic invasion in our cohort. Although the possibility cannot be ruled out that lymph node metastasis was overlooked because of a technical problem associated with eLND or pathological evaluation in some of these patients, we consider microlymphatic invasion to be a premonitory finding of lymph node metastasis and a useful predictor of BCR in patients who underwent RARP and eLND for high-risk PC.

Table 5. Association between lymph node metastasis (pN) and microlymphatic invasion (ly).

		Lymph Node Metastasis, *n*		
		pN0	**pN1**	**Total**
Micro-lymphatic invasion, *n*	ly0	131	5	136
	ly1	35	12	47
	Total	166	17	183

The current study is subject to several limitations. First, despite the advantage of being a prospective study, the sample was relatively small because the subjects were limited to patients who underwent RARP and eLND for high-risk PC. Second, the follow-up period after surgery was relatively short. Nonetheless, we believe that our study provides important insights into BCR after RARP and eLND for high-risk PC. To overcome these limitations and verify our results, a further large-scale prospective study with a long follow-up period is required.

5. Conclusions

Lymphatic invasion was shown to be a significant independent predictor of BCR after RARP and eLND in patients with high-risk PC. Even in patients without lymph node metastasis, lymphatic invasion was independently associated with BCR. Evaluation of lymphatic invasion could be useful for predicting BCR in patients who have undergone RARP and eLND for high-risk PC.

Author Contributions: Conceptualization, S.Y. and Y.K.; methodology, Y.K.; data curation, S.M., T.W. and K.K.; writing—original draft preparation, S.Y.; writing—review and editing, S.Y.; supervision, Y.K. and I.H. All authors have read and agreed to the published version of the manuscript.

Funding: This research received no external funding.

Institutional Review Board Statement: The study was conducted in accordance with the Declaration of Helsinki and approved by the Wakayama Medical University Institutional Review Board (approval number 1670).

Informed Consent Statement: Informed consent was obtained from all subjects involved in the study.

Data Availability Statement: Not applicable.

Acknowledgments: This document was proofread and edited by Benjamin Phillis at the Clinical Study Support Center, Wakayama Medical University.

Conflicts of Interest: The authors declare no conflict of interest.

References

1. Ferlay, J.; Colombet, M.; Soerjomataram, I.; Mathers, C.; Parkin, D.M.; Piñeros, M.; Znaor, A.; Bray, F. Estimating the global cancer incidence and mortality in 2018: GLOBOCAN sources and methods. *Int. J. Cancer* **2019**, *144*, 1941–1953. [CrossRef] [PubMed]
2. Bill-Axelson, A.; Holmberg, L.; Ruutu, M.; Garmo, H.; Stark, J.R.; Busch, C.; Nordling, S.; Häggman, M.; Andersson, S.O.; Bratell, S.; et al. Radical prostatectomy versus watchful waiting in early prostate cancer. *N. Engl. J. Med.* **2011**, *364*, 1708–1717. [CrossRef] [PubMed]
3. Robertson, C.; Close, A.; Fraser, C.; Gurung, T.; Jia, X.; Sharma, P.; Vale, L.; Ramsay, C.; Pickard, R. Relative effectiveness of robot-assisted and standard laparoscopic prostatectomy as alternatives to open radical prostatectomy for treatment of localised prostate cancer: A systematic review and mixed treatment comparison meta-analysis. *BJU Int.* **2013**, *112*, 798–812. [CrossRef]
4. Cao, L.; Yang, Z.; Qi, L.; Chen, M. Robot-assisted and laparoscopic vs. open radical prostatectomy in clinically localized prostate cancer: Perioperative, functional, and oncological outcomes: A Systematic review and meta-analysis. *Medicine* **2019**, *98*, e15770. [CrossRef]

5. Grivas, N.; Zachos, I.; Georgiadis, G.; Karavitakis, M.; Tzortzis, V.; Mamoulakis, C. Learning curves in laparoscopic and robot-assisted prostate surgery: A systematic search and review. *World J. Urol.* **2021**, *40*, 929–949. [CrossRef] [PubMed]
6. Novara, G.; Ficarra, V.; Mocellin, S.; Ahlering, T.E.; Carroll, P.R.; Graefen, M.; Guazzoni, G.; Menon, M.; Patel, V.R.; Shariat, S.F.; et al. Systematic review and meta-analysis of studies reporting oncologic outcome after robot-assisted radical prostatectomy. *Eur. Urol.* **2012**, *62*, 382–404. [CrossRef] [PubMed]
7. Liss, M.A.; Lusch, A.; Morales, B.; Beheshti, N.; Skarecky, D.; Narula, N.; Osann, K.; Ahlering, T.E. Robot-assisted radical prostatectomy: 5-year oncological and biochemical outcomes. *J. Urol.* **2012**, *188*, 2205–2210. [CrossRef]
8. Sooriakumaran, P.; Haendler, L.; Nyberg, T.; Gronberg, H.; Nilsson, A.; Carlsson, S.; Hosseini, A.; Adding, C.; Jonsson, M.; Ploumidis, A.; et al. Biochemical recurrence after robot-assisted radical prostatectomy in a European single-centre cohort with a minimum follow-up time of 5 years. *Eur. Urol.* **2012**, *62*, 768–774. [CrossRef]
9. Suardi, N.; Ficarra, V.; Willemsen, P.; De Wil, P.; Gallina, A.; De Naeyer, G.; Schatteman, P.; Montorsi, F.; Carpentier, P.; Mottrie, A. Long-term biochemical recurrence rates after robot-assisted radical prostatectomy: Analysis of a single-center series of patients with a minimum follow-up of 5 years. *Urology* **2012**, *79*, 133–138. [CrossRef]
10. Sukumar, S.; Rogers, C.G.; Trinh, Q.D.; Sammon, J.; Sood, A.; Stricker, H.; Peabody, J.O.; Menon, M.; Diaz-Insua, M. Oncological outcomes after robot-assisted radical prostatectomy: Long-term follow-up in 4803 patients. *BJU Int.* **2014**, *114*, 824–831. [CrossRef]
11. Abdollah, F.; Dalela, D.; Sood, A.; Sammon, J.; Jeong, W.; Beyer, B.; Fossati, N.; Rogers, C.G.; Diaz-Insua, M.; Peabody, J.; et al. Intermediate-term cancer control outcomes in prostate cancer patients treated with robotic-assisted laparoscopic radical prostatectomy: A multi-institutional analysis. *World J. Urol.* **2016**, *34*, 1357–1366. [CrossRef] [PubMed]
12. Pound, C.R.; Partin, A.W.; Eisenberger, M.A.; Chan, D.W.; Pearson, J.D.; Walsh, P.C. Natural history of progression after PSA elevation following radical prostatectomy. *JAMA* **1999**, *281*, 1591–1597. [CrossRef] [PubMed]
13. Pompe, R.S.; Karakiewicz, P.I.; Tian, Z.; Mandel, P.; Steuber, T.; Schlomm, T.; Salomon, G.; Graefen, M.; Huland, H.; Tilki, D. Oncologic and Functional Outcomes after Radical Prostatectomy for High or Very High Risk Prostate Cancer: European Validation of the Current NCCN® Guideline. *J. Urol.* **2017**, *198*, 354–361. [CrossRef]
14. Hashimoto, T.; Nakashima, J.; Inoue, R.; Komori, O.; Yamaguchi, Y.; Kashima, T.; Satake, N.; Nakagami, Y.; Namiki, K.; Nagao, T.; et al. The significance of micro-lymphatic invasion and pathological Gleason score in prostate cancer patients with pathologically organ-confined disease and negative surgical margins after robot-assisted radical prostatectomy. *Int. J. Clin. Oncol.* **2020**, *25*, 377–383. [CrossRef]
15. Cheng, L.; Zincke, H.; Blute, M.L.; Bergstralh, E.J.; Scherer, B.; Bostwick, D.G. Risk of prostate carcinoma death in patients with lymph node metastasis. *Cancer* **2001**, *91*, 66–73. [CrossRef]
16. Masterson, T.A.; Bianco, F.J., Jr.; Vickers, A.J.; DiBlasio, C.J.; Fearn, P.A.; Rabbani, F.; Eastham, J.A.; Scardino, P.T. The association between total and positive lymph node counts, and disease progression in clinically localized prostate cancer. *J. Urol.* **2006**, *175*, 1320–1324. [CrossRef]
17. Boorjian, S.A.; Thompson, R.H.; Siddiqui, S.; Bagniewski, S.; Bergstralh, E.J.; Karnes, R.J.; Frank, I.; Blute, M.L. Long-term outcome after radical prostatectomy for patients with lymph node positive prostate cancer in the prostate specific antigen era. *J. Urol.* **2007**, *178*, 864–870. [CrossRef]
18. Briganti, A.; Blute, M.L.; Eastham, J.H.; Graefen, M.; Heidenreich, A.; Karnes, J.R.; Montorsi, F.; Studer, U.E. Pelvic lymph node dissection in prostate cancer. *Eur. Urol.* **2009**, *55*, 1251–1265. [CrossRef]
19. Fossati, N.; Willemse, P.M.; Van den Broeck, T.; van den Bergh, R.C.N.; Yuan, C.Y.; Briers, E.; Bellmunt, J.; Bolla, M.; Cornford, P.; De Santis, M.; et al. The Benefits and Harms of Different Extents of Lymph Node Dissection During Radical Prostatectomy for Prostate Cancer: A Systematic Review. *Eur. Urol.* **2017**, *72*, 84–109. [CrossRef]
20. Lestingi, J.F.P.; Guglielmetti, G.B.; Trinh, Q.D.; Coelho, R.F.; Pontes, J., Jr.; Bastos, D.A.; Cordeiro, M.D.; Sarkis, A.S.; Faraj, S.F.; Mitre, A.I.; et al. Extended Versus Limited Pelvic Lymph Node Dissection During Radical Prostatectomy for Intermediate- and High-risk Prostate Cancer: Early Oncological Outcomes from a Randomized Phase 3 Trial. *Eur. Urol.* **2021**, *79*, 595–604. [CrossRef]
21. Wilczak, W.; Wittmer, C.; Clauditz, T.; Minner, S.; Steurer, S.; Büscheck, F.; Krech, T.; Lennartz, M.; Harms, L.; Leleu, D.; et al. Marked Prognostic Impact of Minimal Lymphatic Tumor Spread in Prostate Cancer. *Eur. Urol.* **2018**, *74*, 376–386. [CrossRef]
22. Yamashita, S.; Kawabata, H.; Deguchi, R.; Ueda, Y.; Higuchi, M.; Muraoka, S.; Koike, H.; Kikkawa, K.; Kohjimoto, Y.; Hara, I. Myosteatosis as a novel predictor of urinary incontinence after robot-assisted radical prostatectomy. *Int. J. Urol.* **2022**, *29*, 34–40. [CrossRef] [PubMed]
23. Koike, H.; Kohjimoto, Y.; Iba, A.; Kikkawa, K.; Yamashita, S.; Iguchi, T.; Matsumura, N.; Hara, I. Health-related quality of life after robot-assisted radical prostatectomy compared with laparoscopic radical prostatectomy. *J. Robot. Surg.* **2017**, *11*, 325–331. [CrossRef] [PubMed]
24. Seiler, R.; Studer, U.E.; Tschan, K.; Bader, P.; Burkhard, F.C. Removal of limited nodal disease in patients undergoing radical prostatectomy: Long-term results confirm a chance for cure. *J. Urol.* **2014**, *191*, 1280–1285. [CrossRef] [PubMed]
25. Briganti, A.; Karnes, J.R.; Da Pozzo, L.F.; Cozzarini, C.; Gallina, A.; Suardi, N.; Bianchi, M.; Freschi, M.; Doglioni, C.; Fazio, F.; et al. Two positive nodes represent a significant cut-off value for cancer specific survival in patients with node positive prostate cancer. A new proposal based on a two-institution experience on 703 consecutive N+ patients treated with radical prostatectomy, extended pelvic lymph node dissection and adjuvant therapy. *Eur. Urol.* **2009**, *55*, 261–270. [CrossRef]

26. Touijer, K.A.; Sjoberg, D.D.; Benfante, N.; Laudone, V.P.; Ehdaie, B.; Eastham, J.A.; Scardino, P.T.; Vickers, A. Limited versus Extended Pelvic Lymph Node Dissection for Prostate Cancer: A Randomized Clinical Trial. *Eur. Urol. Oncol.* **2021**, *4*, 532–539. [CrossRef]
27. Morizane, S.; Honda, M.; Shimizu, R.; Tsounapi, P.; Teraoka, S.; Yumioka, T.; Yamaguchi, N.; Kawamoto, B.; Iwamoto, H.; Hikita, K.; et al. Extent of pelvic lymph node dissection improves early oncological outcomes for patients with high-risk prostate cancer without lymph node involvement after robot-assisted radical prostatectomy. *Int. J. Clin. Oncol.* **2022**, *27*, 781–789. [CrossRef]
28. Yang, G.; Xie, J.; Guo, Y.; Yuan, J.; Wang, R.; Guo, C.; Peng, B.; Yao, X.; Yang, B. Identifying the Candidates Who Will Benefit from Extended Pelvic Lymph Node Dissection at Radical Prostatectomy Among Patients with Prostate Cancer. *Front. Oncol.* **2021**, *11*, 790183. [CrossRef]
29. Yuh, B.; Artibani, W.; Heidenreich, A.; Kimm, S.; Menon, M.; Novara, G.; Tewari, A.; Touijer, K.; Wilson, T.; Zorn, K.C.; et al. The role of robot-assisted radical prostatectomy and pelvic lymph node dissection in the management of high-risk prostate cancer: A systematic review. *Eur. Urol.* **2014**, *65*, 918–927. [CrossRef]
30. Briganti, A.; Larcher, A.; Abdollah, F.; Capitanio, U.; Gallina, A.; Suardi, N.; Bianchi, M.; Sun, M.; Freschi, M.; Salonia, A.; et al. Updated nomogram predicting lymph node invasion in patients with prostate cancer undergoing extended pelvic lymph node dissection: The essential importance of percentage of positive cores. *Eur. Urol.* **2012**, *61*, 480–487. [CrossRef]
31. Gandaglia, G.; Ploussard, G.; Valerio, M.; Mattei, A.; Fiori, C.; Fossati, N.; Stabile, A.; Beauval, J.B.; Malavaud, B.; Roumiguié, M.; et al. A Novel Nomogram to Identify Candidates for Extended Pelvic Lymph Node Dissection Among Patients with Clinically Localized Prostate Cancer Diagnosed with Magnetic Resonance Imaging-targeted and Systematic Biopsies. *Eur. Urol.* **2019**, *75*, 506–514. [CrossRef] [PubMed]
32. Cagiannos, I.; Karakiewicz, P.; Eastham, J.A.; Ohori, M.; Rabbani, F.; Gerigk, C.; Reuter, V.; Graefen, M.; Hammerer, P.G.; Erbersdobler, A.; et al. A preoperative nomogram identifying decreased risk of positive pelvic lymph nodes in patients with prostate cancer. *J. Urol.* **2003**, *170*, 1798–1803. [CrossRef] [PubMed]
33. D'Amico, A.V.; Whittington, R.; Malkowicz, S.B.; Schultz, D.; Blank, K.; Broderick, G.A.; Tomaszewski, J.E.; Renshaw, A.A.; Kaplan, I.; Beard, C.J.; et al. Biochemical outcome after radical prostatectomy, external beam radiation therapy, or interstitial radiation therapy for clinically localized prostate cancer. *JAMA* **1998**, *280*, 969–974. [CrossRef] [PubMed]
34. Mohler, J.; Bahnson, R.R.; Boston, B.; Busby, J.E.; D'Amico, A.; Eastham, J.A.; Enke, C.A.; George, D.; Horwitz, E.M.; Huben, R.P.; et al. NCCN clinical practice guidelines in oncology: Prostate cancer. *J. Natl. Compr. Cancer Netw.* **2010**, *8*, 162–200. [CrossRef] [PubMed]
35. Jiang, W.; Zhang, L.; Wu, B.; Zha, Z.; Zhao, H.; Jun, Y.; Jiang, Y. The impact of lymphovascular invasion in patients with prostate cancer following radical prostatectomy and its association with their clinicopathological features: An updated PRISMA-compliant systematic review and meta-analysis. *Medicine* **2018**, *97*, e13537. [CrossRef]
36. Huang, Y.; Huang, H.; Pan, X.W.; Xu, D.F.; Cui, X.G.; Chen, J.; Hong, Y.; Gao, Y.; Yin, L.; Ye, J.Q.; et al. The prognostic value of lymphovascular invasion in radical prostatectomy: A systematic review and meta-analysis. *Asian J. Androl.* **2016**, *18*, 780–785. [CrossRef]
37. Okubo, Y.; Sato, S.; Osaka, K.; Yamamoto, Y.; Suzuki, T.; Ida, A.; Yoshioka, E.; Suzuki, M.; Washimi, K.; Yokose, T.; et al. Clinicopathological Analysis of the ISUP Grade Group and Other Parameters in Prostate Cancer: Elucidation of Mutual Impact of the Various Parameters. *Front. Oncol.* **2021**, *11*, 695251. [CrossRef]

cancers

MDPI

Article

Role of Brachytherapy Boost in Clinically Localized Intermediate and High-Risk Prostate Cancer: Lack of Benefit in Patients with Very High-Risk Factors T3b–4 and/or Gleason 9–10

Hideya Yamazaki [1,*], Gen Suzuki [1], Koji Masui [1], Norihiro Aibe [1], Daisuke Shimizu [1], Takuya Kimoto [1], Kei Yamada [1], Koji Okihara [2], Takashi Ueda [2], Tsukasa Narukawa [2], Takumi Shiraishi [2], Atsuko Fujihara [2], Ken Yoshida [3], Satoaki Nakamura [3], Takashi Kato [4], Yasutoshi Hashimoto [4] and Haruumi Okabe [4]

1 Department of Radiology, Graduate School of Medical Science, Kyoto Prefectural University of Medicine, 465 Kajiicho Kawaramachi Hirokoji, Kamigyo-ku, Kyoto 602-8566, Japan; gensuzu@koto.kpu-m.ac.jp (G.S.); mc0515kj@koto.kpu-m.ac.jp (K.M.); a-ib-n24@koto.kpu-m.ac.jp (N.A.); dshimizu@koto.kpu-m.ac.jp (D.S.); t-kimoto@koto.kpu-m.ac.jp (T.K.); kyamada@koto.kpu-m.ac.jp (K.Y.)

2 Department of Urology, Graduate School of Medical Science, Kyoto Prefectural University of Medicine, 465 Kajiicho Kawaramachi Hirokoji, Kamigyo-ku, Kyoto 602-8566, Japan; kokihara@koto.kpu-m.ac.jp (K.O.); t-ueda@koto.kpu-m.ac.jp (T.U.); tnarukaw@koto.kpu-m.ac.jp (T.N.); takumi14@koto.kpu-m.ac.jp (T.S.); fujihara@koto.kpu-m.ac.jp (A.F.)

3 Department of Radiology, Kansai Medical University, Hirakata 573-1010, Japan; yoshidaisbt@gmail.com (K.Y.); satoaki@nakamura.pro (S.N.)

4 Department of Radiology, Ujitakeda Hospital, Uji-City, Kyoto 611-0021, Japan; hymed_housya@yahoo.co.jp (T.K.); yasu06340829@yahoo.co.jp (Y.H.); h-okabe@takedahp.or.jp (H.O.)

* Correspondence: hideya10@hotmail.com; Tel.: +81-(752)-515-111

Citation: Yamazaki, H.; Suzuki, G.; Masui, K.; Aibe, N.; Shimizu, D.; Kimoto, T.; Yamada, K.; Okihara, K.; Ueda, T.; Narukawa, T.; et al. Role of Brachytherapy Boost in Clinically Localized Intermediate and High-Risk Prostate Cancer: Lack of Benefit in Patients with Very High-Risk Factors T3b–4 and/or Gleason 9–10. *Cancers* **2022**, *14*, 2976. https://doi.org/10.3390/cancers14122976

Academic Editor: Kouji Izumi

Received: 17 May 2022
Accepted: 14 June 2022
Published: 16 June 2022

Simple Summary: In general, brachytherapy (BT) improves biochemical control in intermediate-to high-risk prostate cancer. We previously reported that importance of very high-risk factors (VHR: T3b–4 or Gleason score 9–10) and patients with double VHR (VHR-2) showed the worst prognosis among high-risk groups. We explored the role of BT-boost in patients with VHR and compared it to intermediate- and other high-risk groups. We confirmed that BT-boost improved prostate-specific antigen (PSA) control but resulted in equivalent overall survival rates for the intermediate- and high-risk groups, except for the patients with VHR. In the VHR-1 group (single VHR), BT-boost showed superior PSA control to conventional-dose RT (EQD2 $\leq$ 72 Gy) but not to the dose-escalated radiotherapy group (EQD2 $\geq$ 74 Gy). In the VHR-2 group, BT-boost did not improve the biochemical control rate of either Conv RT or DeRT. BT-boost showed no benefit over modern DeRT in the patients with VHR.

Abstract: This study examined the role of brachytherapy boost (BT-boost) and external beam radiotherapy (EBRT) in intermediate- to high-risk prostate cancer, especially in patients with very high-risk factors (VHR: T3b–4 or Gleason score 9–10) as patients with double very high-risk factors (VHR-2: T3b–4 and Gleason score 9–10) previously showed worst prognosis in localized prostate cancer. We retrospectively reviewed multi-institutional data of 1961 patients that were administered radiotherapy (1091 BT-boost and 872 EBRT: 593 conventional-dose RT (Conv RT: equivalent to doses of 2 Gy per fraction = EQD2 $\leq$ 72 Gy) and 216 dose-escalating RT (DeRT = EQD2 $\geq$ 74 Gy). We found that BT boost improved PSA control and provided an equivalent overall survival rate in the intermediate- and high-risk groups, except for patients within the VHR factor group. In the VHR-1 group (single VHR), BT-boost showed a superior biochemical control rate to the Conv RT group but not to the DeRT group. In the VHR-2 group, BT-boost did not improve outcomes of either Conv RT or DeRT groups. In conclusion, BT-boost showed no benefit to modern DeRT in the patients with VHR; therefore, they are not good candidates for BT-boost to improve outcome and may be amenable to clinical trials using multimodal intensified systemic treatments.

Keywords: radiotherapy; brachytherapy boost; very high-risk; T3b–4; Gleason 9–10; prostate cancer

1. Introduction

Dose escalation in radiotherapy is an established strategy to improve the biochemical control rate in clinically localized through intermediate- and high-risk localized prostate cancer [1–4]. Brachytherapy boost (BT-boost) combined with external beam radiotherapy (EBRT) is a good option to elevate the prescribed dose of radiotherapy without increasing the toxicity due to the superior character of the BT; the rapid falloff of the dose gradient enables us to treat tumors at high doses while maintaining low doses to the surrounding organs at risk. Retrospective [4–8] and prospective analyses, including three randomized controlled trials [9–12], as well as meta-analysis, confirmed the benefit of biochemical control for BT-boost [13].

Recent exploration of risk stratification has introduced a new concept of very high-risk factors (VHR). The most widely used risk classification system in clinics is the National Comprehensive Cancer Network (NCCN) [14], in which the VHR includes a >4 biopsy cores with a Gleason score of 8–10, clinical stage T3b–T4 or primary Gleason score of 5, [14]. For risk stratification including VHR, summation of the number of VHRs (T3b–4 and Gleason score 9–10) was a useful system to identify the worst oncological population [15]. As data were scarce regarding the merits of dose escalation in patients with VHR, the present study examined the role of dose escalation with BT-boost in patients with intermediate- to high-risk cancer as well as VHR. In addition, the NCCN Clinical Practice Guidelines in Oncology stated that doses of $\leq$70 Gy in conventional fractions are not sufficient for the treatment of intermediate- or high-risk prostate cancer [14,15]. Therefore, we divided the control group into conventional dose (Conv RT, doses $\leq$ 72 Gy) and dose-escalated radiotherapy (DeRT, prescribed dose of $\geq$74 Gy, equivalent to doses of 2 Gy per fraction [EQD2]) groups.

Therefore, this study examined the role of BT-boost in patients with VHR for the prognostication of clinically localized high-risk prostate cancer.

2. Materials and Methods

2.1. Patients

We used freely available public data to analyze a large cohort of 1961 patients; among these, 1145 BT-boost (1091 patients administered high-dose BT (HDR-BT) boost from open data for public use [16] and 63 patients treated with low-dose BT (LDR-BT) boost at the Kyoto Prefectural Medical School) [17]. This study included a total of 809 patients administered EBRT (388 administered Conv RT as identified from open data) and 421 patients [16] administered DeRT using intensity-modulated radiotherapy [IMRT] from open data [16] at Uji Takeda Hospital [18] (Table 1). Patients eligible for this study were treated with EBRT with BT-boost or EBRT alone; had histology-proven adenocarcinoma with clinical TNM stage T1–T4N0M0 disease; and had accessible and available data on T classification, Gleason score sum, and initial PSA [iPSA] level. The patients categorized as intermediate or high risks were eligible according to the NCCN risk classification [14]. A simple VHR index was calculated and applied by summing the number of VHR factors in the high-risk group: VHR-0, no VHR; VHR-1, Gleason score 9–10 or T3b–T4; VHR-2, Gleason score = 9–10 and T3b–T4 [19].

We defined PSA failure according to the Phoenix definitions (nadir, +2 ng/mL).

Prostate cancer-specific mortality (PCSM) was defined when prostate cancer was the primary cause of death. Biochemical disease-free survival (bDFS), PCSM, overall survival (OS), and metastasis-free survival (MFS) rates were defined as the intervals from the start of RT to bDFS, distant metastasis, PCSM, and death, respectively.

Table 1. Patients' characteristics.

Factor	Group	Subgroup	BT Boost	EBRT	p-Value
			n = 1152	n = 809	
Age			70 [49, 86]	72 [52, 89]	***<0.001***
iPSA (ng/mL)			13.60 [2.68, 500.00]	14.49 [2.91, 1454.00]	0.087
Gleason score	≤ 6		93 (8.1)	76 (9.4)	0.5443
	7		566 (49.1)	403 (49.8)	
	$8 \leq$		493 (42.8)	330 (40.8)	
T	1		242 (21.0)	176 (21.8)	***0.031***
	2		418 (36.3)	293 (36.3)	
	3		483 (41.9)	319 (39.5)	
	4		9 (0.8)	19 (2.4)	
NCCN risk classification	Intermediate-risk		299 (25.9)	251 (31.0)	***<0.001***
	High-risk	VHR-0: No T3b-4 nor G9–10	519 (45.1)	273 (33.7)	
		VHR-1: T3b-4 or G9–10	295 (25.6)	224 (27.7)	
		VHR-2: T3b-4 and G9–10	39 (3.4)	61 (7.5)	
Modality	BT-boost	LDR-BT	61 (5.3)	0 (0.0)	***<0.001***
		HDR-BT	1091 (94.5)	0 (0.0)	
	EBRT	DeRT (High BED)	0 (0.0)	421 (52.0)	
		Conv RT (Low BED)	0 (0.0)	388 (48.0)	
ADT	Yes		1076 (93.2)	683 (84.4)	***<0.001***
	No		78 (6.8)	126 (15.6)	
	Duration	(month)	42.00 [0.00, 128.00]	8.00 [0.00, 140.00]	***<0.001***
Follow-up		(month)	70.00 [2.00, 177.00]	68.00 [6.37, 145.63]	0.083

EBRT = external beam radiotherapy. De RT; Dose-escalated radiotherapy = EQD2 $\geq$ 74 Gy. Conv RT; Conventional radiotherapy = EQD2 $\leq$ 72 Gy.

Patients included in the public data provided informed consent during the process of building the database and all patients from Uji Takeda Hospital and Kyoto Prefectural Medical School provided written informed consent [19]. This study was approved by the Institutional Review Board of the Kyoto Prefectural University of Medicine (ERB-C-1403) and conducted by the principles of the Declaration of Helsinki.

2.2. Treatment Planning

2.2.1. BT-Boost

The BT-boost groups included HDR-BT and LDR-BT. A multi-institution data of HDR-BT was provided from an open data source [16], and details of treatment have been described elsewhere [20,21]. In brief, the median dose of HDR-BT was 31.5 Gy (range, 10.5–31.5 Gy) in median fraction size 6.3 Gy (range, 5–11 Gy) combined with EBRT in various dose and fractions (median 3 Gy; range, 1.9–3.1 Gy) (Supplemental Table S1). The detailed treatment schedule for LDR-BT (Iodine-125 implantation) was described previously [17]. We included patients with T3a disease or Gleason score sum $\leq$ 8 or a summed Gleason score of 7 (4 + 3), but not for those with a summed Gleason score of 7 (3 + 4) [17] using prescription dose 110 Gy (LDR-BT) with EBRT by three-dimensional conformal radiotherapy (3D-CRT) 40 Gy/20 fractions (Supplemental Table S1). Whole pelvic RT were used in several institutions as a part of EBRT (Supplemental Table S1).

2.2.2. External Beam Radiotherapy (EBRT)

The EBRT group consisted of conventional two-dimensional treatment, 3D-CRT, and IMRT. Supplemental Table S1 depicted the details of patient backgrounds. A freely accessible dataset (n = 417) was used to draw some of EBRT data [16]; 141 image-guided IMRTs using helical TomoTherapy were performed at the Department of Radiology, Uji Takeda Hospital, and detailed technique has been described elsewhere [18]. In brief, the prescribed dose was 74 Gy/37 fractions (2 Gy/fraction, n = 79) or 74.8 Gy/34 fractions (2.2 Gy/fraction, n = 62) for the intermediate-risk and high-risk and groups [18]. We divided a control group into conventional dose group (Conv RT) using does up to 72 Gy and dose-escalated radiotherapy (DeRT) using dose 74 Gy or more in equivalent to doses of 2 Gy per fraction (EQD2). Detail of treatment schedules was depicted in Supplemental Table S1.

2.3. Statistical Analysis

EZR stat package [22] and StatView 5.0 (SAS Institute, Inc., Cary, NC, USA) were used to perform the statistical analyses. Percentages were analyzed using Fisher's exact tests for two groups and chi-square tests for three or more groups. To compare means or medians, Student *t*-tests were used for normally distributed data, and Mann–Whitney U- and Kruskal–Wallis tests for skewed data (i.e., PSA values) [22]. To analyze the biochemical disease-free survival rate (bDFS), distant metastasis-free survival (DMSF), overall survival (OS), and prostate cancer-specific survival rate (PCS), the Kaplan–Meier method was used. Log-rank tests and Bonferroni correction comparisons were performed in analysis of statistically significance. Cox's proportional hazard model for bDFS was used for univariate and multivariate analyses. Statistical significance was set at $p < 0.05$. The propensity score was the probability of being assigned to each group and was calculated using a logistic regression model constructed with the baseline covariates shown in Table 2 (age, T classification, GS, pretreatment PSA, and hormonal therapy history). We used propensity score matching to reduce the selection bias for BT-boost or EBBT (a 1:1 matched cohort was made for comparison of BT-boost and EBRT in the total population and BT-boost versus DeRT).

Table 2. Detailed patient characteristics among subgroups.

			BT Boost		**EBRT**	
Factor	**Group**	**Subgroup**	**HDR + EBRT**	**LDR + EBRT**	**Conv RT**	**DeRT**
			n = 1091	**n = 61**	**n = 593**	**n = 216**
Age			70.00 [49.00, 86.00]	68.00 [52.00, 79.00]	72.00 [52.00, 89.00]	72.00 [54.00, 86.00]
T1234 (%)	1		230 (21.1)	12 (19.7)	121 (20.5)	55 (25.5)
	2		379 (34.7)	39 (63.9)	194 (32.8)	99 (45.8)
	3		473 (43.4)	10 (16.4)	258 (43.7)	61 (28.2)
	4		9 (0.8)	0 (0.0)	18 (3.0)	1 (0.5)
iPSA (ng/ml)			14.39 [2.68, 500.00]	7.70 [3.20, 46.00]	16.83 [2.91, 1454.00]	11.18 [4.00, 265.00]
Gleason score	−6		84 (7.7)	9 (14.8)	41 (6.9)	35 (16.2)
	7		534 (48.9)	32 (52.5)	325 (54.8)	78 (36.1)
	8−		473 (43.4)	20 (32.8)	227 (38.3)	103 (47.7)
ADT (%)	Yes		1041 (95.4)	26 (42.6)	522 (88.0)	161 (74.5)
	No		50 (4.6)	35 (57.4)	71 (12.0)	55 (25.5)
ADT duration	(months)		43.00 [0.00, 128.00]	5.00 [0.00, 14.00]	9.00 [0.00, 140.00]	6.00 [0.00, 80.00]
Risk classification (%)	Intermediate		269 (24.7)	30 (49.2)	176 (29.7)	75 (34.7)
	High		822 (75.3)	31 (50.8)	417 (70.3)	141 (65.3)
		VHR-0	487 (59.3)	31 (50.8)	199 (47.7)	74 (52.5)
		VHR-1	295 (35.9)	0 (0.0)	165 (39.6)	59 (41.8)
		VHR-2	39 (4.8)	0 (0.0)	53 (12.7)	8 (5.7)
Follow-up	(months)		68.00 [2.00, 177.00]	78.00 [17.00, 148.00]	60.37 [6.37, 145.63]	74.00 [23.17, 92.67]

3. Results

3.1. Patient and Disease Characteristics

All 1961 patients with intermediate-to-high-risk prostate cancer were treated with either BT-boost ($n = 1152$) or EBRT ($n = 809$). The median patient age was 71 years (range, 49–89 years). The median initial PSA value was 14.0 ng/mL (range, 2.682–1454 ng/mL). The clinical characteristics of the patients are summarized in Table 1. The median follow-up duration was 69.0 (range: 2–177) months.

3.2. Biochemical Control Rates (Biochemical Disease-Free Survival Rate; bDFS)

The actuarial 5-year bDFS rates were 89.9% (95% confidence interval [CI]: 88.3–91.2%) at 5 years and 78.2% (95% CI: 74.9–81.2%) at 10 years. The bDFS differed significantly among the four risk groups ($p < 0.0001$; Figure 1a).

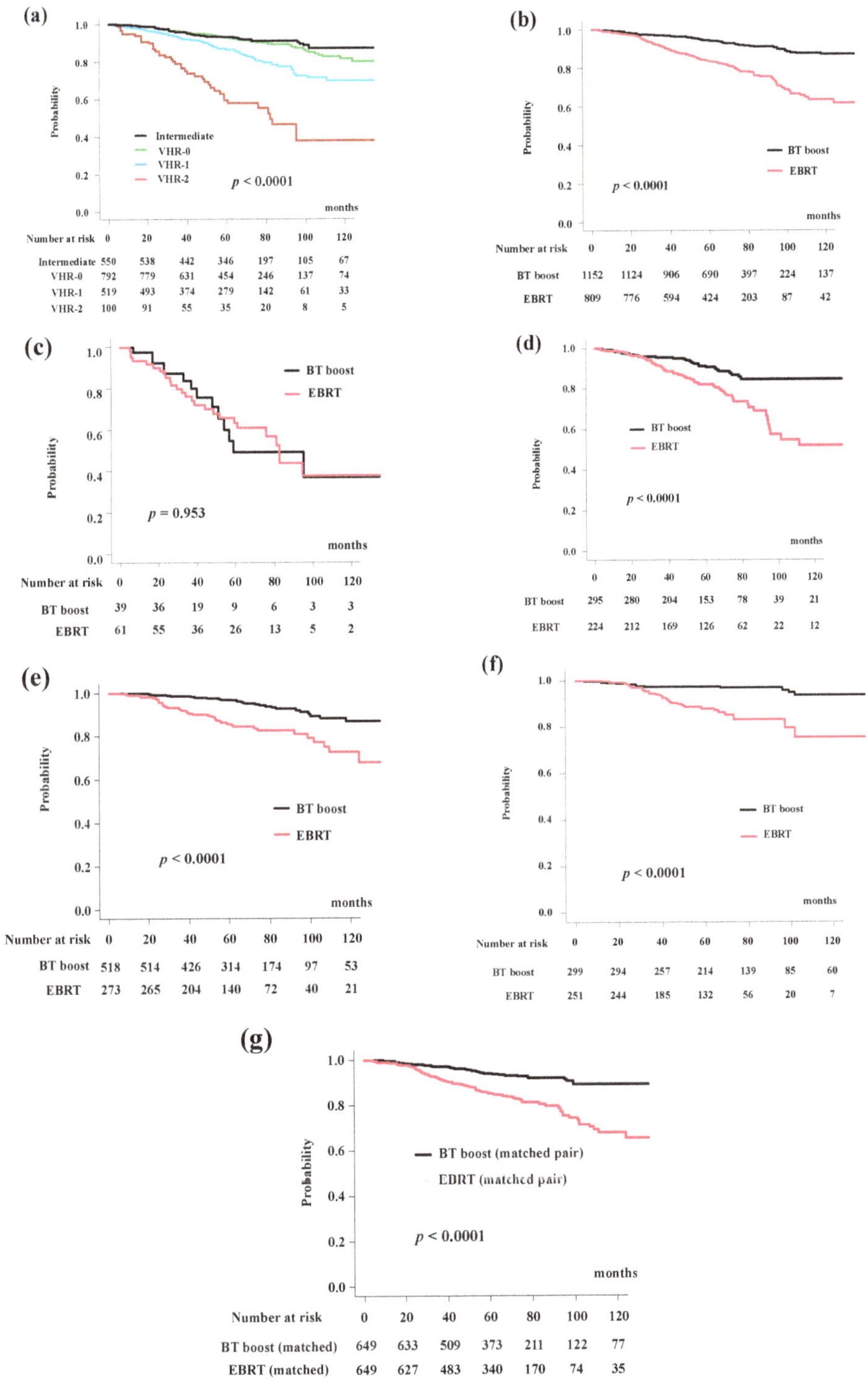

Figure 1. Biochemical control rates (biochemical disease-free survival rate; bDFS). (**a**) bDFS according

to risk stratification. bDFS rates were 59.6% (95% CI: 47.5–69.7%), 86.8% (95% CI: 83.1–89.7%), 93.0% (95% CI: 90.8%–94.8%), 93.3% (95% CI: 90.7%–95.2%) at 5 years in the VHR-2, VHR-1, VHR-0, and intermediate groups, respectively ($p < 0.0001$). (**b**) Comparison of bDFS between EBRT and BT-boost. (**c**) Comparison of bDFS between EBRT and BT-boost in VHR-2 group. (**d**) Comparison of bDFS between EBRT and BT-boost in VHR-1 group. (**e**) Comparison of bDFS between EBRT and BT-boost in VHR-0 group, (**f**) Comparison of bDFS between EBRT and BT-boost in intermediate-risk group. (**g**) Comparison of bDFS between EBRT and BT-boost using matched pair analysis.

BT-boost improved the bDFS to 94.2% (95% CI: 92.5–95.5%) at 5 years and 86.9% (95% CI: 83.4–89.8%) at 10 years compared to those in the EBRT group (83.7%, 95% CI: 80.7–86.3% at 5 years and 63.7%, 95% CI: 56.8–69.7% at 10 years) (Figure 1b, $p < 0.0001$).

The BT-boost group showed superior bDFS compared to that for EBRT in all groups, except for the VHR-2. The BT-boost group had bDFS rates of 49.1% (95% CI: 27.0–67.9%), 90.5% (95% CI: 85.8–93.8%), 96.9% (95% CI: 94.7–98.1%), 97.3% (95% CI: 94.6–98.6%) at 5 years in the VHR-2, VHR-1, VHR-0, and intermediate groups, respectively. The EBRT group had bDFS rates of 63.4% (95% CI: 48.8–74.8%, $p = 0.953$, Figure 1c), 82.2% (95% CI: 76.1–86.9%, $p < 0.0001$, Figure 1d), 85.8% (95% CI: 80.5–89.7%, $p < 0.0001$, Figure 1e), 87.9% (95% CI: 82.5–91.7%, $p < 0.0001$, Figure 1f) at 5-years in the VHR-2, VHR-1, VHR-0, and intermediate groups, respectively.

We applied propensity score matching to generate well-matched pairs (649 and 649 patients; background comparisons are shown in Supplemental Table S1b). The actuarial 5-year biochemical control rates were 93.9% (95% CI: 91.5–95.7%) and 85.3% (95% CI: 82.0–88.0%, $p < 0.0001$, Figure 1g) in the BT-boost and EBRT groups, respectively.

3.3. *Subgroup Analysis (DeRT, Conv RT vs. BT-Boost)*

After dividing EBRT into the Conv RT and DeRT groups (Table 2), the bDFS for each group were 94.2% (95% CI: 92.5%–95.5%), 89.1% (95% CI: 85.2–92.0%), and 79.0% (95% CI: 74.3–82.9%) at 5 years and 86.9% (95% CI: 83.4–89.8%), not available (86.4% at 74 months; 95% CI: 81.5–90.0%), 58.0% (95% CI: 50.9–64.5) at 10 years in the BT-boost group, DeRT and Conv RT group (Figure 2a). BT-boost showed the best outcome among the three groups, with a statistically significant difference not only between the Conv and BT-boost groups but also between the DeRT and BT-boost groups (Figure 2a).

In detailed analysis, BT-boost showed the better outcome not only than Conv RT but also DeRT, except in patients with VHR. The BT-boost group had bDFS rates of 49.1% (95% CI: 27.0–67.9%), 90.5% (95% CI: 85.8–93.8%,), 96.9% (95% CI: 94.7–98.1%), and 97.3% (95% CI: 94.6–98.6%) at 5 years for the VHR-2, VHR-1, VHR-0 and intermediate groups, respectively, while the Conv RT and DeRT group had rates of 54.2% (95% CI: 37.7–68.0%, $p = 1.0$ in comparison to BT-boost, Figure 2b), 80.8% (95% CI: 72.2–86.9%, $p < 0.0001$, Figure 2c), 83.2% (95% CI: 74.8–89.0%, $p < 0.0001$, Figure 2d), 82.9% (95% CI: 72.9–89.5%, $p < 0.0001$, Figure 2e) and 93.7% (95% CI: 63.2–99.1%, $p = 0.086$, Figure 2b), 84.5% (95% CI: 74.6–90.8%, $p = 0.71$, Figure 2c), 89.2% (95% CI: 82.3–93.5%, $p = 0.0008$, Figure 2d), 91.4% (95% CI: 84.8–95.3%, $p = 0.038$, Figure 2e), at 5 years. We generated well-matched pairs for the comparison between BT-boost and DeRT (356 patients each; the background comparisons are shown in Supplemental Table S2) using propensity score matching. The actuarial 5-year biochemical control rates in the BT-boost and DeRT groups were 96.3% (95% CI: 93.5–97.9%) and 89.6% (95% CI: 85.5–92.6%, $p = 0.000588$, Figure 2f), respectively.

As shown in Table 3, the predictors of biochemical control on multivariate analysis included age, treatment modality (BT-boost vs. EBRT or DeRT or Conv RT), iPSA, T classification, and Gleason score sum.

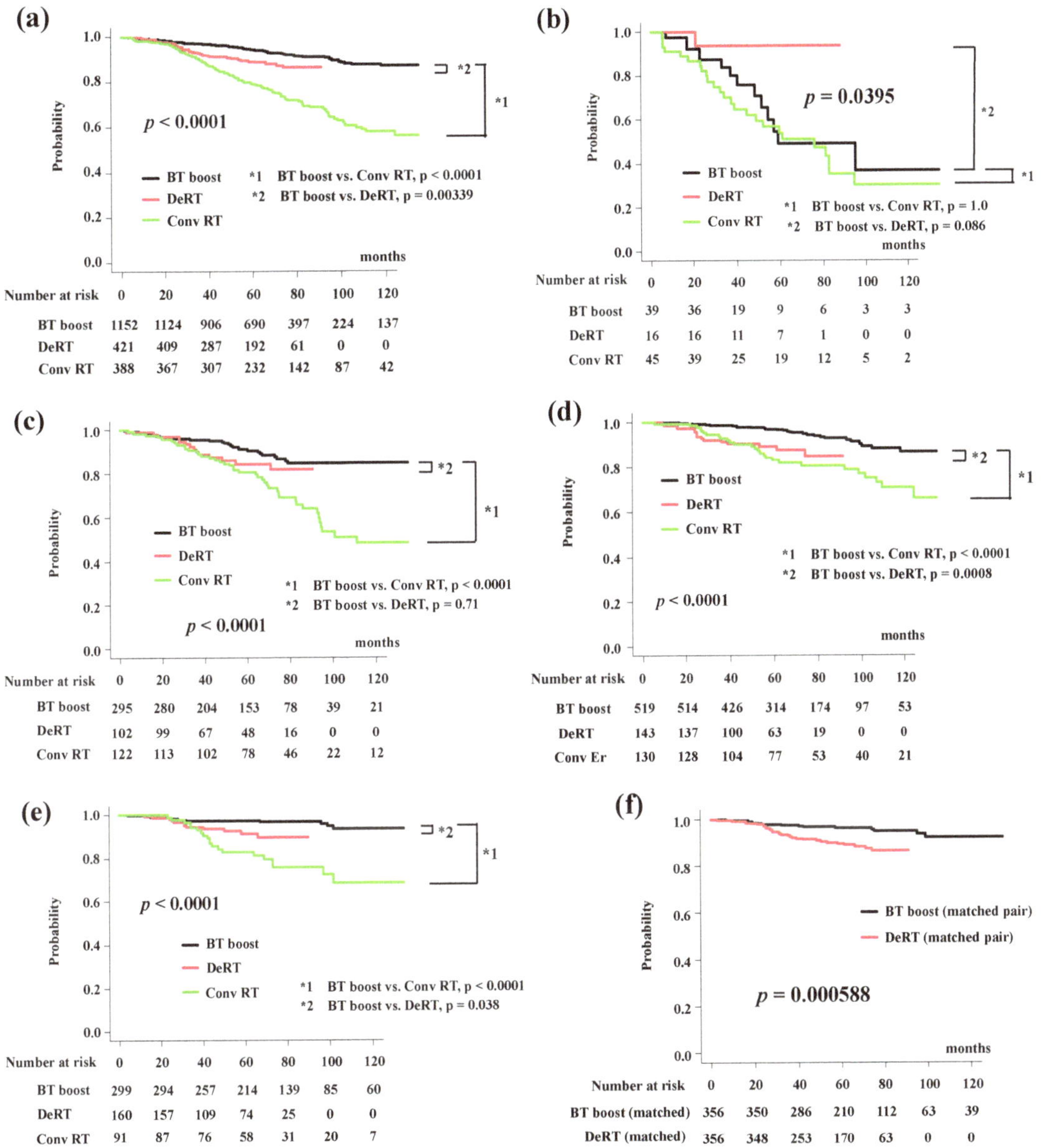

Figure 2. Biochemical control rates among three groups (BT-boost vs. Conv RT vs. DeRT). (**a**) Comparison of bDFS among three groups. (**b**) Comparison of bDFS among three groups in VHR-2 group. (**c**) Comparison of bDFS among three groups in VHR-1 group. (**d**) Comparison of bDFS among three groups in VHR-0 group. (**e**) Comparison of bDFS among three groups in intermediate-risk group. (**f**) Comparison of bDFS between dose escalated radiotherapy (DeRT) and BT-boost using matched pair analysis. bDFS = biochemical disease-free survival rate.

Table 3. Multivariate analysis for PSA control.

Factor	Strata	Hazard Ratio	*p*-Value
Age	Sequential value	0.97 (0.95–1.00)	***0.028***
BT-boost vs. EBRT	BT-boost vs. EBRT	2.83 (2.15–3.72)	***<0.0001***
	BT-boost vs. DeRT	2.05 (1.40–3.01)	***0.00023***
	BT-boost vs. Conv RT	3.32 (2.47–4.45)	***<0.0001***
iPSA	0–9.9 vs. 10–20 vs. 20.1-(ng/mL)	1.33 (1.11–1.59)	***0.0018***
T classification	T1 vs. 2 vs. 3 vs. 4	1.38 (1.14–1.66)	***0.0009***
Gleason score sum	GS-6 vs. 7 vs. 8-	1.57 (1.25–1.97)	***0.00011***
ADT usage	Yes vs. No	0.66 (0.39–1.11)	*0.12*
Age	Sequential value	0.97 (0.95–1.00)	***0.028***

3.4. Distant Metastasis-Free Survival (DMFS) Rates

The DMFS rates were 97.2% (95% CI: 96.3–97.9%) at 5 years and 93.3% (95% CI: 90.9–95.0%) at 10 years. The BT-boost group had DMSF rates of 96.9% (95% CI: 95.5–97.8%) at 5 years and 93.1% (95% CI: 90.1–95.2%) at 10 years. The DMFS rates differed significantly among the four risk groups ($p < 0.0001$; Figure 3a). The EBRT group had PCSM rates of 97.7% (95% CI: 96.2–98.6%) at 5 years and 93.4% (95% CI: 88.9%–96.1%) at 10 years ($p = 0.647$, Figure 3b).

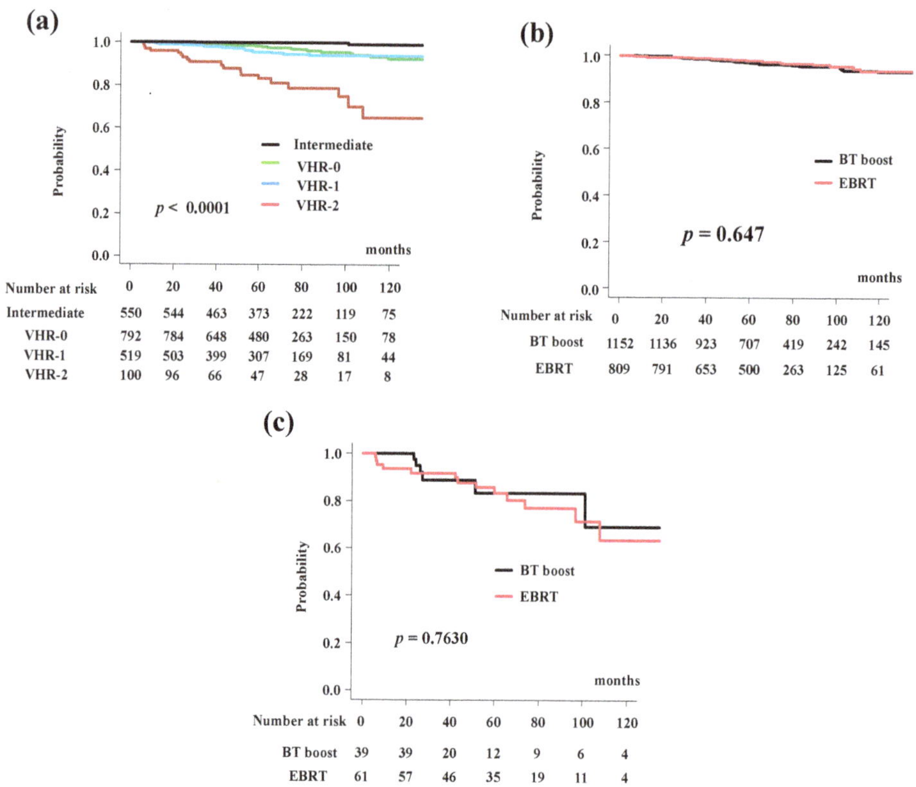

Figure 3. Distant metastasis-free survival rate (DMFS). (**a**) DMFS according to risk stratification. DMSF were 83.2% (95% CI: 72.9–89.8%), 95.4% (95% CI: 92.9–97.1%), 98.2% (95% CI: 96.8%–99.0%), 99.8% (95% CI: 94.8%–100%) at 5 years in the VHR-2, VHR-1, VHR-0, and intermediate groups, respectively ($p < 0.0001$). (**b**) Comparison of DMFS between EBRT and BT-boost. (**c**) Comparison of DMFS between EBRT and BT-boost in VHR-2 group.

The BT-boost group showed DMSF equivalent to EBRT in all groups. The BT-boost group had DMSF rates of 96.9% (95% CI: 62.7–93.2%), 93.7% (95% CI: 89.5–96.3%), 97.7% (95% CI: 95.6–99.7%), 99.7% (95% CI: 97.6–100%) at 5 years in the VHR-2, VHR-1, VHR-0 and intermediate groups, respectively, while the rates in the EBRT were 83.3% (95% CI: 70.1%–91.0%, $p = 0.7630$, Figure 3c), 97.4% (95% CI: 93.8–98.9%, $p = 0.0696$, Supplemental Figure S1a), 99.6% (95% CI: 97.4–99.9%, $p = 0.3840$, Supplemental Figure S1b), and 100% ($p = 0.304$, Supplemental Figure S1c) at 5 years.

3.5. Prostate Cancer-Specific Mortality (PCS)

The cumulative incidence for PCS was 99.2% (95% CI: 98.6–99.5%) at 5 years and 97.5% (95% CI: 95.9–98.5%) at 10 years in the total population. The BT-boost group in the present study had PCS rates of 99.2% (95% CI: 98.4–99.6%) at 5 years and 97.6% (95% CI: 95.4–98.8%) at 10 years. The PCS rates in the EBRT group were 99.1% (95% CI: 98.0–99.6%) at 5 years and 97.4% (95% CI: 94.9–98.6%) at 10 years (Figure 4a, $p = 0.334$). The PCS rates differed significantly among the four risk groups ($p < 0.0001$; Figure 4b).

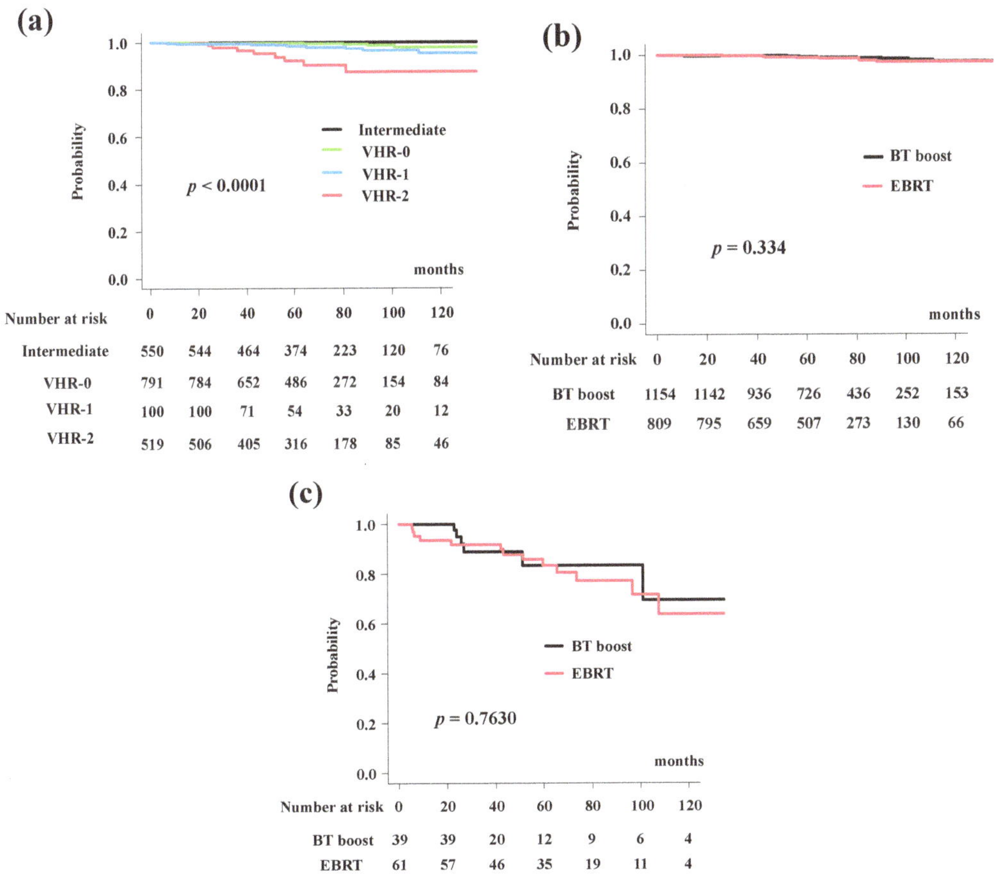

Figure 4. Prostate cancer specific survival rate (PCS). (**a**) PCS according to risk stratification. PCS were 93.8% (95% CI: 85.6–97.4), 98.5% (95% CI: 96.6–99.3%), 99.9% (95% CI: 98.5%–99.9%), and 100%

at 5 years in the VHR-2, VHR-1, VHR-0, and intermediate groups, respectively ($p < 0.0001$). (**b**) Comparison of PCS between EBRT and BT-boost. (**c**) Comparison of PCS between EBRT and BT-boost in VHR-2 group. The BT-boost group showed equivalent PCS to EBRT in all groups.

In detail, the BT-boost group had PCS rates of 92.3% (95% CI: 70.6–98.2%), 97.6% (95% CI: 64.2–99.0%), 100%, and 100% at 5 years for VHR-2, VHR-1, VHR-0 and intermediate groups, while the EBRT group had a PCS of 92.2% (95% CI: 80.4–97.0%, Figure 4c), 99.5% (95% CI: 96.3–99.9%, p = 0.499, Supplemental Figure S2a), 99.6% (95% CI: 97.4–99.9%, p = 0.877, Supplemental Figure S2b), and 100% at 5-years (Supplemental Figure S2c).

3.6. Overall Survival (OS)

The BT-boost group showed equivalent OS rates of 96.3% (CI: 94.9–97.3%) at 5 years and 91.0% (95% CI: 87.8–93.4%) at 10 years. In the EBRT group, the OS was 98.0% (95% CI: 96.6%–98.9%) at 5 years and 92.8% (95% CI: 89.2–95.2%) at 10 years (Figure 5a, p = 0.35). The OS differed significantly among the four risk groups ($p < 0.0001$; Figure 5b).

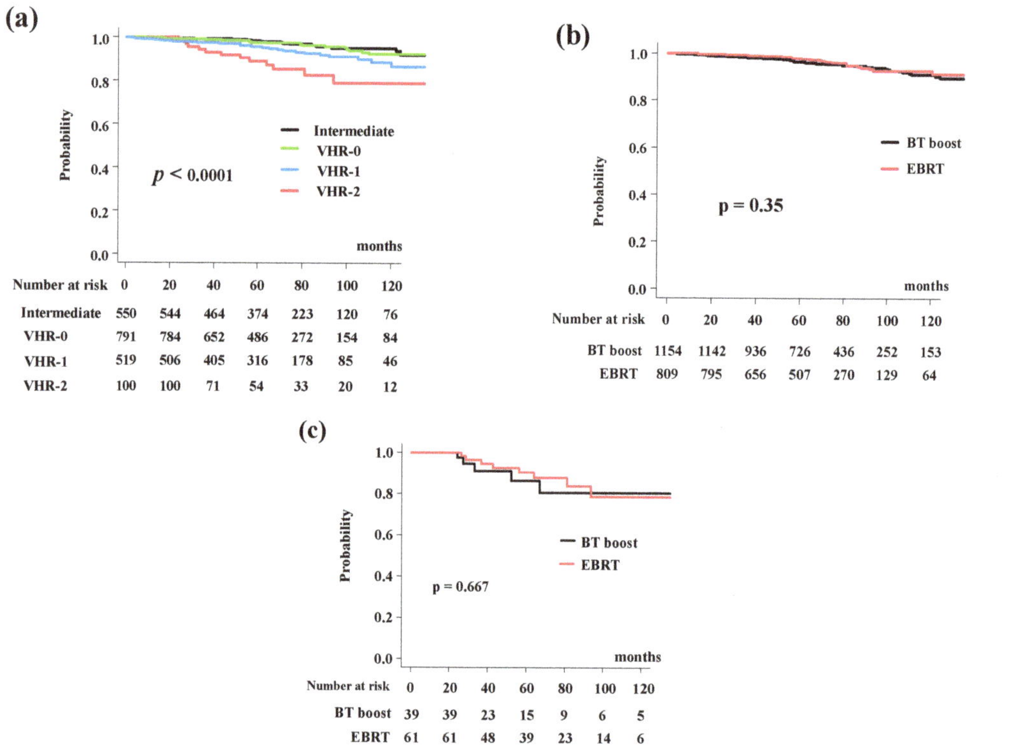

Figure 5. Overall survival rate (OS). (**a**) OS according to risk stratification. OS were 89.0% (95% CI: 79.7–94.2%), 95.9% (95% CI: 93.6–97.4%), 97.6% (95% CI: 96.1%–98.6%), 98.5% (95% CI: 96.9%–99.3%) at 5 years in the VHR-2, VHR-1, VHR-0, and intermediate groups, respectively ($p < 0.0001$). (**b**) Comparison of bDFS between EBRT and BT-boost. (**c**) Comparison of bDFS between EBRT and BT-boost in VHR-2 group. The BT-boost group showed an equivalent OS to those for EBRT in all groups.

In detail, the BT-boost group had an OS of 86.3% (95% CI: 66.4–94.8%), 93.6% (95% CI: 89.6–96.1%), 97.6% (95% CI: 95.6–98.7%), and 97.7% (95% CI: 95.0–99.0%), at 5 years for the VHR-2, VHR-1, VHR-0, and intermediate groups. The EBRT group had OS rates of 90.5% (95% CI: 78.5–95.9%, p = 0.667, Figure 5c), 98.9% (95% CI: 95.5–99.7%, p = 0.177,

Supplemental Figure S3a), 97.7% (95% CI: 994.6–99.1%, $p = 0.322$, Supplemental Figure S3b), and 99.6% (95% CI: 97.2–99.9%. $p = 0.587$, Supplemental Figure S3c), at 5-years.

4. Discussion

The present study explored the role of BT-boost in intermediate- to high-risk prostate cancer. The results demonstrated that BT-boost showed superior bDFS compared to that in the EBRT group except for the VHR-2 group. To our knowledge, this is the first report to show the merits and limitations of BT-boost in patients with intermediate-to high-risk prostate cancer, with a focus on the VHR-2 group. In their meta-analysis of three randomized control trials (RCTs), Kee et al. reported a significant benefit in 5-year bDFS in favor of BT-boost versus EBRT but not in OS and grade $\geq$ 3 late toxicities [12]. However, two of the RCTs [9–11] had a major bias in their methodologies, as the EBRT arm was not the standard care of treatment (too few doses were delivered in the EBRT arm) and their findings could not be translated into modern clinical situations. However, the recent Androgen Suppression Combined with Elective Nodal and Dose Escalated Radiation Therapy (ASCENDE-RT) trial showed that even with escalated EBRT, BT-boost provided better benefits in terms of biochemical control [9]. Our data were also consistent with their data demonstrating superior bDFS for BT-boost compared to both Conv RT and DeRT in patients without VHR. The use of androgen deprivation therapy (ADT) and its optimal duration was another confounding factor for bDFS analysis. The bDFS was significantly better regardless of the BT technique used (low or high dose rates) in these three RCTs, independent of the ADT duration. Higher BED delivered by BT (12–38%) with the better dose distribution due to the steep dose gradient, which delivered a non-homogeneous dose escalation [12,13], was an important factor to improve the outcomes. Furthermore, several studies have reported the superior efficacy of BT-boost not only in terms of bDFS but also in PCS and OS [7,8]. Therefore, BT-boost for intermediate- and high-risk prostate cancer was an attractive technique in numerous retrospective and prospective studies.

The concept of VHR was recently introduced. High-risk prostate cancer has been subdivided according to VHR in several ways. The NCCN used clinical stage T3b–T4 lesions, primary Gleason score = 5, or > 4 biopsy cores with Gleason scores of 8–10 [14]. After the initial estimation [23], a confirmation study was conducted, despite different definitions of VHR [14,24,25]. We also confirmed the importance of VHR factors, in which VHR-2 showed a higher hazard risk for DMSF, PCS, and OS than VHR-0 (hazard ratio = 8.81, 11.99, and 4.644, respectively) and VHR-1 (hazard ratio = 5.268, 2.359, and 2.896, respectively), and was a potentially better stratification system than the previous ones [15]. Our results add additional evidence of VHR-2 in a population at very high risk for recurrence outside the prostate (i.e., distant metastasis), even with the highest intensification of local radiotherapy with BT-boost. Our data could provoke a controversy regarding the indication for BT-boost in the patients with VHR, who may not be good candidates for BT-boost. These VHR criteria may be beneficial for better treatment choice for individual patients according to prognosis of the high-risk disease predisposing a risk of aggressive oncological outcomes, which may require intensive follow-up for metastasis using modern technologies; prostate-specific membrane antigen positron emission tomography scan [26] and earlier and/or adjuvant systemic therapy; or longer periods of ADT use in addition to abiraterone, docetaxel, and enzalutamide [27–30], which could be in a multimodal treatment clinical trial setting.

The present study has several limitations. First, the role of the biopsy core in the VHR system could not be analyzed because the public database did not contain these data. In addition, recent image-guided biopsy techniques made it impossible to assess older data as it was not compatible with recent systems. Second, the retrospective nature, limited follow-up time, and small sample size (especially in the VHR-2 group) in this study may limit the application of its findings. Thus, studies with longer follow-up and larger samples are needed to obtain concrete conclusions; although it could be difficult to perform, an RCT is anticipated.

5. Conclusions

BT-boost improved bDFS in intermediate- and higher risk groups, except for the patients with very high-risk factors (VHR-2: T3b-4 and Gleason 9–10). In the VHR-1 group (single VHR), BT-boost showed a superior biochemical control rate to the Conv RT group but not the DeRT group. In the VHR-2 group (double VHR), BT-boost did not improve outcomes of either the Conv RT or DeRT group. BT-boost showed no benefit to modern DeRT in the patients with VHR; therefore, they are not good candidates for BT-boost to improve outcome and may be amenable to clinical trials using multimodal intensified systemic treatments.

Supplementary Materials: The following are available online at https://www.mdpi.com/article/10.3390/cancers14122976/s1, Figure S1: Distant metastasis-free survival rate (DMFS), (**a**) Comparison of DMFS between EBRT and BT-boost in VHR-1 group. (**b**) Comparison of DMFS between EBRT and BT-boost in VHR-0 group. (**c**) Comparison of DMFS between EBRT and BT-boost in intermediate-risk group. Figure S2: Prostate cancer specific survival rate (PCS), (**a**) Comparison of PCS between EBRT and BT-boost in VHR-1 group. (**b**) Comparison of PCS between EBRT and BT-boost in VHR-0 group. (**c**) Comparison of PCS between EBRT and BT-boost in intermediate-risk group. Figure S3: Overall survival rate (OS), (**a**) Comparison of bDFS between EBRT and BT-boost in VHR-1 group. (**b**) Comparison of bDFS between EBRT and BT-boost in VHR-0 group. (**c**) Comparison of bDFS between EBRT and BT-boost in intermediate-risk group. Table S1: Detailed treatment schedule, Table S2: Comparison of background of Patient characteristics after propensity score matching, Table S3: Background Comparison between BT-boost and DeRT after propensity score matching.

Author Contributions: Data curation, H.Y., K.M., T.N. and T.S.; Formal analysis, G.S.; Investigation, D.S., T.K. (Takuya Kimoto), K.O. and A.F.; Methodology, K.M.; Project administration, H.Y.; Resources, T.U.; Software, N.A. and Y.H.; Supervision, H.O.; Validation, S.N. and T.K. (Takashi Kato); Visualization, K.Y. (Ken Yoshida); Writing—original draft, H.Y.; Writing—review & editing, K.Y. (Kei Yamada). All authors have read and agreed to the published version of the manuscript.

Funding: This work was supported by JSPS KAKENHI Grant Number JP21K07600.

Institutional Review Board Statement: The study was conducted according to the guidelines of the Declaration of Helsinki and approved by the Institutional Review Board of Kyoto Prefectural University of Medicine: ERB-C-1403.

Informed Consent Statement: Informed consent was obtained from all subjects involved in the study.

Data Availability Statement: The data of HDR-BT and part of EBRT for this manuscript can be obtained from the public database [19] and another part of EBRT and LDR-BT can be obtained from the author upon reasonable request.

Acknowledgments: We appreciate the participants and physicians for building big, free data of treatment outcomes [19].

Conflicts of Interest: The authors declare no conflict of interest.

References

1. Dearnaley, D.P.; Sydes, M.R.; Graham, J.D.; Aird, E.G.; Bottomley, D.; Cowan, R.A.; Huddart, R.A.; Jose, C.C.; Matthews, J.H.; Millar, J.; et al. Escalated-dose versus standard-dose conformal radiotherapy in prostate cancer: First results from the MRC RT01 randomized controlled trial. *Lancet Oncol.* **2007**, *8*, 475–487. [CrossRef]
2. Peeters, S.T.H.; Heemsbergen, W.D.; Koper, P.C.M.; van Putten, W.L.J.; Slot, A.; Dielwart, M.F.H.; Bonfrer, J.M.; Incrocci, L.; Lebesque, J.V. Dose-response in radiotherapy for localized prostate cancer: Results of the Dutch multicenter randomized phase III trial comparing 68 Gy of radiotherapy with 78 Gy. *J. Clin. Oncol.* **2006**, *24*, 1990–1996. [CrossRef] [PubMed]
3. Zietman, A.L.; DeSilvio, M.L.; Slater, J.D.; Rossi, C.J.; Miller, D.W.; Adams, J.A.; Shipley, W.U. Comparison of conventional-dose vs high-dose conformal radiation therapy in clinically localized adenocarcinoma of the prostate: A randomized controlled trial. *JAMA* **2005**, *294*, 1233–1239. [CrossRef] [PubMed]
4. Spratt, D.E.; Zumsteg, Z.S.; Ghadjar, P.; Kollmeier, M.A.; Pei, X.; Cohen, G.; Polkinghorn, W.; Yamada, Y.; Zelefsky, M.J. Comparison of high-dose (86.4 Gy) IMRT vs combined brachytherapy plus IMRT for intermediate-risk prostate cancer. *BJU Int.* **2014**, *114*, 360–367. [CrossRef]

5. Viani, G.A.; Stefano, E.J.; Afonso, S.L. Higher-than-conventional radiation doses in localized prostate cancer treatment: A metaanalysis of randomized, controlled trials. *Int. J. Radiat. Oncol. Biol. Phys.* **2009**, *74*, 1405–1418. [CrossRef] [PubMed]
6. Villalba, S.R.; Denia, P.M.; Pérez-Calatayud, M.J.; Sancho, J.R.; Pérez-Calatayud, J.; Escrivá, A.F.; Tendero, P.T.; Ortega, M.S. Low-/high-dose-rate brachytherapy boost in patients with intermediate-risk prostate cancer treated with radiotherapy: Long-term results from a single institution team experience. *J. Contemp. Brachyther.* **2021**, *13*, 135–144. [CrossRef] [PubMed]
7. Kent, A.R.; Matheson, B.; Millar, J.L. Improved survival for patients with prostate cancer receiving a high-dose-rate brachytherapy boost to EBRT compared with EBRT alone. *Brachytherapy* **2019**, *18*, 313–321. [CrossRef]
8. Wedde, T.B.; Smastuen, M.C.; Brabrand, S.; Fossa, S.D.; Kaasa, S.; Tafjord, G.; Russnes, K.M.; Hellebust, T.P.; Lilleby, W. Ten-year survival after high-dose-rate brachytherapy combined with external beam radiation therapy in high-risk prostate cancer: A comparison with the Norwegian SPCG-7 cohort. *Radiother. Oncol.* **2019**, *132*, 211–217. [CrossRef]
9. Morris, W.J.; Tyldesley, S.; Rodda, S.; Halperin, R.; Pai, H.; McKenzie, M.; Duncan, G.; Morton, G.; Hamm, J.; Murray, N. Androgen Suppression Combined with Elective Nodal and Dose Escalated Radiation Therapy (the ASCENDE-RT Trial): An Analysis of Survival Endpoints for a Randomized Trial Comparing a Low-Dose-Rate Brachytherapy Boost to a Dose-Escalated External Beam Boost for High- and Intermediate-risk Prostate Cancer. *Int. J. Radiat. Oncol. Biol. Phys.* **2017**, *98*, 275–285.
10. Hoskin, P.J.; Rojas, A.M.; Ostler, P.J.; Bryant, L.; Lowe, G.J. Randomised trial of external-beam radiotherapy alone or with high-dose-rate brachytherapy for prostate cancer: Mature 12-year results. *Radiother. Oncol.* **2021**, *154*, 214–219. [CrossRef]
11. Sathya, J.R.; Davis, I.R.; Julian, J.A.; Guo, Q.; Daya, D.; Dayes, I.S.; Lukka, H.R.; Levine, M. Randomized trial comparing iridium implant plus external-beam radiation therapy with external beam radiation therapy alone in node-negative locally advanced cancer of the prostate. *J. Clin. Oncol.* **2005**, *23*, 1192–1199. [CrossRef] [PubMed]
12. Chin, J.; Rumble, R.B.; Kollmeier, M.; Heath, E.; Efstathiou, J.; Dorff, T.; Berman, B.; Feifer, A.; Jacques, A.; Loblaw, D.A. Brachytherapy for Patients With Prostate Cancer: American Society of Clinical Oncology/Cancer Care Ontario Joint Guideline Update. *J. Clin. Oncol.* **2017**, *35*, 1737–1743. [CrossRef] [PubMed]
13. Kee, D.L.C.; Gal, J.; Falk, A.T.; Schiappa, R.; Chand, M.-E.; Gautier, M.; Doyen, J.; Hannoun-Levi, J.-M. Brachytherapy versus external beam radiotherapy boost for prostate cancer: Systematic review with meta-analysis of randomized trials. *Cancer Treat. Rev.* **2018**, *70*, 265–271. [CrossRef] [PubMed]
14. The National Comprehensive Cancer Network Clinical Practice Guidelines in Oncology. Prostate Cancer-Version 4. 2019. Available online: http://www.nccn.org/professionals/physician_gls/pdf/prostate.pdf (accessed on 2 February 2020).
15. Kuban, D.A.; Levy, L.B.; Cheung, M.R.; Lee, A.K.; Choi, S.; Frank, S.; Pollack, A. Long-term failure patterns and survival in a randomized dose-escalation trial for prostate cancer. Who dies of disease? *Int. J. Radiat. Oncol. Biol. Phys.* **2011**, *79*, 1310–1317. [CrossRef] [PubMed]
16. An Open Data of Multicenter Data Collection: Outcome of Radiation Therapy for Prostate Cancer to Establish a Prognostic Prediction System by Machine Learning (B17–278). Available online: https://www.khp.kitasato-u.ac.jp/ska/radiotherapy/arcivements/#results (accessed on 2 February 2020).
17. Okihara, K.; Kobayashi, K.; Iwata, T.; Naitoh, Y.; Kamoi, K.; Kawauchi, A.; Yamada, K.; Miki, T. Assessment of permanent brachytherapy combined with androgen deprivation therapy in an intermediate-risk prostate cancer group without a Gleason score of 4 + 3: A single Japanese institutional experience. *Int. J. Urol.* **2014**, *21*, 271–276. [CrossRef]
18. Sasaki, N.; Yamazaki, H.; Shimizu, D.; Suzuki, G.; Masui, K.; Nakamura, S.; Okabe, H.; Nishikawa, T.; Yoshida, K. Long-term Outcomes of a Dose–reduction Trial to Decrease Late Gastrointestinal Toxicity in Patients with Prostate Cancer Receiving Soft Tissue-matched Image-guided Intensity-modulated Radiotherapy. *Anticancer Res.* **2018**, *38*, 385–391.
19. Yamazaki, H.; Suzuki, G.; Masui, K.; Aibe, N.; Shimizu, D.; Kimoto, T.; Yamada, K.; Shiraishi, T.; Fujihara, A.; Okihara, K.; et al. Novel Prognostic Index of High-Risk Prostate Cancer Using Simple Summation of Very High-Risk Factors. *Cancers* **2021**, *13*, 3486. [CrossRef]
20. Ishiyama, H.; Satoh, T.; Kitano, M.; Tabata, K.-I.; Komori, S.; Ikeda, M.; Soda, I.; Kurosaka, S.; Sekiguchi, A.; Kimura, M.; et al. High-dose-rate brachytherapy and hypofractionated external beam radiotherapy combined with long-term hormonal therapy for high-risk and very high-risk prostate cancer: Outcomes after 5-year follow-up. *J. Radiat. Res.* **2014**, *55*, 509–517. [CrossRef]
21. Kasahara, T.; Ishizaki, F.; Kazama, A.; Yuki, E.; Yamana, K.; Maruyama, R.; Oshikane, T.; Kaidu, M.; Aoyama, H.; Bilim, V.; et al. High-dose-rate brachytherapy and hypofractionated external beam radiotherapy combined with long-term androgen deprivation therapy for very high-risk prostate cancer. *Int. J. Urol.* **2020**, *27*, 800–806. [CrossRef]
22. Kanda, Y. Investigation of the freely available easy-to-use software 'EZR' for medical statistics. *Bone Marrow Transplant.* **2013**, *48*, 452–458. [CrossRef]
23. Sundi, D.; Tosoian, J.J.; Nyame, Y.A.; Alam, R.; Achim, M.; Reichard, C.A.; Li, J.; Wilkins, L.; Schwen, Z.; Han, M.; et al. Outcomes of very high-risk prostate cancer after radical prostatectomy: Validation study from 3 centers. *Cancer* **2019**, *125*, 391–397. [CrossRef] [PubMed]
24. Sundi, D.; Wang, V.M.; Pierorazio, P.M.; Han, M.; Bivalacqua, T.J.; Ball, M.W.; Antonarakis, E.S.; Partin, A.W.; Schaeffer, E.M.; Ross, A.E. Very-high-risk localized prostate cancer: Definition and outcomes. *Prostate Cancer Prostatic Dis.* **2014**, *17*, 57–63. [CrossRef] [PubMed]
25. Narang, A.K.; Gergis, C.; Robertson, S.P.; He, P.; Ram, A.N.; McNutt, T.R.; Griffith, E.; Deweese, T.A.; Honig, S.; Singh, H.; et al. Very High-Risk Localized Prostate Cancer: Outcomes Following Definitive Radiation. *Int. J. Radiat. Oncol.* **2016**, *94*, 254–262. [CrossRef] [PubMed]

26. Perera, M.; Papa, N.; Roberts, M.; Williams, M.; Udovicich, C.; Vela, I.; Christidis, D.; Bolton, D.; Hofman, M.S.; Lawrentschuk, N.; et al. Gallium-68 Prostate-specific Membrane Antigen Positron Emission Tomography in Advanced Prostate Can-cer-Updated Diagnostic Utility, Sensitivity, Specificity, and Distribution of Prostate-specific Membrane Antigen-avid Lesions: A Systematic Review and Meta-analysis. *Eur. Urol.* **2020**, *77*, 403–417.
27. Komura, K.; Sweeney, C.J.; Inamoto, T.; Ibuki, N.; Azuma, H.; Kantoff, P.W. Current treatment strategies for advanced prostate cancer. *Int. J. Urol.* **2018**, *25*, 220–231. [CrossRef]
28. Burgess, L.; Roy, S.; Morgan, S.; Malone, S. A Review on the Current Treatment Paradigm in High-Risk Prostate Cancer. *Cancers* **2021**, *13*, 4257. [CrossRef]
29. Stattin, P.; Sandin, F.; Thomsen, F.B.; Garmo, H.; Robinson, D.; Lissbrant, I.F.; Jonsson, H.; Bratt, O. Association of Radical Local Treatment with Mortality in Men with Very High-risk Prostate Cancer: A Semiecologic, Nationwide, Population-based Study. *Eur. Urol.* **2017**, *72*, 125–134. [CrossRef]
30. Fukagai, T.; Namiki, T.S.; Carlile, R.G.; Yoshida, H.; Namiki, M. Comparison of the clinical outcome after hormonal therapy for prostate cancer between Japanese and Caucasian men. *BJU Int.* **2006**, *97*, 1190–1193. [CrossRef]

cancers

MDPI

Article

Comparison of Clinical Outcomes of Radical Prostatectomy versus IMRT with Long-Term Hormone Therapy for Relatively Young Patients with High- to Very High-Risk Localized Prostate Cancer

Hung-Jen Shih [1,2,3,†], Shyh-Chyi Chang [4,5,†], Chia-Hao Hsu [4,5], Yi-Chu Lin [4], Chu-Hsuan Hung [4] and Szu-Yuan Wu [6,7,8,9,10,11,12,13,*]

1 Division of Urology, Department of Surgery, Changhua Christian Hospital, Changhua 500, Taiwan; 106385@w.tmu.edu.tw
2 Department of Recreation and Holistic Wellness, MingDao University, Changhua 500, Taiwan
3 Department of Urology, School of Medicine, College of Medicine, Taipei Medical University, Taipei 110, Taiwan
4 Department of Urology, Lo-Hsu Medical Foundation, Lotung Poh-Ai Hospital, Yilan 265, Taiwan; mork2747@gmail.com (S.-C.C.); c095001@mail.pohai.org.tw (C.-H.H.); ret7988@mail.pohai.org.tw (Y.-C.L.); c857026@mail.pohai.org.tw (C.-H.H.)
5 Faculty of Medicine, National Yang-Ming University School of Medicine, Taipei 11221, Taiwan
6 Department of Food Nutrition and Health Biotechnology, College of Medical and Health Science, Asia University, Taichung 413, Taiwan
7 Big Data Center, Lo-Hsu Medical Foundation, Lotung Poh-Ai Hospital, Yilan 265, Taiwan
8 Division of Radiation Oncology, Lo-Hsu Medical Foundation, Lotung Poh-Ai Hospital, Yilan 265, Taiwan
9 Department of Healthcare Administration, College of Medical and Health Science, Asia University, Taichung 413, Taiwan
10 Cancer Center, Lo-Hsu Medical Foundation, Lotung Poh-Ai Hospital, Yilan 265, Taiwan
11 Graduate Institute of Business Administration, College of Management, Fu Jen Catholic University, Taipei 242062, Taiwan
12 Department of Management, College of Management, Fo Guang University, Yilan 262307, Taiwan
13 Centers for Regional Anesthesia and Pain Medicine, Wan Fang Hospital, Taipei Medical University, Taipei 110, Taiwan
* Correspondence: szuyuanwu5399@gmail.com
† These authors have contributed equally to this study (coauthors).

Citation: Shih, H.-J.; Chang, S.-C.; Hsu, C.-H.; Lin, Y.-C.; Hung, C.-H.; Wu, S.-Y. Comparison of Clinical Outcomes of Radical Prostatectomy versus IMRT with Long-Term Hormone Therapy for Relatively Young Patients with High- to Very High-Risk Localized Prostate Cancer. *Cancers* **2021**, *13*, 5986. https://doi.org/10.3390/cancers13235986

Academic Editor: Kouji Izumi

Received: 29 September 2021
Accepted: 24 November 2021
Published: 28 November 2021

Simple Summary: That the definitive optimal treatments for relatively young men (aged ≤ 65 years) with high- or very high-risk localized prostate cancer (HR/VHR-LPC) are radical prostatectomy (RP) or radiation plus antiandrogen therapy (RT-ADT) is controversial. To the best of our knowledge, our study is the first and largest to examine biochemical failure (BF), all-cause death, locoregional recurrence, and distant metastasis in relatively young men with HR/VHR-LPC as defined by National Comprehensive Cancer Network risk strata. After head-to-head propensity score matching was used to balance the potential confounders, a multivariable Cox proportional hazards regression model was used to analyze oncologic outcomes. In relatively young men with HR/VHR-LPC, RP and RT-ADT yielded similar oncologic outcomes and RP reduced the risk of BF compared with RT-ADT.

Abstract: That intensity-modulated radiotherapy (IMRT) plus antiandrogen therapy (IMRT-ADT) and radical prostatectomy (RP) are the definitive optimal treatments for relatively young patients (aged ≤ 65 years) with high- or very high-risk localized prostate cancer (HR/VHR-LPC), but remains controversial. We conducted a national population-based cohort study by using propensity score matching (PSM) to evaluate the clinical outcomes of RP and IMRT-ADT in relatively young patients with HR/VHR-LPC. *Methods*: We used the Taiwan Cancer Registry database to evaluate clinical outcomes in relatively young (aged ≤ 65 years) patients with HR/VHR-LPC, as defined by the National Comprehensive Cancer Network risk strata. The patients had received RP or IMRT-ADT (high-dose, ≥72 Gy plus long-term, 1.5–3 years, ADT). Head-to-head PSM was used to balance potential confounders. A Cox proportional hazards regression model was used to analyze oncologic outcomes. *Results*: High-dose IMRT-ADT had a higher risk of biochemical failure (adjusted hazard ratio [aHR] = 2.03, 95% confidence interval [CI] 1.56–2.65, $p < 0.0001$) compared with RP; IMRT-ADT did not have an increased risk of all-cause death (aHR = 1.2, 95% CI 0.65–2.24, $p = 0.564$), locoregional recurrence (aHR = 0.88, 95% CI 0.67–1.06, $p = 0.3524$), or distant metastasis (aHR = 1.03, 95% CI 0.56–1.9, $p = 0.9176$) compared with RP. *Conclusion*: In relatively young patients with HR/VHR-LPC, RP and IMRT-ADT yielded similar oncologic outcomes and RP reduced the risk of biochemical failure compared with IMRT-ADT.

Keywords: prostate cancer; radical prostatectomy; intensity-modulated radiotherapy; young men

1. Introduction

According to estimates from Global Cancer Statistics 2020, prostate cancer (PC) is the second most common cancer (1,414,259 new cases) and the fifth leading cause of cancer-related deaths (375,304 deaths) in men worldwide [1]. According to the Taiwan Cancer Registry database (TCRD), PC is the fifth most common cancer and the sixth leading cause of cancer-related deaths in men in Taiwan [2,3]. Increased treatment efficacy and decreased treatment-related side effects are the most critical concerns for patients with PC [4], especially younger patients whose survival is expected to be relatively long. For localized PC (LPC), therapeutic treatment decision-making is based on the LPC risk stratification and health status of the patient [5–7]. Several risk stratification systems, such as those of D'Amico, the American Urological Association (AUA), the European Association of Urology (EAU), and the National Comprehensive Cancer Network (NCCN) [8] include various factors such as prostate-specific antigen (PSA), biopsy Gleason score, or clinical T stage, which are used to classify patients and provide crucial data for treatment modality decision-making [5–7]. The NCCN risk stratification system [8] is used by most physicians in Taiwan. Patients with high-risk or very high-risk LPC (HR/VHR-LPC) have poor oncologic outcomes compared with very low-, low-, favorable-intermediate-, or unfavorable-intermediate-risk LPC, and consequently, these patients require definitive therapy such as external beam radiotherapy (EBRT) or radical prostatectomy (RP) rather than watchful waiting unless the expected survival of the patient is less than five years and they are asymptomatic [8–10]. Recently, the proportional rate of high-risk LPC (HRLPC) has increased (from 11.8% in 2004 to 20.4% in 2016) [11]. However, no consensus has been reached yet on the optimal treatment recommendation for HR/VHR-LPC to be included in clinical guidelines [5,7].

According to the European Association of Urology–European Society for Radiotherapy and Oncology–International Society of Geriatric Oncology 2020 guidelines on PC, a reasonable first-step treatment for patients with HRLPC includes RP or dose-escalated intensity-modulated radiotherapy (IMRT) plus long-term (2–3 years) androgen-deprivation therapy (ADT) [7]. The NCCN version 2.2021 guidelines [8] indicate that the treatment of choice for patients with HR/VHPC with a life expectancy > 5 years is EBRT plus 1.5–3 years of ADT, EBRT plus brachytherapy, including 1–3 years of ADT or RP [8]. However, no randomized clinical trials (RCTs) have yet to evaluate high-dose IMRT plus ADT versus RP regarding oncologic outcomes. Current recommendations for deciding on a treatment modality are based on the results of retrospective population-based studies or meta-analyses [8–10]. However, the comparisons in these studies [8–10] of the oncologic outcomes of RP and high-dose IMRT plus ADT for patients with HR/VHR-LPC are subject to some concerns, with their analyses of relatively young patients with expected long-term survival being particularly questionable. The most common concern is selection bias among patients who are receiving RP and RT because of differing backgrounds, inconsistent irradiation doses, varying durations of ADT use, and distinct RT techniques [8–10]. For retrospective population studies, an effort should be made to balance baseline patient characteristics and maintain consistency in risk classifications and treatment protocols.

For relatively young patients with HRLPC who received definitive treatment, more favorable oncologic outcomes were noted in patients who received RP than in those who received RT [12,13]. However, the results of these studies should be cautiously interpreted because the proportion of ADT used was not recorded in these studies [12,13], and patients who received RP were younger and had fewer comorbidities and less advanced tumors compared with patients who received RT in retrospective studies [14,15]. Furthermore, detailed comparative studies of all-cause death, locoregional recurrence (LRR), biochemical failure (BF), and distant metastasis (DM) associated with standard treatments (RP versus RT plus long-term ADT) in relatively young patients with HRLPC are still lacking. High-dose IMRT plus long-term ADT or RP is one of the treatment recommendations for patients with NCCN HR/VHR-LPC according to the NCCN guidelines [8]. Administering the treatment that can provide the optimal survival benefit is the paramount concern when treating relatively healthy younger (aged $\leq$ 65 years) patients with PC. Patients with PC aged < 65 years were defined as young in our study because the mean age of patients diagnosed as having PC is 69 years in Taiwan [3], and the mean age of patients diagnosed with PC is 66 years in the United States [16]. Several studies have compared RP and EBRT with or without ADT in relatively young and healthy patients, and the results have demonstrated that RP provides superior survival outcomes compared with EBRT [12,13,17]. However, varying definitions of risk stratification, various ADT duration, and inconsistent radiation dosages are concerns that militate against applying the results of these studies in current clinical suggestions [12,13,17]. Therefore, a head-to-head propensity score matching (PSM) analysis was conducted in this study to evaluate these oncologic outcomes of RP and compare them with high-dose IMRT plus long-term ADT for patients with HR/VHR-LPC according to the NCCN risk stratification system [8].

2. Patients and Methods

2.1. Database

A population-based cohort study using Taiwan's National Health Insurance Research Database (NHIRD), which is linked to the TCRD, was conducted. The TCRD contains data of nearly 100% of cancer patients in Taiwan, which was established in 1979 [18]. The NHIRD includes de-identified basic demographic information, disease diagnoses, drugs, and procedures of all beneficiaries [19]. To verify the cause of death and vital status of each patient, The TCRD death registry was additionally linked to the NHIRD. The detailed data on LPC, such as the American Joint Committee on Cancer (AJCC) stage, surgical procedures, techniques, RT dose, hormone treatments, and pathologic stages, were included in TCRD [2,20–23].

2.2. The Cohort

We enrolled patients identified from the TCRD to establish a cohort. Relatively young patients (aged $\leq$ 65 years) who had received a diagnosis of NCCN HR/VHR-LPC and received high-dose IMRT and long-term (1.5–3 years) ADT or RP between 1 January 2011 and 31 December 2016 were included. In this cohort, the relatively young men with HR/VHR-LPC and a life expectancy > years received combination IMRT and long-term ADT or RP in accordance with NCCN guidelines [8]. The index date was defined as the date of LPC diagnosis by pathological confirmation. The patients were followed from the index date to 31 December 2018. Our protocols were reviewed and approved by the Institutional Review Board (IRB109-015-B). The specific method is stated in our previous paper [2].

2.2.1. Inclusion Criteria

(1) Tumor staging from cT1 to T3a, pretreatment PSA levels from 0 to more than 20 ng/mL, or grade group from 1 to 5 were defined as NCCN HR/VHR-LPC.
(2) A newly diagnosed NCCN HR/VHR-LPC who received RP or IMRT.

(3) No other cancer, clinical lymph node metastasis, or distant metastasis were named as LPC.
(4) Removal of the entire prostate gland, seminal vesicles, and the surrounding lymph nodes was defined as standard surgical procedures of RP [24].
(5) Standard IMRT was defined that pelvic lymph nodes receiving prophylactic doses of 45 Gy in 1.8 Gy per fraction, the seminal vesicles having 54 Gy, and the prostate receiving boost radiation dose to 72–81 Gy.

2.2.2. Exclusion Criteria

(1) Doses less than 72 Gy of IMRT were defined as insufficient irradiation doses based on previous reports and NCCN guidelines [8,25–27].
(2) IMRT without long-term (<1.5 years) ADT.
(3) Patients with PC who did not receive standard RP or doses of IMRT after LPC diagnosis.

BF after RP was defined as a serum PSA level of ≥0.2 ng/mL according to the definition of BF of the AUA [28]. BF was defined as a PSA nadir plus ≥2 ng/mL after having reached a PSA nadir after treatment of IMRT based on the Radiation Therapy Oncology Group-ASTRO Phoenix Consensus [29]. However, the possible treatments (such as salvage irradiation after RP, salvage prostatectomy, high-intensity focused ultrasound after IMRT, or systemic therapy after BF) were allowed and did not disqualify patients from our inclusion. The clinical outcomes (BF, LRR, DM, and all-cause death) were compared between patients who received RP (group 1) and high-dose IMRT-ADT (group 2). The LRR or DM was defined clinically or radiologically as overt local recurrence or distant failure. Local recurrence was confirmed by prostate biopsy through pathological diagnosis.

2.3. Covariates

The covariates, which might be associated with all-cause death, are shown in Table 1. Comorbidities were scored by the Charlson comorbidity index (CCI) scores [30,31] and special comorbidities associated with all-cause death. Comorbidities censored 12 months before the index date were included in our study. If the primary diagnostic code, using the *International Classification of Diseases, Ninth Revision, Clinical Modification* (*ICD-9-CM*), upon visit to the first admission or the outpatient department, was repeated more than twice, comorbidities were included and verified in our study. We removed peripheral vascular disease, cerebrovascular disease, chronic pulmonary disease, myocardial infarction, congestive heart failure, diabetes, and hypertension from CCI scores to prevent repeated adjustment.

Table 1. Propensity score-matched demographic and clinic characteristics of young patients with high- to very high-risk prostate adenocarcinoma.

		Prostatectomy N = 481		High-Dose IMRT + Long-Term ADT N = 215		
		n	(%)	N	(%)	*p*-Value
Age	Mean (SD)	62.6	(2.3)	62.3	(2.3)	0.3378
	Median (IQR, Q1–Q3)	63	(58–65)	63	(59–65)	
	20–59	73	(15.2)	29	(13.5)	0.9833
	60–65	408	(84.8)	186	(86.5)	
Years of diagnosis	2011–2012	67	(13.9)	30	(14.0)	0.9953
	2013	79	(16.4)	32	(14.9)	
	2014	96	(20.0)	42	(19.5)	
	2015	120	(24.9)	54	(25.1)	
	2016	119	(24.7)	57	(26.5)	
CCI scores	0	220	(45.7)	99	(46.0)	0.9279
	1	124	(25.8)	53	(24.7)	
	2+	137	(28.5)	63	(29.3)	
Myocardial infarction		5	(1.0)	4	(1.9)	0.7702
Congestive heart failure		20	(4.2)	8	(3.7)	0.4891

Table 1. *Cont.*

		Prostatectomy N = 481		High-Dose IMRT + Long-Term ADT N = 215		
		n	(%)	N	(%)	*p*-Value
Peripheral vascular disease		10	(2.1)	5	(2.3)	0.8838
Cerebrovascular disease		26	(5.4)	18	(8.4)	0.3550
Chronic pulmonary disease		60	(12.5)	24	(11.2)	0.5333
Diabetes		132	(27.4)	56	(26.0)	0.5507
Hypertension		244	(50.7)	115	(53.5)	0.7777
Income	Very low	155	(32.2)	68	(31.6)	0.6764
	Low	175	(36.4)	81	(37.7)	
	Middle	98	(20.4)	38	(17.7)	
	High	53	(11.0)	28	(13.0)	
Hospital area	North	259	(53.8)	109	(50.7)	0.9569
	Central	103	(21.4)	45	(20.9)	
	South	110	(22.9)	54	(25.1)	
	East	9	(1.9)	7	(3.3)	
Hospital level	Medical center	289	(60.1)	113	(52.6)	0.5018
	Others	192	(39.9)	102	(47.4)	
cT-stage	cT1	176	(36.6)	75	(34.9)	0.9798
	cT2a	115	(23.9)	52	(24.2)	
	cT2b	24	(5.0)	10	(4.7)	
	cT2c	139	(28.9)	57	(26.5)	
	cT3a	27	(5.6)	21	(9.8)	
Gleason score	≤5	5	(1.0)	6	(2.8)	0.6573
	6	58	(12.1)	54	(25.1)	
	7	289	(60.1)	106	(49.3)	
	8	86	(17.9)	31	(14.4)	
	9+	33	(6.9)	13	(6.0)	
	Missing	10	(2.1)	5	(2.3)	
Grade group	1–2	12	(2.5)	5	(2.3)	0.2556
	3	60	(12.5)	59	(27.4)	
	4	360	(74.8)	134	(62.3)	
	5	49	(10.2)	17	(7.9)	
Preoperative PSA (ng/mL)	0–5	81	(16.8)	31	(14.4)	0.6906
	5–10	148	(30.8)	56	(26.0)	
	10–20	160	(33.3)	65	(30.2)	
	20+	45	(9.4)	43	(20.0)	
	Missing	47	(9.8)	20	(9.3)	
EAU risk group	Localized intermediate	203	(42.2)	77	(35.8)	0.8815
	Localized high	242	(50.3)	111	(51.6)	
	Localized advanced	36	(7.5)	27	(12.6)	
Follow-up time, months	Mean (SD)	60.2	(17.6)	59.9	(17.3)	
All-cause death		27	(5.6)	12	(5.6)	0.5704
Biochemical recurrence		102	(21.2)	84	(39.1)	<0.0001
Locoregional recurrence		27	(5.6)	14	(6.5)	0.9982
Distant metastasis		31	(6.4)	16	(7.4)	1.0000

IQR, interquartile range; SD, standard deviation; RP, radical prostatectomy; T, tumor; cT, clinical tumor stage; PSA, prostate-specific antigen; EAU, European Association of Urology; IMRT, intensity-modulated radiotherapy; ADT, antiandrogen therapy; N, numbers; AJCC, American Joint Committee on Cancer; CCI, Charlson comorbidity index.

2.4. Endpoints

All-cause death between RP and high-dose IMRT plus long-term ADT is our primary endpoint. BF, LRR, and DM between young men with HR/VHR-LPC who underwent RP and those who underwent high-dose IMRT plus long-term ADT were our secondary endpoints.

2.5. Propensity Score Matching

We used optimal matching in our study as a 1:4 ratio to reach a sufficient sample size for further analysis [32]. If the sample size was insufficient for a 1:4 ratio, we used a 1:3 ratio to increase the sample size for analysis. Nevertheless, not all covariates were 1:3 matched between the RP and IMRT groups; some covariates were matched 1:2 or 1:1 between the RP and IMRT groups. Thus, an exact 3:1 ratio between the RP and IMRT groups was not attained.

2.6. Statistics

In modeling the study duration from the index date to all-cause mortality, a cox proportional hazards model was applied with the control for confounders in young patients with NCCN HR/VHR-LPC. To minimize the influences of potential confounders, head-to-head PSM was conducted during comparisons of treatment outputs between those two treatment groups. A width equal to 0.2 of the standard deviation of the logit of the propensity score was balanced in the logit of the propensity score using calipers [33,34]. In order to reduce any discrepancy between the two treatment groups, the controls with similar background covariates to the case patients were opted for [35]. A strong and robust predictor was applied to account for clustering within matched sets, and a Cox model was applied to regress endpoints on the treatment status. Thereafter, the multivariable Cox regression analysis was used to calculate the hazard ratios (HRs) to define whether the covariates were required to be re-adjusted to diminish any confounding effects if there was an unbalance in conditions existing after PSM was performed. Potential prognosis factors were also tightly controlled during the analysis, and the endpoint was all factors associated with the mortality in the treatment group.

The risk of all-cause death was calculated for young men with HR/VHR-LPC. The other secondary endpoints, such as BF, LRR, and DM, were assessed and estimated by applying a proportional subdistribution hazard regression model to cope with the competing risk of death in the analysis of time-to-event data. All statistical analyses were conducted using SAS version 9.3. $p < 0.05$ was considered as significant in a two-tailed Wald test. The risk of all-cause death was also estimated by applying the Kaplan-Meier method, and differences among high-dose IMRT + HT or RP were defined using the stratified log-rank test to compare survival curves (stratified on matched sets). A p-value less than 0.05 was considered statistically significant.

3. Results

3.1. Study Cohort after Propensity Scores Matching

We included 696 young men with NCCN HR/VHR-LPC (Table 1), 481 receiving RP, and 215 receiving high-dose IMRT-ADT groups, respectively. The mean follow-up duration for the RP and IMRT + long-term HT groups were 60.2 and 59.9 months after the index dates, successively. After PSM was performed, there were no statistically significant differences ($p > 0.05$) noticed between groups of covariates (Table 1). Most p-values were more than 0.5, suggesting that the matching variables' distribution was close (Table 1).

3.2. Clinical Outcomes between the Two Therapeutic Groups

Treatment was not a significant predictor of all-cause mortality based on the multivariate Cox regression analysis (Table 2). RP was not associated with higher overall survival (OS) compared with the definitive high-dose IMRT-ADT in young patients with NCCN HR/VHR-LPC through multivariate Cox regression analysis. No significant differences were found in the descriptive covariates, except for hospital level and EAU risk group, because PSM was conducted accurately (Table 2). The adjusted hazard ratio (aHR; 95% confidence interval [CI]) of BF for IMRT-ADT compared with RP was 2.03 (1.56–2.65, $p < 0.0001$; Table 3). In younger patients with NCCN HR/VHR-LPC, RP did not significantly affect LRR compared with IMRT-ADT (Table 4). There were no significant differences for DM between IMRT-ADT and RP in younger patients with NCCN

HR/VHR-LPC (Table 5). Taken together, IMRT-ADT was not a significant risk factor of all-cause death (aHR = 1.2, 95% CI 0.65–2.24, $p = 0.564$), LR (aHR = 0.88, 95% CI 0.67–1.06, $p = 0.3524$), or DM (aHR = 1.03, 95% CI 0.56–1.9, $p = 0.9176$) compared with RP. Hospital level and EAU risk group were significant prognostic factors for mortality, BF, and LRR by multivariate analysis (Tables 2–4). Moreover, through multivariate analysis, the EAU risk group was also a significant prognostic factor for DM (Table 5).

Table 2. Multivariate Cox proportional hazards regression analysis of all-cause death of young patients with high- to very high-risk prostate adenocarcinoma.

Covariates		Adjusted HR *	(95% CI)	*p*-Value
Curative treatment	Radical prostatectomy	ref		0.5640
	High-dose IMRT + long-term ADT	1.20	(0.65–2.24)	
Age	20–59	ref		0.6834
	60–65	1.18	(0.54–2.58)	
Years of diagnosis	2011–2012	ref		0.4500
	2013	1.30	(0.59–2.87)	
	2014	0.55	(0.21–1.45)	
	2015	0.92	(0.37–2.26)	
	2016	0.82	(0.31–2.18)	
CCI scores	0	ref		0.1043
	1	1.10	(0.51–2.38)	
	2+	2.30	(0.96–5.54)	
Congestive heart failure		1.37	(0.44–4.32)	0.5865
Peripheral vascular disease		0.00	-	0.9797
Cerebrovascular disease		1.10	(0.48–2.53)	0.8199
Chronic pulmonary disease		0.60	(0.22–1.69)	0.3353
Diabetes		1.20	(0.59–2.45)	0.6142
Hypertension		1.37	(0.78–2.40)	0.2762
Income	Very low	ref		0.3395
	Low	1.41	(0.74–2.68)	
	Middle	0.94	(0.43–2.08)	
	High	0.64	(0.24–1.69)	
Hospital level	Academic centers	ref		0.0129
	Nonacademic centers	2.01	(1.16–3.50)	
Hospital area	North	ref		0.0026
	Central	1.64	(0.82–3.28)	
	South	2.20	(1.13–4.31)	
	East	7.68	(2.51–23.55)	
cT-stage	cT1	ref		0.2690
	cT2a	1.02	(0.51–2.02)	
	cT2b	0.67	(0.22–2.02)	
	cT2c	0.47	(0.21–1.07)	
	cT3a	0.38	(0.08–1.74)	
EAU risk group	Localized intermediate	ref		0.0454
	Localized high	1.57	(0.81–3.06)	
	Localized advanced	2.55	(1.36–5.18)	

RP, radical prostatectomy; T, tumor; cT, clinical tumor stages; PSA, prostate-specific antigen; EAU, European Association of Urology; IMRT, intensity-modulated radiotherapy; ADT, antiandrogen therapy; AJCC, American Joint Committee on Cancer; CCI, Charlson comorbidity index; CI, confidence interval, aHR, adjusted hazard ratio; Ref, reference group; NTD, New Taiwan Dollars. * All covariates in Table 2 were adjusted.

Table 3. Multivariate Cox proportional hazards regression analysis of biochemical recurrence in young patients with high- to very high-risk of prostate adenocarcinoma.

Covariates		Adjusted HR *	(95% CI)	*p*-Value
Curative treatment	Radical prostatectomy	ref		<0.0001
	IMRT + long-term ADT	2.03	(1.56–2.65)	
Age	20–59	ref		0.6054
	60–69	1.08	(0.82–1.42)	
	70–80			
	80+			
Years of diagnosis	2011–2012	ref		0.3193
	2013	0.81	(0.56–1.16)	
	2014	0.89	(0.62–1.27)	
	2015	0.85	(0.59–1.22)	
	2016	0.67	(0.45–0.98)	
CCI scores	0	ref		0.6576
	1	1.12	(0.83–1.52)	
	2+	1.20	(0.79–1.83)	
Congestive heart failure		0.74	(0.38–1.44)	0.3760
Peripheral vascular disease		0.51	(0.16–1.64)	0.2569
Cerebrovascular disease		1.07	(0.67–1.70)	0.7711
Chronic pulmonary disease		0.92	(0.58–1.45)	0.7106
Diabetes		0.97	(0.68–1.37)	0.8568
Hypertension		0.93	(0.73–1.17)	0.5365
Income	Low	ref		0.6583
	Very Low	1.06	(0.78–1.43)	
	Middle	1.13	(0.82–1.55)	
	High	0.91	(0.66–1.26)	
Hospital level	Academic centers	ref		0.0073
	Nonacademic centers	1.37	(1.09–1.73)	
Hospital area	North	ref		0.1560
	Central	1.05	(0.93–1.79)	
	South	1.11	(0.83–1.49)	
	East	1.50	(0.70–3.18)	
cT-stage	cT1	ref		0.4036
	cT2a	1.04	(0.78–1.39)	
	cT2b	1.08	(0.71–1.64)	
	cT2c	1.18	(0.41–1.81)	
	cT3a	1.26	(0.24–1.99)	
EAU risk group	Localized intermediate	ref		<0.0001
	localized-high	2.18	(1.63–2.91)	
	Localized advanced	3.41	(1.59–7.32)	

RP, radical prostatectomy; T, tumor; cT, clinical tumor stage; PSA, prostate-specific antigen; EAU, European Association of Urology; IMRT, intensity-modulated radiotherapy; ADT, antiandrogen therapy; AJCC, American Joint Committee on Cancer; CCI, Charlson comorbidity index; CI, confidence interval; aHR, adjusted hazard ratio; Ref, reference group; NTD, New Taiwan Dollars. * All covariates mentioned in Table 2 were adjusted.

Table 4. Multivariate Cox proportional hazards regression analysis of locoregional recurrence in young patients with high- to very high-risk prostate adenocarcinoma.

Covariates		Adjusted HR *	(95% CI)	*p*-Value
Curative treatment	Radical prostatectomy	ref		0.3524
	IMRT + long-term ADT	0.88	(0.67–1.06)	
Age	20–59	ref		0.5068
	60–65	0.87	(0.57–1.32)	
Years of diagnosis	2011–2012	ref		0.6379
	2013	1.57	(0.81–3.03)	
	2014	1.26	(0.66–2.41)	
	2015	1.38	(0.72–2.63)	
	2016	1.08	(0.53–2.20)	

Table 4. *Cont.*

Covariates		Adjusted HR *	(95% CI)	p-Value
CCI scores	0	ref		0.1806
	1	0.58	(0.33–1.04)	
	2+	0.66	(0.32–1.36)	
Congestive heart failure		2.10	(0.73–6.01)	0.1665
Peripheral vascular disease		0.90	(0.67–1.31)	0.4021
Cerebrovascular disease		1.61	(0.70–3.71)	0.2584
Chronic pulmonary disease		0.90	(0.37–2.20)	0.8124
Diabetes		1.32	(0.75–2.33)	0.3324
Hypertension		0.80	(0.54–1.20)	0.2893
Income	Very Low	ref		0.1690
	Low	0.74	(0.44–1.27)	
	Middle	1.05	(0.63–1.72)	
	High	0.61	(0.36–1.04)	
Hospital level	Academic centers	ref		0.0456
	Nonacademic centers	1.05	(1.00–1.42)	
Hospital area	North	ref		0.9213
	Central	0.90	(0.58–1.40)	
	South	1.04	(0.62–1.76)	
	East	0.62	(0.08–4.54)	
cT-stage	cT1	ref		0.2812
	cT2a	1.00	(0.63–1.60)	
	cT2b	1.03	(0.43–1.60)	
	cT2c	1.06	(0.40–1.63)	
	cT3a	1.11	(0.51–1.78)	
EAU risk group	Localized intermediate	ref		0.0077
	Localized high	1.68	(1.08–2.62)	
	Localized advanced	5.32	(1.44–19.72)	

RP, radical prostatectomy; T, tumor; cT, clinical tumor stage; PSA, prostate-specific antigen; EAU, European Association of Urology; IMRT, intensity-modulated radiotherapy; ADT, antiandrogen therapy; AJCC, American Joint Committee on Cancer; CCI, Charlson comorbidity index; CI, confidence interval; aHR, adjusted hazard ratio; Ref, reference group; NTD, New Taiwan Dollars. * All covariates mentioned in Table 2 were adjusted.

Table 5. Multivariate Cox proportional hazards regression analysis of distant metastasis in patients with high- to very high-risk of prostate adenocarcinoma.

Covariates		Adjusted HR *	(95% CI)	p-Value
Curative treatment	Radical prostatectomy	ref		0.9176
	IMRT + long-term ADT	1.03	(0.56–1.90)	
Age	20–59	ref		0.7536
	60–69	1.10	(0.62–1.95)	
	70–80			
	80+			
Years of diagnosis	2011–2012	ref		0.2664
	2013	1.66	(0.83–3.31)	
	2014	0.91	(0.42–1.95)	
	2015	0.76	(0.35–1.67)	
	2016	0.97	(0.44–2.16)	
CCI scores	0	ref		0.4698
	1	1.22	(0.63–2.36)	
	2+	1.70	(0.72–4.02)	
Congestive heart failure		0.57	(0.14–2.40)	0.4450
Peripheral vascular disease		1.45	(0.39–5.42)	0.5775
Cerebrovascular disease		1.21	(0.56–2.60)	0.6237
Chronic pulmonary disease		0.98	(0.43–2.25)	0.9626
Diabetes		1.64	(0.85–3.19)	0.1424
Hypertension		1.16	(0.73–1.84)	0.5247
Income	Very Low	ref		0.8722

Table 5. *Cont.*

Covariates		Adjusted HR *	(95% CI)	*p*-Value
	Low	1.29	(0.69–2.41)	
	Middle	1.23	(0.63–2.40)	
	High	1.20	(0.60–2.41)	
Hospital level	Medical center	ref		0.1107
	Others	1.49	(0.91–2.43)	
Hospital area	North	ref		0.2710
	Central	1.59	(0.92–2.75)	
	South	2.07	(0.88–3.62)	
	East	3.85	(0.81–4.71)	
cT-stage	cT1	ref		0.4248
	cT2a	1.00	(0.55–1.67)	
	cT2b	1.03	(0.51–1.12)	
	cT2c	1.08	(0.69–1.61)	
	cT3a	1.09	(0.67–2.82)	
EAU risk group	Localized intermediate	ref		0.0114
	localized high	1.26	(1.08–3.17)	
	Localized advanced	3.43	(1.58–4.43)	

RP, radical prostatectomy; T, tumor; cT, clinical tumor stage; PSA, prostate-specific antigen; EAU, European Association of Urology; IMRT, intensity-modulated radiotherapy; ADT, antiandrogen therapy; AJCC, American Joint Committee on Cancer; CCI, Charlson comorbidity index; CI, confidence interval; aHR, adjusted hazard ratio; Ref, reference group; NTD, New Taiwan Dollars. * All covariates mentioned in Table 2 were adjusted.

Kaplan–Meier survival curves for the PSM cohort of younger patients with NCCN HR/VHR-LPC who received high-dose IMRT-ADT or RP are presented in Figure 1. The survival curve for RP was not significantly better than that for high-dose IMRT-ADT in younger patients with NCCN HR/VHR-LPC. The 5-year survival rates for RP and high-dose IMRT-ADT were 94.7% and 95.9% (p = 0.9983), respectively.

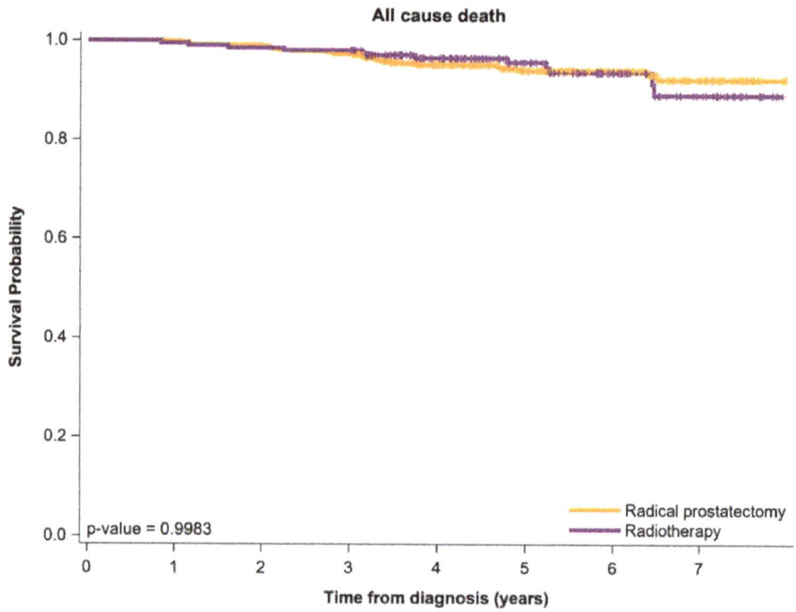

Figure 1. Survival curves for endpoints by Kaplan–Meier method for propensity score-matched young patients with NCCN high- to very high-risk prostate adenocarcinoma receiving various curative-intent treatments NCCN, National Comprehensive Cancer Network.

4. Discussion

A well-designed study to compare the oncological outcomes between RP and high-dose IMRT plus long-term ADT in relatively young ($\leq$ 65 years) men with NCCN HR/VHR-LPC based on the commonly used NCCN risk classifications remains lacking. Our study included patients with HR/VHR-LPC diagnosed according to the definition in the NCCN version 2.2021 guidelines [8] who received adequate long-term ADT and a sufficient radiation dosage in this well-designed PSM study. The findings of our study revealed that either RP or high-dose IMRT plus long-term ADT yield the same rate of all-cause death, LRR, and DM for relatively young men with NCCN HR/VHR-LPC after a mean 5-year follow-up duration. However, BF-free survival (BFFS) in the young men with NCCN HR/VHR-LPC who were receiving RP was superior to that of those patients receiving high-dose IMRT plus long-term ADT.

BF is a crucial endpoint when evaluating the efficacy of primary treatment, and patients with BF should receive salvage treatment to prevent or delay disease progression [36]. Patients with BF have an increased likelihood of experiencing substantial anxiety and negative moods and a decreased quality of life after salvage treatment [37,38]. Although the impact of BF on subsequent PC mortality remains unknown, an observational study found that BF was associated with an increased risk of PC mortality [39]. For relatively young healthy patients, therapy with low BF is a superior choice because of those patients' relatively long life expectancy, according to the results of our study (Table 3). Relatively young patients with HR/VHR-LPC who were treated with high-dose IMRT plus long-term ADT experienced a 2.03-fold BF increase compared with those treated with RP. Although the effect of local treatment on BF was not observed in all-cause death, LRR, or DM after PSM (Tables 2–5), this may be attributable to salvage treatment improving survival outcomes after BF of primary treatment and a long natural disease history to mortality of LPC [40–44]. Our study is compatible with the previous studies, which demonstrated no significant differences in all-cause death between RP or RT-ADT in men with HR/VHR-LPC [45,46]. Initial treatment with RP as compared with EBRT and ADT was not associated with an increased risk of prostate cancer-specific mortality in men with a Gleason score of 8-10 for prostate cancer [45]. Evidence demonstrating definitive superiority of either modality is lacking [46]. In our novel findings, in relatively young men with HR/VHR-LPC and a life expectancy > 5 years, RP and RT-ADT still yielded similar all-cause death, LRR, and DM, although RP reduced the risk of BF compared with RT-ADT. Given the possible complications and mood adverse effects after salvage treatment [40–44], RP may be the superior choice for relatively young healthy patients with HR/VHR-LPC (Table 3). However, this suggestion should be confirmed by the results of a well-designed RCT.

Several risk classification tools are available for classifying patients with localized PC and provide data for treatment decisions [5,6,8,47–49]. However, the most commonly used risk classification for PC in Taiwan is the NCCN risk classification [8]. In one population-based comparison study, the NCCN risk group system exhibited superior discriminatory ability for predicting PC-specific mortality compared with the EAU risk group system [50]. In our study, we used the NCCN risk group system to classify the patients with LPC. However, reclassification of patients with NCCN HR/VHR-LPC by the EAU risk group system may have the potential to determine the patients with the highest risk of disease progression. If the patients with NCCN HR/VHR-LPC were stratified by the EAU risk group system, 7.5% of the patients in the RP group and 12.6% of the patients in the IMRT plus long-term ADT group would be classified as locally advanced (Table 1). After multivariate Cox proportional hazards regression analysis, EAU-locally advanced PC was a risk factor for disease progression (Tables 2–5). This finding indicated that if the patients with NCCN HR/VHR-LPC were classified as EAU-locally advanced, these patients would require more aggressive therapy and close follow-up.

Our results demonstrated that patients treated at academic centers experienced lower all-cause death, BF, and LRR than those treated at nonacademic centers (Tables 2–4). This finding is compatible with a relevant study that focused on RP for patients with PC [20].

Additional studies have compared the PSA recurrence rate in patients with PC treated with RP between high-volume and low-volume centers, and these studies have found that fewer PSA recurrences and distant metastases were identified in high-volume centers regardless of whether the treatment was IMRT or RP [21,51]. For patients treated with EBRT plus ADT, the patients who received treatment at a center with a high-volume radiation facility had longer overall survival [52]. The same finding was demonstrated in patients with diffuse large B-cell lymphoma; high-risk patients treated at academic centers had longer overall survival [53]. These data highlight the essential role of facility volume for oncological outcomes in patients with PC. Multivariate Cox proportional hazards regression analysis of all-cause death (Table 2) showed a statistically significant difference ($p = 0.0026$) among patients treated at different hospitals (hospital areas). The hospital areas in Taiwan were associated with rural and urbanized regions in Taiwan. The urbanization grades in Taiwan are North, Central, South, and East Taiwan, in order. In other words, North Taiwan is the most urbanized area in Taiwan. Our results showed that the mortality rate of relatively young men with HR/VHR-LPC and a life expectancy > 5 years were proportion to urbanization grade, whatever the RP and RT-ADT. Our outcomes were also compatible with the previous studies in which the high urbanization grade was associated with low mortality of prostate cancer [54,55].

On the risk of radiation-induced second cancer, given that the study presented here compares radiotherapy vs. surgery in relatively young men that have a long-enough lifespan to develop such long-term effects. For relatively young age patients with a longer life expectancy, this aspect might further influence treatment-related decisions among prostate cancer patients with a high risk to develop second malignancies after receiving radiation treatment for the primary tumor [56–58]. Moreover, photon exposure (such as IMRT) has a complex radiobiology that influences long-term effects in patients treated for primary cancers. IMRT is likely to almost double the incidence of second malignancies compared with conventional RT [59,60]. The numbers of second malignancies may be larger for longer survival (or for younger patients) using IMRT. Therefore, RP is not only superior to RT-ADT in BF but also results in a low risk of radiation-induced second cancer in these relatively young men with HR/VHR-LPC and a longer life expectancy life.

In comparison to the other National cancer registry-based reports like the Danish Prostate Cancer Registry, Cancer Registry of Norway, and United in Fight against prOstate cancer (UFO) registry [61–63], there was more information, consistent treatments, and the same risk stratification as using the NCCN risk stratification, similar ADT duration, sufficient radiation dosage, and the same radiation technique in our TCRD study. Moreover, there was no PSM design in the previous studies, and the most common concern was selection bias among patients from the aforementioned Cancer Registry database [61–63] who are receiving RP and RT because of differing backgrounds.

The current manuscript includes totally different populations and outcomes from our previous study [2]. The population, cT stages, PSA, Gleason scores grade, treatments, ADT use, surgical difficulties and complications, life expectancy, and numbers of unfavorable intermediate-risk groups are very different from high- to very high-risk groups. For example, the duration of ADT use for the intermediate-risk group (4–6 months) [2] is different from high- to very high-risk group (1.5 years at least). Moreover, the complications and difficulties of RP were also different between the intermediate groups and high-to very high-risk groups. In addition, the indications of curative treatments for intermediate groups and high- to very-high risk groups were also different. Curative treatments are indicated for a life expectancy with > 10 years and > 5 years for intermediate groups and high- to very high-risk groups, respectively [2]. Therefore, to clarify that the optimal therapeutic treatments of RP or IMRT-ADT are very important between different populations, including intermediate-risk groups and high- to very high-risk groups. Finally, the outcomes were also different in the two studies. RP is only superior to IMRT plus long-term ADT in BF for high- to very high-risk groups in the current study, although RP is superior to IMRT plus short-term ADT in overall survival, BF, LRR, and DM for intermediate-risk groups [2].

In summary, the population, treatments, and outcomes were totally different in the two studies. Therefore, we still think the current study is worthy for valuable clinical references for high- to very-high risk groups.

The strength of our study was that it is the largest and first head-to-head PSM study to compare the detailed oncologic outcomes of RP and high-dose IMRT plus long-term ADT for relatively young patients with NCCN HR/VHR-LPC. Moreover, consistent RT techniques, similar irradiation doses, and homogenous durations of ADT use were employed in this study. Additional potential cofounding factors of BF were well-matched through PSM in our study and indicated balance (Table 1). Our study is the first study to demonstrate a statistical difference in BFFS between RP or high-dose IMRT plus long-term ADT for relatively young patients with NCCN HR/VHR-LPC, but no significant differences were observed regarding all-cause death, LRR, or DM. Our findings may be valuable in shared decision-making between physicians and young patients with NCCN HR/VHR-LPC when selecting between RP or high-dose IMRT plus long-term ADT. In future clinical trials, the oncologic outcomes of RP and high-dose IMRT plus long-term ADT determined herein could be referenced for further risk management in young patients with NCCN HR/VHR PC.

Our study has some limitations. First, brachytherapy was not included in this study because of its lack of favor in Taiwan. The mainstream treatments for localized PC in Taiwan are RP and EBRT. Second, our entire study population was Asian. The results should be cautiously extrapolated to other races. Third, this study did not include possible risk factors regarding all-cause death, such as lifestyle, dietary habits, or body mass index, that might contribute to a high incidence of mortality as a competing risk factor of BF. However, only 5% mortality rate was noted between the two groups and did not reach statistical significance. The potential competing risk of all-cause death for BF could be disregarded. Moreover, BF was estimated using a proportional subdistribution hazard regression model to overcome the competing risk of death in the analysis of time-to-event data [64,65]. Thus, in real-world applications, RP might be associated with BFFS rather than high-dose IMRT with long-term ADT for patients with NCCN HR/VHR-LPC. Finally, this study was a retrospective population cohort study. A prospective RCT is recommended to define the optimal localized treatment for patients with NCCN HR/VHR-LPC.

5. Conclusions

Relatively young patients with NCCN HR/VHR-LPC who received either RP or high-dose IMRT plus long-term ADT had similar oncological outcomes. Additionally, RP demonstrated lower BF.

Author Contributions: Conception and design: H.-J.S., S.-C.C., C.-H.H. (Chia-Hao Hsu), Y.-C.L., C.-H.H. (Chu-Hsuan Hung), and S.-Y.W.; collection and assembly of data: H.-J.S., S.-C.C., and S.-Y.W.; data analysis and interpretation: H.-J.S., S.-C.C., and S.-Y.W.; administrative support: S.-Y.W.; manuscript writing: H.-J.S., S.-C.C., and S.-Y.W.; final approval of manuscript: all authors. All authors have read and agreed to the published version of the manuscript.

Funding: Lo-Hsu Medical Foundation, Lotung Poh-Ai Hospital, supports S.-Y.W.'s work (Funding Number: 10908, 10909, 11001, 11002, 11003, 11006, and 11013).

Institutional Review Board Statement: The study protocols were reviewed and approved by the Institutional Review Board of Tzu-Chi Medical Foundation (IRB109-015-B).

Informed Consent Statement: Informed consent was waived because the data sets are covered under the Personal Information Protection Act.

Data Availability Statement: Restrictions apply to the availability of these data. Data was obtained from Taiwan Ministry of Health and Welfare and are available from Szu-Yuan Wu with the permission of Institutional Review Board of Tzu-Chi Medical Foundation (IRB109-015-B).

Conflicts of Interest: The authors have no potential conflict of interest to declare. The data sets supporting the study conclusions are included in the manuscript.

Abbreviations

RP, radical prostatectomy; PC, prostate cancer; BFFS, biochemical failure-free survival; CI, confidence interval; T, tumor; PSA, prostate-specific antigen; AJCC, American Joint Committee on Cancer; SD, standard deviation; HR, hazard ratio; aHR, adjusted hazard ratio; RCT, randomized controlled trial; NCCN, National Comprehensive Cancer Network; RT-ADT, radiation plus antiandrogen therapy; HR/VHR-LPC, high- or very high-risk localized prostate cancer; HRLPC, high-risk localized prostate cancer; TCRD, Taiwan Cancer Registry database; IMRT, intensity-modulated radiotherapy; LPC, localized prostate cancer; EAU, European Association of Urology; AUA, American Urological Association; EBRT, external beam radiotherapy; ADT, antiandrogen therapy; PSM, propensity score matching; NHIRD, National Health Insurance Research Database; CCI, Charlson comorbidity index; *ICD-10-CM, International Classification of Diseases, Ninth Revision, Clinical Modification*; OS, overall survival.

References

1. Sung, H.; Ferlay, J.; Siegel, R.L.; Laversanne, M.; Soerjomataram, I.; Jemal, A.; Bray, F. Global Cancer Statistics 2020: GLOBOCAN Estimates of Incidence and Mortality Worldwide for 36 Cancers in 185 Countries. *CA Cancer J. Clin.* **2021**, *71*, 209–249. [CrossRef]
2. Wu, S.Y.; Chang, S.C.; Chen, C.I.; Huang, C.C. Oncologic Outcomes of Radical Prostatectomy and High-Dose Intensity-Modulated Radiotherapy with Androgen-Deprivation Therapy for Relatively Young Patients with Unfavorable Intermediate-Risk Prostate Adenocarcinoma. *Cancers* **2021**, *13*, 1517. [CrossRef]
3. Health Promotion Administration, Ministry of Health and Welfare. *Taiwan Cancer Registry Annual Report*; Ministry of Health and Welfare: Taipei City, Taiwan, 2018.
4. Gomella, L.G.; Johannes, J.; Trabulsi, E.J. Current prostate cancer treatments: Effect on quality of life. *Urology* **2009**, *73*, S28–S35. [CrossRef]
5. Parker, C.; Castro, E.; Fizazi, K.; Heidenreich, A.; Ost, P.; Procopio, G.; Tombal, B.; Gillessen, S.; ESMO Guidelines Committee. Prostate cancer: ESMO Clinical Practice Guidelines for diagnosis, treatment and follow-up. *Ann. Oncol.* **2020**, *31*, 1119–1134. [CrossRef]
6. Sanda, M.G.; Cadeddu, J.A.; Kirkby, E.; Chen, R.C.; Crispino, T.; Fontanarosa, J.; Freedland, S.J.; Greene, K.; Klotz, L.H.; Makarov, D.V.; et al. Clinically Localized Prostate Cancer: AUA/ASTRO/SUO Guideline. Part I: Risk Stratification, Shared Decision Making, and Care Options. *J. Urol.* **2018**, *199*, 683–690. [CrossRef] [PubMed]
7. Mottet, N.; van den Bergh, R.C.N.; Briers, E.; Van den Broeck, T.; Cumberbatch, M.G.; De Santis, M.; Fanti, S.; Fossati, N.; Gandaglia, G.; Gillessen, S.; et al. EAU-EANM-ESTRO-ESUR-SIOG Guidelines on Prostate Cancer-2020 Update. Part 1: Screening, Diagnosis, and Local Treatment with Curative Intent. *Eur. Urol.* **2021**, *79*, 243–262. [CrossRef]
8. The National Comprehensive Cancer Network: NCCN Clinical Practice Guidelines in Oncology: Prostate Cancer. Available online: https://www.nccn.org/professionals/physician_gls/pdf/prostate.pdf (accessed on 17 February 2021).
9. Narang, A.K.; Gergis, C.; Robertson, S.P.; He, P.; Ram, A.N.; McNutt, T.R.; Griffith, E.; DeWeese, T.A.; Honig, S.; Singh, H.; et al. Very High-Risk Localized Prostate Cancer: Outcomes Following Definitive Radiation. *Int. J. Radiat. Oncol. Biol. Phys.* **2016**, *94*, 254–262. [CrossRef]
10. Rodrigues, G.; Warde, P.; Pickles, T.; Crook, J.; Brundage, M.; Souhami, L.; Lukka, H.; Genitourinary Radiation Oncologists of Canada. Pre-treatment risk stratification of prostate cancer patients: A critical review. *Can. Urol. Assoc. J.* **2012**, *6*, 121–127. [CrossRef] [PubMed]
11. Agrawal, V.; Ma, X.; Hu, J.C.; Barbieri, C.E.; Nagar, H. Trends in Diagnosis and Disparities in Initial Management of High-Risk Prostate Cancer in the US. *JAMA Netw. Open* **2020**, *3*, e2014674. [CrossRef] [PubMed]
12. Berg, S.; Cole, A.P.; Krimphove, M.J.; Nabi, J.; Marchese, M.; Lipsitz, S.R.; Noldus, J.; Choueiri, T.K.; Kibel, A.S.; Trinh, Q.D. Comparative Effectiveness of Radical Prostatectomy Versus External Beam Radiation Therapy Plus Brachytherapy in Patients with High-risk Localized Prostate Cancer. *Eur. Urol.* **2019**, *75*, 552–555. [CrossRef] [PubMed]
13. Huang, H.; Muscatelli, S.; Naslund, M.; Badiyan, S.N.; Kaiser, A.; Siddiqui, M.M. Evaluation of Cancer Specific Mortality with Surgery versus Radiation as Primary Therapy for Localized High Grade Prostate Cancer in Men Younger Than 60 Years. *J. Urol.* **2019**, *201*, 120–128. [CrossRef] [PubMed]
14. Boorjian, S.A.; Karnes, R.J.; Viterbo, R.; Rangel, L.J.; Bergstralh, E.J.; Horwitz, E.M.; Blute, M.L.; Buyyounouski, M.K. Long-term survival after radical prostatectomy versus external-beam radiotherapy for patients with high-risk prostate cancer. *Cancer* **2011**, *117*, 2883–2891. [CrossRef]
15. Moris, L.; Cumberbatch, M.G.; Van den Broeck, T.; Gandaglia, G.; Fossati, N.; Kelly, B.; Pal, R.; Briers, E.; Cornford, P.; De Santis, M.; et al. Benefits and Risks of Primary Treatments for High-risk Localized and Locally Advanced Prostate Cancer: An International Multidisciplinary Systematic Review. *Eur. Urol.* **2020**, *77*, 614–627. [CrossRef]
16. Bray, F.; Ferlay, J.; Soerjomataram, I.; Siegel, R.L.; Torre, L.A.; Jemal, A. Global cancer statistics 2018: GLOBOCAN estimates of incidence and mortality worldwide for 36 cancers in 185 countries. *CA Cancer J. Clin.* **2018**, *68*, 394–424. [CrossRef] [PubMed]

17. Gu, X.; Gao, X.; Cui, M.; Xie, M.; Ma, M.; Qin, S.; Li, X.; Qi, X.; Bai, Y.; Wang, D. Survival outcomes of radical prostatectomy and external beam radiotherapy in clinically localized high-risk prostate cancer: A population-based, propensity score matched study. *Cancer Manag. Res.* **2018**, *10*, 1061–1067. [CrossRef] [PubMed]
18. Chiang, C.J.; You, S.L.; Chen, C.J.; Yang, Y.W.; Lo, W.C.; Lai, M.S. Quality assessment and improvement of nationwide cancer registration system in Taiwan: A review. *Jpn. J. Clin. Oncol.* **2015**, *45*, 291–296. [CrossRef] [PubMed]
19. Wen, C.P.; Tsai, S.P.; Chung, W.S. A 10-year experience with universal health insurance in Taiwan: Measuring changes in health and health disparity. *Ann. Intern. Med.* **2008**, *148*, 258–267. [CrossRef]
20. Chang, S.C.; Chen, H.M.; Wu, S.Y. There Are No Differences in Positive Surgical Margin Rates or Biochemical Failure-Free Survival among Patients Receiving Open, Laparoscopic, or Robotic Radical Prostatectomy: A Nationwide Cohort Study from the National Cancer Database. *Cancers* **2020**, *13*, 106. [CrossRef]
21. Chang, S.C.; Hsu, C.H.; Lin, Y.C.; Wu, S.Y. Effects of 1-Year Hospital Volume on Surgical Margin and Biochemical-Failure-Free Survival in Patients Undergoing Robotic versus Nonrobotic Radical Prostatectomy: A Nationwide Cohort Study from the National Taiwan Cancer Database. *Cancers* **2021**, *13*, 488. [CrossRef]
22. Wu, S.Y.; Chang, S.C.; Chen, C.I.; Huang, C.C. Latest Comprehensive Medical Resource Consumption in Robot-Assisted versus Laparoscopic and Traditional Open Radical Prostatectomy: A Nationwide Population-Based Cohort Study. *Cancers* **2021**, *13*, 1564. [CrossRef]
23. Wu, S.Y.; Fang, S.C.; Shih, H.J.; Wen, Y.C.; Shao, Y.J. Mortality associated with statins in men with advanced prostate cancer treated with androgen deprivation therapy. *Eur. J. Cancer* **2019**, *112*, 109–117. [CrossRef]
24. Lepor, H. A review of surgical techniques for radical prostatectomy. *Rev. Urol.* **2005**, *7* (Suppl. S2), S11–S17.
25. Kupelian, P.A.; Elshaikh, M.; Reddy, C.A.; Zippe, C.; Klein, E.A. Comparison of the efficacy of local therapies for localized prostate cancer in the prostate-specific antigen era: A large single-institution experience with radical prostatectomy and external-beam radiotherapy. *J. Clin. Oncol. Off. J. Am. Soc. Clin. Oncol.* **2002**, *20*, 3376–3385. [CrossRef]
26. Kupelian, P.A.; Potters, L.; Khuntia, D.; Ciezki, J.P.; Reddy, C.A.; Reuther, A.M.; Carlson, T.P.; Klein, E.A. Radical prostatectomy, external beam radiotherapy or < =72 Gy, external beam radiotherapy > or =72 Gy, permanent seed implantation, or combined seeds/external beam radiotherapy for stage T1-T2 prostate cancer. *Int. J. Radiat. Oncol. Biol. Phys.* **2004**, *58*, 25–33. [CrossRef]
27. Kupelian, P.; Kuban, D.; Thames, H.; Levy, L.; Horwitz, E.; Martinez, A.; Michalski, J.; Pisansky, T.; Sandler, H.; Shipley, W.; et al. Improved biochemical relapse-free survival with increased external radiation doses in patients with localized prostate cancer: The combined experience of nine institutions in patients treated in 1994 and 1995. *Int. J. Radiat. Oncol. Biol. Phys.* **2005**, *61*, 415–419. [CrossRef] [PubMed]
28. Cookson, M.S.; Aus, G.; Burnett, A.L.; Canby-Hagino, E.D.; D'Amico, A.V.; Dmochowski, R.R.; Eton, D.T.; Forman, J.D.; Goldenberg, S.L.; Hernandez, J.; et al. Variation in the definition of biochemical recurrence in patients treated for localized prostate cancer: The American Urological Association Prostate Guidelines for Localized Prostate Cancer Update Panel report and recommendations for a standard in the reporting of surgical outcomes. *J. Urol.* **2007**, *177*, 540–545. [CrossRef] [PubMed]
29. Roach, M., 3rd; Hanks, G.; Thames, H., Jr.; Schellhammer, P.; Shipley, W.U.; Sokol, G.H.; Sandler, H. Defining biochemical failure following radiotherapy with or without hormonal therapy in men with clinically localized prostate cancer: Recommendations of the RTOG-ASTRO Phoenix Consensus Conference. *Int. J. Radiat. Oncol. Biol. Phys.* **2006**, *65*, 965–974. [CrossRef]
30. Charlson, M.; Szatrowski, T.P.; Peterson, J.; Gold, J. Validation of a combined comorbidity index. *J. Clin. Epidemiol.* **1994**, *47*, 1245–1251. [CrossRef]
31. Chen, J.H.; Yen, Y.C.; Yang, H.C.; Liu, S.H.; Yuan, S.P.; Wu, L.L.; Lee, F.P.; Lin, K.C.; Lai, M.T.; Wu, C.C.; et al. Curative-Intent Aggressive Treatment Improves Survival in Elderly Patients With Locally Advanced Head and Neck Squamous Cell Carcinoma and High Comorbidity Index. *Medicine* **2016**, *95*, e3268. [CrossRef]
32. Rassen, J.A.; Shelat, A.A.; Myers, J.; Glynn, R.J.; Rothman, K.J.; Schneeweiss, S. One-to-many propensity score matching in cohort studies. *Pharm. Drug Saf.* **2012**, *21* (Suppl. S2), 69–80. [CrossRef]
33. Austin, P.C. Optimal caliper widths for propensity-score matching when estimating differences in means and differences in proportions in observational studies. *Pharm. Stat.* **2011**, *10*, 150–161. [CrossRef]
34. Austin, P.C. The use of propensity score methods with survival or time-to-event outcomes: Reporting measures of effect similar to those used in randomized experiments. *Stat. Med.* **2014**, *33*, 1242–1258. [CrossRef]
35. Liu, W.C.; Liu, H.E.; Kao, Y.W.; Qin, L.; Lin, K.C.; Fang, C.Y.; Tsai, L.L.; Shia, B.C.; Wu, S.Y. Definitive radiotherapy or surgery for early oral squamous cell carcinoma in old and very old patients: A propensity-score-matched, nationwide, population-based cohort study. *Radiother. Oncol.* **2020**, *151*, 214–221. [CrossRef]
36. Simmons, M.N.; Stephenson, A.J.; Klein, E.A. Natural history of biochemical recurrence after radical prostatectomy: Risk assessment for secondary therapy. *Eur. Urol.* **2007**, *51*, 1175–1184. [CrossRef] [PubMed]
37. Ames, S.C.; Tan, W.W.; Ames, G.E.; Stone, R.L.; Rizzo, T.D., Jr.; Heckman, M.G.; Crook, J.E.; Clark, M.M.; Rummans, T.A.; Werch, C.E. Quality of life of men with biochemical recurrence of prostate cancer. *J. Psychosoc. Oncol.* **2008**, *26*, 17–34. [CrossRef] [PubMed]
38. Berge, V.; Baco, E.; Dahl, A.A.; Karlsen, S.J. Health-related quality of life after salvage high-intensity focused ultrasound (HIFU) treatment for locally radiorecurrent prostate cancer. *Int. J. Urol.* **2011**, *18*, 646–651. [CrossRef] [PubMed]
39. Uchio, E.M.; Aslan, M.; Wells, C.K.; Calderone, J.; Concato, J. Impact of biochemical recurrence in prostate cancer among US veterans. *Arch. Intern. Med.* **2010**, *170*, 1390–1395. [CrossRef] [PubMed]

40. Trock, B.J.; Han, M.; Freedland, S.J.; Humphreys, E.B.; DeWeese, T.L.; Partin, A.W.; Walsh, P.C. Prostate cancer-specific survival following salvage radiotherapy vs observation in men with biochemical recurrence after radical prostatectomy. *JAMA* **2008**, *299*, 2760–2769. [CrossRef]
41. Roberts, W.B.; Han, M. Clinical significance and treatment of biochemical recurrence after definitive therapy for localized prostate cancer. *Surg. Oncol.* **2009**, *18*, 268–274. [CrossRef]
42. Artibani, W.; Porcaro, A.B.; De Marco, V.; Cerruto, M.A.; Siracusano, S. Management of Biochemical Recurrence after Primary Curative Treatment for Prostate Cancer: A Review. *Urol. Int.* **2018**, *100*, 251–262. [CrossRef]
43. Ahmed, H.U.; Cathcart, P.; McCartan, N.; Kirkham, A.; Allen, C.; Freeman, A.; Emberton, M. Focal salvage therapy for localized prostate cancer recurrence after external beam radiotherapy: A pilot study. *Cancer* **2012**, *118*, 4148–4155. [CrossRef] [PubMed]
44. Zaorsky, N.G.; Calais, J.; Fanti, S.; Tilki, D.; Dorff, T.; Spratt, D.E.; Kishan, A.U. Salvage therapy for prostate cancer after radical prostatectomy. *Nat. Rev. Urol.* **2021**, *18*, 643–668. [CrossRef] [PubMed]
45. Westover, K.; Chen, M.H.; Moul, J.; Robertson, C.; Polascik, T.; Dosoretz, D.; Katin, M.; Salenius, S.; D'Amico, A.V. Radical prostatectomy vs radiation therapy and androgen-suppression therapy in high-risk prostate cancer. *BJU Int.* **2012**, *110*, 1116–1121. [CrossRef]
46. Greenberger, B.A.; Zaorsky, N.G.; Den, R.B. Comparison of Radical Prostatectomy Versus Radiation and Androgen Deprivation Therapy Strategies as Primary Treatment for High-risk Localized Prostate Cancer: A Systematic Review and Meta-analysis. *Eur. Urol. Focus* **2020**, *6*, 404–418. [CrossRef] [PubMed]
47. Bekelman, J.E.; Rumble, R.B.; Chen, R.C.; Pisansky, T.M.; Finelli, A.; Feifer, A.; Nguyen, P.L.; Loblaw, D.A.; Tagawa, S.T.; Gillessen, S.; et al. Clinically Localized Prostate Cancer: ASCO Clinical Practice Guideline Endorsement of an American Urological Association/American Society for Radiation Oncology/Society of Urologic Oncology Guideline. *J. Clin. Oncol.: Off. J. Am. Soc. Clin. Oncol.* **2018**, *36*, 3251–3258. [CrossRef] [PubMed]
48. Sanda, M.G.; Cadeddu, J.A.; Kirkby, E.; Chen, R.C.; Crispino, T.; Fontanarosa, J.; Freedland, S.J.; Greene, K.; Klotz, L.H.; Makarov, D.V.; et al. Clinically Localized Prostate Cancer: AUA/ASTRO/SUO Guideline. Part II: Recommended Approaches and Details of Specific Care Options. *J. Urol.* **2018**, *199*, 990–997. [CrossRef]
49. Epstein, J.I.; Zelefsky, M.J.; Sjoberg, D.D.; Nelson, J.B.; Egevad, L.; Magi-Galluzzi, C.; Vickers, A.J.; Parwani, A.V.; Reuter, V.E.; Fine, S.W.; et al. A Contemporary Prostate Cancer Grading System: A Validated Alternative to the Gleason Score. *Eur. Urol.* **2016**, *69*, 428–435. [CrossRef]
50. Xie, M.; Gao, X.S.; Ma, M.W.; Gu, X.B.; Li, H.Z.; Lyu, F.; Bai, Y.; Chen, J.Y.; Ren, X.Y.; Liu, M.Z. Population-Based Comparison of Different Risk Stratification Systems Among Prostate Cancer Patients. *Front. Oncol.* **2021**, *11*, 646073. [CrossRef]
51. Barzi, A.; Klein, E.A.; Dorff, T.B.; Quinn, D.I.; Sadeghi, S. Prostatectomy at high-volume centers improves outcomes and lowers the costs of care for prostate cancer. *Prostate Cancer Prostatic Dis.* **2016**, *19*, 84–91. [CrossRef]
52. Patel, S.A.; Goyal, S.; Liu, Y.; Moghanaki, D.; Patel, P.R.; Hanasoge, S.; Dhere, V.R.; Shelton, J.W.; Godette, K.D.; Jani, A.B.; et al. Analysis of Radiation Facility Volume and Survival in Men With Lymph Node-Positive Prostate Cancer Treated With Radiation and Androgen Deprivation Therapy. *JAMA Netw. Open* **2020**, *3*, e2025143. [CrossRef]
53. Ermann, D.A.; Vardell, V.A.; Kallam, A.; Silberstein, P.T.; Armitage, J.O. Academic Centers Compared With Nonacademic Centers for Patients With International Prognostic Index Risk-stratified Diffuse Large B-cell Lymphoma: A Survival Outcomes Analysis. *Clin. Lymphoma Myeloma Leuk.* **2020**, *20*, e174–e183. [CrossRef]
54. Stolzenbach, L.F.; Deuker, M.; Colla-Ruvolo, C.; Nocera, L.; Tian, Z.; Maurer, T.; Tilki, D.; Briganti, A.; Saad, F.; Mirone, V.; et al. Differences between rural and urban prostate cancer patients. *World J. Urol.* **2021**, *39*, 2507–2514. [CrossRef]
55. Walsh, P.C. Geographic patterns of prostate cancer mortality and variations in access to medical care in the United States. *J. Urol.* **2005**, *174*, 1294–1295. [CrossRef]
56. Buwenge, M.; Scirocco, E.; Deodato, F.; Macchia, G.; Ntreta, M.; Bisello, S.; Siepe, G.; Cilla, S.; Alitto, A.R.; Valentini, V.; et al. Radiotherapy of prostate cancer: Impact of treatment characteristics on the incidence of second tumors. *BMC Cancer* **2020**, *20*, 90. [CrossRef] [PubMed]
57. Bezak, E.; Takam, R.; Yeoh, E.; Marcu, L.G. The risk of second primary cancers due to peripheral photon and neutron doses received during prostate cancer external beam radiation therapy. *Phys. Med.* **2017**, *42*, 253–258. [CrossRef] [PubMed]
58. Hegemann, N.S.; Schlesinger-Raab, A.; Ganswindt, U.; Horl, C.; Combs, S.E.; Holzel, D.; Gschwend, J.E.; Stief, C.; Belka, C.; Engel, J. Risk of second cancer following radiotherapy for prostate cancer: A population-based analysis. *Radiat Oncol.* **2017**, *12*, 2. [CrossRef]
59. Hall, E.J.; Wuu, C.S. Radiation-induced second cancers: The impact of 3D-CRT and IMRT. *Int. J. Radiat. Oncol. Biol. Phys.* **2003**, *56*, 83–88. [CrossRef]
60. Marcu, L.G. Photons—Radiobiological issues related to the risk of second malignancies. *Phys. Med.* **2017**, *42*, 213–220. [CrossRef] [PubMed]
61. Uemura, H.; Ye, D.; Kanesvaran, R.; Chiong, E.; Lojanapiwat, B.; Pu, Y.S.; Rawal, S.K.; Abdul Razack, A.H.; Zeng, H.; Chung, B.H.; et al. United in Fight against prOstate cancer (UFO) registry: First results from a large, multi-centre, prospective, longitudinal cohort study of advanced prostate cancer in Asia. *BJU Int.* **2020**, *125*, 541–552. [CrossRef]
62. Nguyen-Nielsen, M.; Moller, H.; Tjonneland, A.; Borre, M. Patient-reported outcome measures after treatment for prostate cancer: Results from the Danish Prostate Cancer Registry (DAPROCAdata). *Cancer Epidemiol.* **2020**, *64*, 101623. [CrossRef]

63. Aas, K.; Berge, V.; Myklebust, T.A.; Fossa, S.D. Comparative Survival Outcomes of High-risk Prostate Cancer Treated with Radical Prostatectomy or Definitive Radiotherapy Regimens. *Eur. Urol. Open Sci.* **2021**, *26*, 55–63. [CrossRef] [PubMed]
64. Berry, S.D.; Ngo, L.; Samelson, E.J.; Kiel, D.P. Competing risk of death: An important consideration in studies of older adults. *J. Am. Geriatr Soc.* **2010**, *58*, 783–787. [CrossRef] [PubMed]
65. Lau, B.; Cole, S.R.; Gange, S.J. Competing risk regression models for epidemiologic data. *Am. J. Epidemiol.* **2009**, *170*, 244–256. [CrossRef] [PubMed]

cancers

MDPI

Article

Novel Prognostic Index of High-Risk Prostate Cancer Using Simple Summation of Very High-Risk Factors

Hideya Yamazaki [1,*], Gen Suzuki [1], Koji Masui [1], Norihiro Aibe [1], Daisuke Shimizu [1], Takuya Kimoto [1], Kei Yamada [1], Takumi Shiraishi [1], Atsuko Fujihara [1], Koji Okihara [1], Ken Yoshida [2], Satoaki Nakamura [2] and Haruumi Okabe [3]

[1] Department of Radiology, and Urology, Graduate School of Medical Science, Kyoto Prefectural University of Medicine, 465 Kajiicho Kawaramachi Hirokoji, Kamigyo-ku, Kyoto 602-8566, Japan; gensuzu@koto.kpu-m.ac.jp (G.S.); mc0515kj@koto.kpu-m.ac.jp (K.M.); a-ib-n24@koto.kpu-m.ac.jp (N.A.); dshimizu@koto.kpu-m.ac.jp (D.S.); t-kimoto@koto.kpu-m.ac.jp (T.K.); kyamada@koto.kpu-m.ac.jp (K.Y.); takumi14@koto.kpu-m.ac.jp (T.S.); fujihara@koto.kpu-m.ac.jp (A.F.); okihara@koto.kpu-m.ac.jp (K.O.)

[2] Department of Department of Radiology, Kansai Medical University, Hirakata 573-1010, Japan; yoshidaisbt@gmail.com (K.Y.); satoaki@nakamura.pro (S.N.)

[3] Department of Radiology, Ujitakeda Hospital, Uji-City 611-0021, Japan; h-okabe@takedahp.or.jp

* Correspondence: hideya10@hotmail.com; Tel.: +81-(752)-515-111

Simple Summary: We explored the role of each very high-risk factor and found that simple summation of the number of very high-risk (VHR) factors (T3b–4 and Gleason score 9–10) is an easy and very high predictive power to separate VHR-2 (both T3b–4 and Gleason score 9–10) and others (VHR-1; T3b–4 or Gleason score 9–10, VHR-0; none of T3b–4 and Gleason score 9–10). The VHR-2 group showed a strikingly lower biochemical control rate and distant metastasis free survival rate than other groups, resulting in higher prostate cancer specific mortality than the VHR-1 and VHR-0 groups.

Citation: Yamazaki, H.; Suzuki, G.; Masui, K.; Aibe, N.; Shimizu, D.; Kimoto, T.; Yamada, K.; Shiraishi, T.; Fujihara, A.; Okihara, K.; et al. Novel Prognostic Index of High-Risk Prostate Cancer Using Simple Summation of Very High-Risk Factors. *Cancers* **2021**, *13*, 3486. https://doi.org/10.3390/cancers13143486

Academic Editor: Kouji Izumi

Received: 29 May 2021
Accepted: 9 July 2021
Published: 12 July 2021

Abstract: This study aimed to examine the role of very high-risk (VHR) factors (T3b–4 and Gleason score 9–10) for prognosis of clinically localized high-risk prostate cancer. We reviewed multi-institutional retrospective data of 1413 patients treated with radiotherapy (558 patients treated with external beam radiotherapy (EBRT) and 855 patients treated with brachytherapy (BT) ± EBRT. We introduced an index by simple summation of the number of VHR factors—VHR-0, VHR-1, and VHR-2. With median follow-up of 69.6 months, the 5-year biochemical disease free survival rate (bDFS), prostate cancer-specific mortality (PCSM), and distant metastasis-free survival (DMSF) rates were 59.4%, 7.65%, and 83.2% for the VHR-2 group, respectively; 86.7%, 1.50%, and 95.4% for the VHR-1 group, respectively; and 93.1%, 0.12%, and 98.2% for the VHR-0 group, respectively. The VHR-2 group had significantly worse bDFS, PCSM, and DMSF than the VHR-0 (hazard ratios: 4.55, 9.607, and 7.904, respectively) and VHR-1 (hazard ratios: 1.723, 2.391, and 1.491, respectively) groups. The VHR-2 group could be identified as a super high-risk group compared with other groups, and could be a good candidate for clinical trials using multimodal intensified treatments. Simple summation of the number of VHR factors is an easy and useful predictive index for bDFS, PCSM, and DMSF.

Keywords: very high-risk; T3b–4; Gleason 9–10; prostate cancer; brachytherapy

1. Introduction

Risk stratification in newly diagnosed prostate cancer is an important diagnostic process for selecting an optimal management approach for both physicians and patients. The most widely used risk classification system is the National Comprehensive Cancer Network (NCCN) [1]. The high-risk category was defined as biopsy Gleason score sum ≥ 8, prostate-specific antigen (PSA) level > 20 ng/mL, or clinical stage ≥T3a, which helps identify patients who have a high risk of recurrence and progression after treatment [1].

There is heterogeneity in the high-risk group: the rates of 10-year freedom from biochemical recurrence (bDFS) after surgery ranged from 25 to 68% [2]. To meticulously select patients for adequate treatment, high-risk prostate cancer was subdivided into the very high-risk (VHR) group, considered to have the worst prognosis, including those with primary Gleason score = 5, >4 biopsy cores with a Gleason score of 8–10, or clinical stage T3b–T4 [1], which comprised a surgical cohort of 753 high-risk patients [2]. The influence of each VHR factor in patients after radiotherapy and the best separation system is unclear because there is insufficient information to determine the outcome of patients with VHR factors after radiotherapy and they are treated with the same protocol as the high-risk group [3–6]. Therefore, we tried to examine the importance of the VHR factors (T3b–4 and Gleason score 9–10) for radiotherapy and developed an easy identification index by simply summing the number of VHR factors while preserving the point-of-care clinical applicability of the existing NCCN risk strata.

To analyze a large cohort, we used freely available public data on high-dose rate brachytherapy (HDR-BT) boost and external beam radiotherapy (EBRT) [7], including low-dose rate (LDR-BT) ± EBRT [8] and intensity-modulated radiotherapy (IMRT) performed in our institution [9]. Therefore, we aimed to examine the role of VHR factors for prognostication of clinically localized high-risk prostate cancer.

2. Materials and Methods

2.1. Patients

We retrospectively examined the data of patients treated with BT + EBRT (822 patients treated with HDR-BT boost identified from open data for public use and 33 patients treated with LDR-BT ± EBRT at Kyoto Prefectural Medical School) [7,8] and EBRT (417 patients treated with EBRT identified from open data and 141 patients treated with intensity modulated radiotherapy [IMRT] at Uji Takeda Hospital) [7,9] (Table 1). Patients treated with BT ± EBRT or EBRT; with clinical TNM stage T1–T4, with N0M0 disease with histology-proven adenocarcinoma; and with available and accessible data on pretreatment PSA (initial PSA [iPSA]) level, Gleason score sum, and T classification were eligible for this study. Patients were staged and were eligible if they were categorized as high-risk patients according to the NCCN risk classification—they have at least one of those high risk factors: (i) T3–4, (ii) Gleason score = 8–10, or (iii) PSA level > 20 ng/mL [1]. In general, pretreatment evaluation included clinical history, physical examination, blood laboratory findings, pelvic computed tomography (CT), and a bone scan. Magnetic resonance imaging (MRI) was recommended on request [6]. We created a simple index by summing the number of VHR factors—VHR-0: no VHR; VHR-1: Gleason score = 9–10 or T3b–T4; VHR-2: Gleason score = 9–10 and T3b–T4. We used cut-off value at Gleason 9–10 because Kuban et al. reported the importance of a Gleason score of 9 or 10 as a predictive factor for prostate cancer-specific mortality (PCSM) [10]. In addition, the new International Society of Urological Pathology grading system separates Gleason score 9–10 disease as a distinct entity with poorer outcomes [11].

PSA failure was defined using the Phoenix definition (nadir, +2 ng/mL). Prostate cancer specific mortality (PCSM) was defined based on either clinical documentation or inclusion of prostate cancer as a primary cause of death on a death certificate. Patients were classified as having distant metastasis when they had imaging evidence of lesions that were clinically or pathologically diagnosed as metastatic. Typically, imaging to detect distant metastasis was performed at the time of PSA failure or for subsequent PSA increases after an initial PSA failure. Outcomes of interest included bDFS, PCSM, OS, and MFS, which were defined by intervals from the start of radiotherapy to PSA failure, distant metastasis, PCSM, and death, respectively. All patients from Kyoto Prefectural Medical School and Uji Takeda Hospital provided written informed consent, and patients whose information were included in the public data provided an informed consent during the process of building public data. This study was conducted in accordance with the Declaration of Helsinki and was approved by the institutional review board of Kyoto Prefectural University of Medicine (ERB-C-1403).

Table 1. Characteristics of patients.

Variables	Strata	Total	
		(n = 1413)	
		No. or Median (range)	(%)
Age		71 (60–89)	
T Category	≤2	583	(41%)
	3a	587	(41%)
	3b	215	(15%)
	4	28	(2%)
iPSA (ng/mL)	≤20	684	(48%)
	20<	474	(33%)
	50<	151	(11%)
	100<	104	(7%)
Gleason score	≤7	591	(42%)
	8≤	346	(24%)
	9≤	436	(31%)
	10≤	40	(3%)
Modality	EBRT	558	(39%)
	BT ± EBRT	855	(60%)
Hormonal therapy	Yes	1348	(95%)
Duration	(Months)	40 (1–140)	
	No	65	(5%)
Neoadjuvant	Yes	1200	(85%)
Duration	(Month)	9 (1–92)	
Adjuvant	Yes	921	(65%)
Duration	(Month)	36 (1–134)	
Follow-up	(Months)	69.6 (2–177)	

BT = brachytherapy, EBRT = external beam radiotherapy, PSA = prostate-specific antigen.

2.2. *Treatment Planning*

2.2.1. Brachytherapy with or without External Beam Radiotherapy (BT ± EBRT)

BT ± EBRT groups consist of high dose rate brachytherapy (HDR-BT) with external beam radiotherapy (EBRT) or low dose rate brachytherapy (LDR-BT) with or without EBRT. We used multi-institution data from an open data source for HDR-BT [7], and details of the treatment have been described elsewhere [6]. All HDR-BT treatments used a combination of HDR-BT (median dose 31.5 Gy, range, 10.5–31.5 Gy) and EBRT in various fractions (Supplemental Table S1). The median fraction size of HDR-BT was 6.3 Gy (range, 5–11 Gy), while that of EBRT was 3 Gy (range, 2–3 Gy). For details of the treatment for LDR, the implant technique was previously described in detail [8]. We performed permanent intraoperative Iodine-125 implantation. We used combination therapy for patients with T3 disease or Gleason score sum ≤ 8 or Gleason score sum of 7 (4 + 3), but not for those with Gleason score sum of 7 (3 + 4) [8]. The prescription dose for the clinical target volume (prostate) was 145 Gy (LDR-BT alone) or 110 Gy (LDR-BT with 40 Gy/20 fractions EBRT by three-dimensional conformal radiotherapy (3D-CRT); Supplemental Table S1. For LDR and almost HDR cases, we used localized CTV; prostate + base of seminal vesicle in EBRT. However, several institutions used whole pelvic radiotherapy for the initial part of EBRT. Please refer to Table S1. We used planned follow-up by PSA blood test carried out every 3 months for the first 2 years, and every 6 months thereafter.

2.2.2. External Beam Radiotherapy (EBRT)

The EBRT group received conventional two-dimensional treatment, 3D-CRT, and IMRT. The details are shown in Table S1. Some EBRT data were obtained from a freely accessible dataset (n = 417) [7] and 141 image-guided IMRTs using helical TomoTherapy were performed at the Department of Radiology, Uji Takeda Hospital. The detailed technique of image-guided IMRT using helical TomoTherapy has been described elsewhere [9]. The prescribed dose was 74.8 Gy/34 fractions (2.2 Gy/fraction, n = 62) between June 2007 and 2009, with 95% of the planning target volume (PTV) receiving at the least prescribed dose (D95), and was reduced to 74 Gy/37 fractions (2 Gy/fraction, n = 79) for the high-risk and intermediate-risk groups from June 2009 to September 2013 [9].

2.3. Statistical Analysis

StatView 5.0 and EZR stat package were used for statistical analyses [12]. EZR stat package was used to competing risk analysis (Gray analysis and Fine–Gray model). Percentages were analyzed using chi-square tests and Student's t-tests were used for normally distributed data. Mann–Whitney U-tests and Kruskal–Wallis test for skewed data (i.e., PSA value) were used to compare means or medians. The Kaplan–Meier method was used to analyze the biochemical disease free survival rate (bDFS), distant metastasis free survival (DMSF), overall survival (OS), and Gray analysis for prostate cancer-specific survival rate (PCSM), and comparisons were made using log-rank tests or Gray analysis. Cause-specific manner (died of other cause of cancer was assigned as a censor) was applied to the bDFS, OS, and DMSF and competing risk analysis for PCSM. Cox's proportional hazard model for bDFS, DMSF, and OS, and the Fine–Gray model for PCSM, were used for uni- and multivariate analyses. $p < 0.05$ was considered statistically significant.

3. Results

3.1. Patient and Tumor Characteristics

All 1413 patients with high-risk prostate cancer were treated with either BT ± EBRT (n = 855) or EBRT (n = 558). The median age was 71 years (range, 60–89 years). The median value of iPSA was 20.5 ng/mL (range, interquartile range = 2682−1454 ng/mL, 9.86–39.4 ng/mL). The clinical characteristics of the patients are presented in Table 1. The median follow-up duration for the entire cohort was 69.6 (range: 2–177) months, with a minimum of 1 year for surviving patients or until death.

Table 2 shows the patient characteristics of the VHR-0, VHR-1, and VHR-2 groups. The VHR-2 group tended to be treated with more EBRT and ADT than the VHR-0 and -1 groups. The median value of iPSA was 20.7 ng/mL (range, interquartile range = 2682–1454 ng/mL, 9.2–34.68 ng/mL), 17.7 ng/mL (3.09–500 ng/mL, 9.45–43.9 ng/mL), and 36.5 ng/mL (5.3–391 ng/mL, 18.7–73.7 ng/mL) for the VHR-0, VHR-1, and VHR-2 groups, respectively.

Table 2. Comparison among three groups stratified with the very high-risk (VHR) index.

Variables	Strata	VHR-0 (n = 794)		VHR-1 (n = 519)		VHR-2 (n = 100)		p-Value
		No. or Median (Range)	(%)	No. or Median (Range)	(%)	No. or Median (Range)	(%)	
Age		70 (60–86)		71 (60–86)		70 (60–89)		0.02202
T Category	≤2	386	(49%)	197	(38%)	0	(0%)	**<0.0001**
	3a	408	(51%)	179	(34%)	0	(0%)	
	3b	0	(0%)	130	(25%)	85	(85%)	
	4	0	(0%)	13	(3%)	15	(15%)	
iPSA (ng/mL)	≤20	373	(47%)	281	(54%)	30	(30%)	**<0.0001**
	20<	306	(39%)	135	(26%)	33	(33%)	
	50<	74	(9%)	51	(10%)	26	(26%)	
	100<	41	(5%)	52	(10%)	11	(11%)	
Gleason score	−7	480	(60%)	111	(21%)	0	(0%)	**<0.0001**
	8	314	(40%)	32	(6%)	0	(0%)	
	9	0	(0%)	346	(67%)	90	(90%)	
	10	0	(0%)	30	(6%)	10	(10%)	
Modality	EBRT	273	(34%)	224	(43%)	61	(61%)	**<0.0001**
	BT ± EBRT	521	(66%)	295	(57%)	39	(39%)	
Hormonal Therapy	Yes	746	(94%)	503	(97%)	99	(99%)	**0.0088**
	(Months)	41 (1–112)		33 (2–140)		25 (4–128)		0.0777
	No	48	(6%)	16	(3%)	1	(1%)	

Table 2. *Cont.*

Variables	Strata	VHR-0 (n = 794)		VHR-1 (n = 519)		VHR-2 (n = 100)		p-Value
		No. or Median (Range)	(%)	No. or Median (Range)	(%)	No. or Median (Range)	(%)	
Neoadjuvant	Yes	669		438		93		
Duration	(Month)	10 (1–89)		9 (1–92)		8 (4–24)		0.0696
Adjuvant	Yes	526		334		61		
Duration	(Month)	36 (1–114)		36 (1–134)		36 (1–49)		**0.0171**
Follow-up	(Months)	68.2 (9–177)		67 (2–158)		62.9 (20.4–153)		0.2253
Prostate cancer-specific mortality(PCSM)	No	787	(99%)	508	(98%)	92	(92%)	**<0.0001**
	Yes	7	(1%)	11	(2%)	8	(8%)	
PSA failure	No	720	(91%)	435	(84%)	60	(60%)	**<0.0001**
	Yes	74	(9%)	84	(16%)	40	(40%)	
Overall survival	Alive	765	(96%)	486	(94%)	87	(87%)	**0.0002**
	Death	29	(4%)	33	(6%)	13	(13%)	
Distant metastasis	No	769	(97%)	497	(96%)	81	(81%)	**<0.0001**
	Yes	25	(3%)	22	(4%)	19	(19%)	

Bold values indicate statistically significance, NA; not available. BT = brachytherapy, EBRT = external beam radiotherapy. VHRF-0, -1, and -2 indicate no VHRF, one VHRF, and two VHRF.

3.2. *Biochemical Disease-Free Survival Rate (bDFS)*

The actuarial 5-year bDFS rate was 88.5% (95% confidence interval (CI): 86.2–82.2%) in all patients. The VHR-2 group showed worst bDFS (59.4%, 95% CI: 47.8–97.6%) at 5 years compared with the VHR-1 group (86.7%, 95% CI: 83.0–69.6%); and the VHR-0 group showed a 5-year bDFS of 93.1% (90.8–94.8%). There was a significant difference among the three groups ($p < 0.0001$; Figure 1).

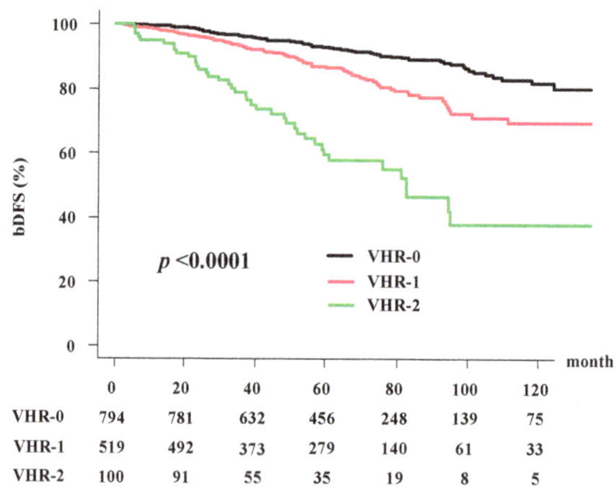

Figure 1. Biochemical disease-free survival rate (bDFS) according to the very-high risk (VHR) index.

As shown in Table 3, the predictors of bDFS in univariate analysis included treatment modality, T classification, Gleason score, baseline PSA level, and ADT duration. In multivariate Cox regression analysis (Table 4), treatment modality (BT ± EBRT) showed superior outcomes compared with EBRT; hazard ratio (HRa) = 0.447, 95% CI: 0.315–633, $p < 0.0001$) and VHR index (VHR-1 vs. VHR-0; HRa = 1.723, 95% CI: 1.256–2.362, $p < 0.0001$, VHR-2 vs. VHR-0; HRa = 4.55, 95% CI: 3.065–6.755, $p < 0.0001$) still had a significant influence on bDFS.

Table 3. Uni-variate analysis for biochemical, overall, prostate cancer-specific, and metastasis-free survival rate using the Cox proportional hazards model or the Fine–Gray model.

Variable	Strata	bDFS HRa	bDFS 95% CI	bDFS *p*	PCSM HRa	PCSM 95% CI	PCSM *p*	OS HRa	OS 95% CI	OS *p*	MFS HRa	MFS 95% CI	MFS *p*
Age	–70 vs. 71-	1.106	0.836–1.464	0.4817	0.6257	0.281–1.39	0.25	1.493	0.9374–2.377	0.091	0.7179	0.4392–1.173	0.1862
T Classification	≤2 vs. 3a≤	2.234	1.625–3.071	**<0.0001**	4.013	1385–11.62	**0.01**	1.95	1.169–3.254	**0.01057**	4.645	2.299–9.382	**<0.0001**
	≤3a vs. 3b≤	2.819	2.101–3.783	**<0.0001**	3.1887	1.454–6.988	**0.0038**	2.074	1.261–3.411	**0.004**	3.144	1.911–5.173	**<0.0001**
	≤3b vs. 4≤	4.837	2.855–8.195	**<0.0001**	5.699	1.632–19.9	**0.0064**	1.747	0.5496–5.552	0.3444	7.153	3.41–15	**<0.0001**
Gleason Score	≤7 vs. 8≤	1.652	1.227–2.224	**0.0009**	2.227	0.934–5.308	**0.0708**	1.794	1.097–2.933	**0.01989**	1.848	1.141–3.319	**0.0145**
	≤8 vs. 9≤	2.219	1.679–2.934	**<0.0001**	3.833	1.591–8.295	**0.0022**	1.978	1.257–3.114	**0.0032**	2.376	1.464–3.855	**0.0005**
	≤9 vs. 10≤	1.316	0.619–2.799	0.475	4.94	1.435–17.0	**0.011**	2.769	1.115–6.874	**0.0281**	1.82	0.571–5.801	0.3111
Pretreatment PSA (ng/mL)	≤20 vs. 20<	1.635	1.223–2.187	**0.0009**	1.393	0.6331–3.065	0.41	0.7676	0.4818–1.223	0.2655	1.508	0.9127–2.492	0.1088
	≤50 vs. 50<	2.001	1.482–2.701	**<0.0001**	1.774	0.7739–4.068	0.18	1.758	1.075–2.875	**0.02454**	2.074	1.242–3.461	**0.005**
	≤100 vs. 100<	1.621	1.097–2.576	**0.0171**	2.316	0.3038–17.65	0.42	1.135	0.520–2.475	0.7498	1.371	0.6254–3.006	0.4304
ADT duration (months)	≤40 vs. 41-	0.5067	0.372–0.689	**<0.0001**	0.9922	0.9746–1.01	0.39	1.193	0.7545–1.888	0.4497	0.8925	0.5434–1.466	0.6531
Modality	EBRT vs. BT ± EBRT	0.355	0.266–0.474	**<0.0001**	1.128	0.5181–2.467	0.76	0.9053	0.566–1.447	0.6775	0.9109	0.5537–1.498	0.7133
No. of very-high risk factors	VHR-0	1	(referent)	-	1	(referent)	-	1	(referent)	-	1	(referent)	-
	VHR-1	1.93	1.412–2.639	**<0.0001**	2.408	0.9297–6.244	**0.07**	1.8	1.092–2.966	**0.021**	1.41	0.795–2.502	0.24
	VHR-2	5.989	4.072–8.808	**<0.0001**	10.07	3.659–27.74	**<0.0001**	3.756	1.952–7.228	**<0.0001**	7.045	3.878–12.798	**<0.0001**

Competing risks regression model of prostate cancer-specific survival using the Fine–Gray model, treating other-cause mortality as a competing risk. BT = brachytherapy, EBRT = external beam radiotherapy VHRF-0, -1, and -2 indicate no, one, and two VHR factors, respectively. bDFS = biohemical failure-free survival, PCSM = prostate cancer specified mortality, OS = overall survival, MFSR = metastasis-free survival rate. Bold values indicate statistically significance.

Table 4. Multi-variate analysis for biochemical, overall, prostate cancer-specific, and metastasis-free survival rate using the Cox proportional hazards model or the Fine–Gray model.

Variable	Strata	bDFS HRa	bDFS 95% CI	bDFS *p*	PCSM HRa	PCSM 95% CI	PCSM *p*	OS HRa	OS 95% CI	OS *p*	MFS HRa	MFS 95% CI	MFS *p*
Age	≤70 vs. 71-	0.798	0.601–1.059	0.1182	0.6676	0.2844–1.567	0.35	1.572	0.982–2.518	0.0597	0.772	0.469–1.270	0.308
ADT Duration (months)	≤40 vs. 41-	0.87	0.606–1.250	0.4516	0.4535	0.1528–1.346	0.15	1.212	0.709–2.073	0.4823	0.825	0.466–1.463	0.5113
Modality	EBRT vs, BT ± EBRT	0.447	0.315–0.633	**<0.0001**	0.6297	0.2433–1.630	0.34	1.314	0.750–2.301	0.3401	1.53	0.876–2.888	0.1277
No. of very high-risk factors	VHR-0	1	(referent)	-	1	(referent)	-	1	(referent)	-	1	(referent)	-
	VHR-1	1.723	1.256–2.362	**0.0007**	2.391	0.8974–6.373	**0.081**	1.88	1.137–3.109	**0.0139**	1.491	0.837–2.656	0.1756
	VHR-2	4.55	3.065–6.755	**<0.0001**	9.607	3.29–28.05	**<0.0001**	4.327	2.206–8.487	**<0.0001**	7.904	4.251–14.696	**<0.0001**

Competing risks regression model was applied for prostate cancer-specific mortality using the Fine–Gray model, treating other-cause mortality as a competing risk. BT = brachytherapy, EBRT = external beam radiotherapy. VHRF-0, −1, and −2 indicate no VHRF, one VHRFs, and two VHRFs, respectively. bDFS = biohemical failure-free survival, PCSM = prostate cancer specified mortality, OS = overall survival, MFSR = metastasis-free survival rate. Bold values indicate statistically significance.

3.3. *Distant Metastasis-Free Survival Rate (DMFS)*

The distant metastasis-free survival rates (DMFS) were 96.1% (95% CI: 94.1%–97.1%) at 5 years and 90.8% (95% CI: 87.5%–90.2%) at 10 years (Figure 2). The VHR-2 group had the worst DMSF of 83.2% (95% CI: 72.9%–89.8%) at 5 years and 65.0% (95% CI: 46.0%–78.7%) at 10 years; the VHR-1 group was 95.4% (95% CI: 92.9%–97.1%) at 5 years and 94.0% (95% CI: 90.8%–96.1%) at 10 years; and the VHR-0 group was 98.2% (95% CI: 96.8%–99.0%) at 5 years and 92.4% (95% CI: 87.5%–95.4%) at 10 years. A significant difference was observed among the three groups ($p < 0.0001$; Figure 2).

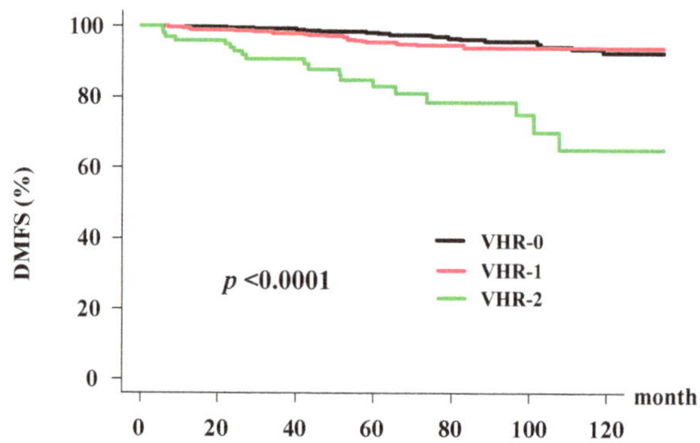

	0	20	40	60	80	100	120
VHR-0	794	786	650	482	265	152	80
VHR-1	519	503	399	307	169	81	44
VHR-2	100	96	66	47	28	17	8

Figure 2. Distant metastasis-free survival rate (DMFS) according to the VHR index.

As shown in Table 3, the predictors of DMSF survival rate on univariate analysis included treatment modality, T classification, Gleason score, baseline PSA level (−50 vs. 50<), and VHR index. In multivariate Cox regression analysis (Table 4), the VHR index between VHR-2 and VHR-0 (HRa = 7.904, 95% CI: 4.251–14.696, $p < 0.0001$) had a significant influence on OS.

3.4. *Prostate Cancer-Specific Morality (PCSM)*

The cumulative incidence of prostate cancer-specific mortality (PCSM) was 1.14% (95% CI: 0.9–1.9%) at 5 years and 3.12% (95% CI: 1.5–3.8%) at 10 years in the total population. The VHR-2 group had PCSM rates of 7.65% (95% CI: 3.1–15.0%) at 5 years and 11.8% (95% CI: 5.9–21.2%) at 10 years; the VHR-1 group had PCSM rates of 1.5% (95% CI: 0.6–3.1%) at 5 years and 3.9% (95% CI: 1.8–7.5%) at 10 years; and the VHR-0 group had PCSM rates of 0.12% (95% CI: 0.0–0.7%) at 5 years and 1.5% (95% CI: 0.5–3.6%) at 10 years. Significant differences in PCSM were observed among the three groups ($p < 0.0001$; Figure 3).

As shown in Table 3, VHR indices showed a significant ability to stratify the risk of PCSM, and the predictors of PCSM in univariate analysis were T classification, Gleason score, and VHR index. In the multivariate Fine–Gray model (Table 3), the VHR remained a significant factor for PCSM between VHR-2 and VHR-0 (HRa = 9.067; 95% CI: 3.29–28.05, $p < 0.0001$).

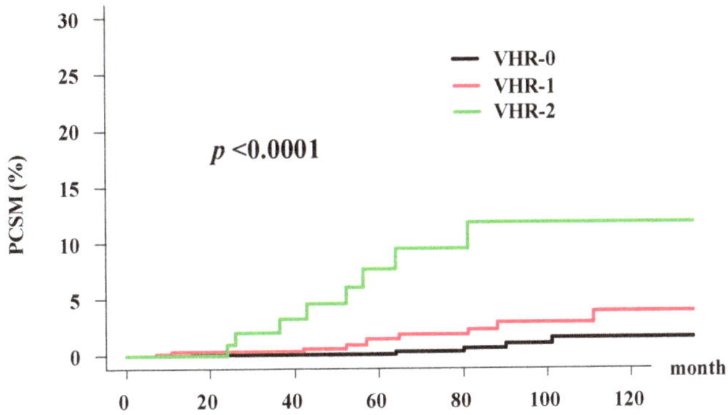

VHR-0	**794**	**787**	**654**	**489**	**275**	**157**	**84**
VHR-1	**519**	**506**	**404**	**316**	**176**	**85**	**46**
VHR-2	**100**	**100**	**71**	**54**	**32**	**20**	**11**

Figure 3. Prostate cancer-specific mortality (PCSM) according to the VHR index.

3.5. Overall Survival Rate (OS)

The overall survival (OS) rates were 96.4% (95% CI = 95.2–96.4%) at 5 years and 89.7% (86.2–96.2%) at 10 years in the total population. The VHR-2 group had worst OS rates of 88.9% (95% CI: 79.5–94.1%) at 5 years and 78.9% (95% CI: 64.7–87.9%) at 10 years; in the VHR-1 group, the rates were 95.9% (95% CI: 93.6–97.4%) at 5 years and 88.2% (95% CI: 82.1–82.3) at 10 years; and in the VHR-0 group, the rates were 97.7% (95% CI: 96.1–98.6%) at 5 years and 92.0% (95% CI: 87.6–94.9%) at 10 years. A significant difference was observed among the three groups ($p = 0.0001$; Figure 4).

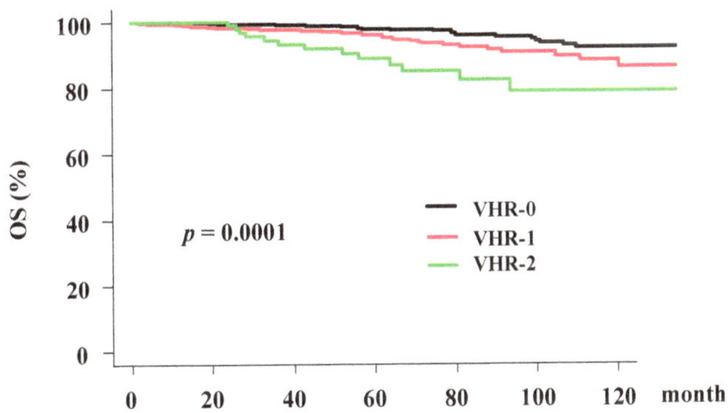

VHR-0	**794**	**787**	**654**	**489**	**275**	**157**	**84**
VHR-1	**519**	**506**	**404**	**316**	**176**	**85**	**46**
VHR-2	**100**	**100**	**71**	**54**	**32**	**20**	**11**

Figure 4. Overall survival rate (OS) according to the VHR index.

As shown in Table 3, the predictors of OS in univariate analysis included treatment modality, T classification, Gleason score, baseline PSA level, and VHR. The results of the multivariate Cox regression analysis (Table 4) revealed that VHR (VHR-2 vs. VHR-0; HRa = 4.327, 95% CI: 2.206–8.487, $p < 0.0001$, VHR-1 vs. VHR-0; HRa = 1.88, 95% CI: 1.137–3.109, $p = 0.013$) remained significant factors for OS.

4. Discussion

Here, we have proposed an easy and useful index for a risk stratum that identifies men with worst oncological outcomes after radiotherapy for localized prostate cancer using a cohort of >1400 patients. These criteria may be beneficial for counseling individual patients regarding the treatment and prognosis of high-risk disease and the risk of requiring subsequent neoadjuvant, concurrent, or post-radiation therapies. The VHR criteria could also be useful as a risk stratification tool in future clinical protocols.

High-risk prostate cancer was subdivided into VHR groups in several ways. The NCCN used clinical stage T3b–T4 lesions, primary Gleason score = 5, or >4 biopsy cores with a Gleason score of 8–10 [1]. One of the initial studies that defined VHR was performed on the patients who underwent surgery [2] at Johns Hopkins, in which the VHR criteria used were multiple high-risk features, >4 biopsy cores with a Gleason score sum of 8–10, or primary Gleason score of 5 to create the risk factor groupings predictive for DMSF and PCSM. Then, they validated the role of VHR in three center cohorts, revealing HRa of 2.78 in DMSF, and 6.77 in PCSM to other NCCN high-risk men [13]. Narang et al. confirmed the role of VHR in high-risk patients undergoing radiotherapy plus androgen deprivation therapy at Johns Hopkins (HRa = DMSF: 2.49, PCMS: 3.19, and OS: 1.87, respectively) [14]. Our analysis confirmed the importance of VHR factors, in which VHR-2 showed the highest hazard risk for DMSF, PCSM, and OS compared with VHR-0 (HRa = 8.81, 11.99, and 4.644, respectively) and VHR-1 (HRa = 5.268, 2.359, and 2.896, respectively), and was distinctly better than the previous stratification system. The summation of the number of high risk factors has been explored in several studies including the above mentioned studies [2,4,6,13–15]. Wattson et al. reported a HRa of 4.8 for PCSM for those with at least two high risk factors compared with those with one high risk factor [16]. Our data may concur with this result; the VHR index also showed a significant difference. In addition, the VHR index showed an interesting characteristic—a significant difference (i.e., threshold) was only observed between VHR-2 and others in DMFS; therefore, it is useful to separate high-risk patients into VHR-2 and others. Rodrigues et al. reported ProCaRS classification [17]. They divided high risk patients by % core and iPSA value, and 40% of 5-year bDFS was found in extremely high-risk group. Although we could not compare our result directly to their outcome because we did not have information about % core, we could provide data for node 5 category (iPSA > 32.5 ng/mL, part of extremely high-risk group), in which 5-year bDFS was 83.5%. Therefore, Japanese patients tend to show a superior outcome to the Canadian population [17]. We used long term ADT, which could be one of the reasons of our good outcome compared with previous studies. Furthermore, good efficiency of ADT was found in Japanese men and is explained by the Japanese-specific high sensitivity to hormonal therapy [18].

The Gleason score is reported to be one of the most important factors for prognosis. Kuban et al. cited the importance of a Gleason score of 9 or 10, which was predictive of PCSM [10]. Sabolch et al. also reported that the presence of Gleason score of 5 on the biopsy specimen was the strongest prognostic factor for all clinical outcomes, including PCSM and OS after EBRT (≥75 Gy) with T1–T4 prostate cancer [19]. Our data partly concurred with their data because a significant threshold to separate PCSM with the highest hazard ratio was obtained between T3a and T3b and Gleason score sum 8 and 9, but not in iPSA (Table 3). Tsumura et al. reported similar results that stage T3b patients with grade group 5 may have a greater risk for PCSM [20].

BT ± EBRT showed superior efficacy in terms of bDFS compared with EBRT. This finding is typical because BT has a unique characteristic that allows it to deliver higher doses of radiation to the target lesion without excessive irradiation of the adjacent organs and is considered to be one of the best radiotherapy options [21]. Therefore, a number of studies and randomized controlled trials demonstrated the superiority of treatment by increasing the prescribed dose for localized prostate cancer in bDFS [22], especially with BT boost [22,23]. Our results are in line with the findings of a previous study, which indicated that BT improves bDFS. Furthermore, several studies found superior efficacy of dose escalation in terms not only of bDFS, but also of PCSM and OS [24–26]. At present, however, our data indicated that the combination of BT improved bDFS, but did not improve the PCSM or OS, and this discussion should be left for further studies.

Following advancements of treatment including long term ADT use, distant metastasis occurred only in 66 patients (4.6%) and PCSM in 26 patients (1.8%) out of more than 1400 patients. Of these, the lowest DMFS and highest PCMS ratio were found in the VHR-2 group compared with the other VHR groups, resulting in worst OS. Therefore, men with VHR-2 prostate cancer experience unusually aggressive oncologic outcomes and should be considered for intensive follow-up for metastasis using state-of-the-art technologies such as prostate-specific membrane antigen positron emission tomography scan [27] and/or adjuvant/earlier intervention with effective systemic therapy, such as docetaxel Abiraterone and Enzalutamide, in addition to longer periods of ADT use [28], that is, clinical trial settings using multimodal treatment.

There are several limitations to the present study. First, we could not examine the role of the biopsy core because the public database did not contain these data, and advancement in image-guided biopsy techniques made it impossible to assess for old data owing to its incompatibility with recent systems; high-grade tumor nodules were either undersampled or oversampled, and lacked a central pathologic review. Second, our study had limitations owing to its retrospective nature, limited follow-up time, and small sample size for reflecting the total prostate cancer patient population, which may limit the application of its findings. Thus, a longer follow-up with a larger sample is needed to obtain concrete conclusions. The authors should discuss the results and how they can be interpreted from the perspective of previous studies and of the working hypotheses. The findings and their implications should be discussed in the broadest context possible. Future research directions may also be highlighted.

5. Conclusions

A simple summation of the number of VHR factors is an easy and useful predictive index not only for bDFS, but also for PCSM and DMSF. These VHR-2 patients could be good candidates for more intense treatment with systemic agents.

Supplementary Materials: The following are available online at https://www.mdpi.com/article/10.3390/cancers13143486/s1, Table S1: Detailed Treatment schedule.

Author Contributions: Conceptualization, H.Y.; Data curation, G.S., K.M., D.S., T.K., T.S., K.Y. (Ken Yoshida) and H.O.; Formal analysis, H.Y.; Investigation, G.S., D.S., and A.F.; Methodology, N.A. and S.N.; Resources, K.O.; Supervision, K.Y. (Kei Yamada); Validation, K.M. and K.O.; Writing—original draft, H.Y.; Writing—review & editing, K.Y. (Kei Yamada). All authors have read and agreed to the published version of the manuscript.

Funding: This research received no external funding.

Institutional Review Board Statement: The study was conducted according to the guidelines of the Declaration of Helsinki, and approved by the Institutional Review Board of Kyoto Prefectural University of Medicine (protocol code ERB-C-1403, 6 September 2017).

Informed Consent Statement: Informed consent was obtained from all subjects involved in the study.

Data Availability Statement: The data of HDR-BT for this manuscript can be obtained from the public data base [7] and LDR-BT can be obtained from the author upon reasonable request.

Acknowledgments: The authors appreciate the participants and physicians for building big free data of treatment outcome [7].

Conflicts of Interest: The authors declare no conflict of interest.

References

1. The National Comprehensive Cancer Network Clinical Practice Guidelines in Oncology. Prostate Cancer-Version 4. 2019. Available online: http://www.nccn.org/professionals/physician_gls/pdf/prostate.pdf (accessed on 2 February 2020).
2. Sundi, D.; Wang, V.M.; Pierorazio, P.M.; Han, M.; Bivalacqua, T.J.; Ball, M.W.; Antonarakis, E.S.; Partin, A.W.; Schaeffer, E.M.; Ross, A.E. Very-high-risk localized prostate cancer: Definition and outcomes. *Prostate Cancer Prostatic Dis.* **2014**, *17*, 57–63. [CrossRef]
3. Kasahara, T.; Ishizaki, F.; Kazama, A.; Yuki, E.; Yamana, K.; Maruyama, R.; Oshikane, T.; Kaidu, M.; Aoyama, H.; Bilim, V.; et al. High-dose-rate brachytherapy and hypofractionated external beam radiotherapy combined with long-term androgen deprivation therapy for very high-risk prostate cancer. *Int. J. Urol.* **2020**, *27*, 800–806. [CrossRef]
4. Saad, A.; Goldstein, J.; Lawrence, Y.R.; Spieler, B.; Leibowitz-Amit, R.; Berger, R.; Davidson, T.; Urban, D.; Tsang, L.; Alezra, D.; et al. Classifying high-risk versus very high-risk prostate cancer: Is it relevant to outcomes of conformal radiotherapy and androgen deprivation? *Radiat. Oncol.* **2017**, *12*, 5. [CrossRef] [PubMed]
5. Tomita, N.; Soga, N.; Ogura, Y.; Kageyama, T.; Kodaira, T. Very high-risk prostate cancer: Stratification by outcomes of radiotherapy and long-term androgen deprivation therapy. *Asia-Pac. J. Clin. Oncol.* **2017**, *13*, 145–151. [CrossRef]
6. Ishiyama, H.; Satoh, T.; Kitano, M.; Tabata, K.-I.; Komori, S.; Ikeda, M.; Soda, I.; Kurosaka, S.; Sekiguchi, A.; Kimura, M.; et al. High-dose-rate brachytherapy and hypofractionated external beam radiotherapy combined with long-term hormonal therapy for high-risk and very high-risk prostate cancer: Outcomes after 5-year follow-up. *J. Radiat. Res.* **2014**, *55*, 509–517. [CrossRef] [PubMed]
7. An Open Data of Multicenter Data Collection: Outcome of Radiation Therapy for Prostate Cancer to Establish a Prognostic Prediction System by Machine Learning (B17-278). Available online: https://www.khp.kitasato-u.ac.jp/ska/radiotherapy/arcivements/#results (accessed on 2 February 2020).
8. Okihara, K.; Kobayashi, K.; Iwata, T.; Naitoh, Y.; Kamoi, K.; Kawauchi, A.; Yamada, K.; Miki, T. Assessment of permanent brachytherapy combined with androgen deprivation therapy in an intermediate-risk prostate cancer group without a Gleason score of 4 + 3: A single Japanese institutional experience. *Int. J. Urol.* **2014**, *21*, 271–276. [CrossRef] [PubMed]
9. Sasaki, N.; Yamazaki, H.; Shimizu, D.; Suzuki, G.; Masui, K.; Nakamura, S.; Okabe, H.; Nishikawa, T.; Yoshida, K. Long-term Outcomes of a Dose-reduction Trial to Decrease Late Gastrointestinal Toxicity in Patients with Prostate Cancer Receiving Soft Tissue-matched Image-guided Intensity-modulated Radiotherapy. *Anticancer Res.* **2018**, *38*, 385–391. [CrossRef] [PubMed]
10. Kuban, D.A.; Levy, L.B.; Cheung, M.R.; Lee, A.K.; Choi, S.; Frank, S.; Pollack, A. Long-Term Failure Patterns and Survival in a Randomized Dose-Escalation Trial for Prostate Cancer. Who Dies of Disease? *Int. J. Radiat. Oncol. Biol. Phys.* **2011**, *79*, 1310–1317. [CrossRef]
11. Epstein, J.I.; Amin, M.B.; Reuter, V.E.; Humphrey, P.A. Contemporary Gleason Grading of Prostatic Carcinoma: An Update with Discussion on Practical Issues to Implement the 2014 International Society of Urological Pathology (ISUP) Consensus Conference on Gleason Grading of Prostatic Carcinoma. *Am. J. Surg. Pathol.* **2017**, *41*, e1–e7. [CrossRef]
12. Kanda, Y. Investigation of the freely available easy-to-use software 'EZR' for medical statistics. *Bone Marrow Transplant.* **2013**, *48*, 452–458. [CrossRef] [PubMed]
13. Sundi, D.; Tosoian, J.J.; Nyame, Y.A.; Alam, R.; Achim, M.; Reichard, C.A.; Li, J.; Wilkins, L.; Schwen, Z.; Han, M.; et al. Outcomes of very high-risk prostate cancer after radical prostatectomy: Validation study from 3 centers. *Cancer* **2019**, *125*, 391–397. [CrossRef] [PubMed]
14. Narang, A.K.; Gergis, C.; Robertson, S.P.; He, P.; Ram, A.N.; McNutt, T.R.; Griffith, E.; DeWeese, T.A.; Honig, S.; Singh, H.; et al. Very High-Risk Localized Prostate Cancer: Outcomes Following Definitive Radiation. *Int. J. Radiat. Oncol.* **2016**, *94*, 254–262. [CrossRef] [PubMed]
15. Umezawa, R.; Inaba, K.; Nakamura, S.; Wakita, A.; Okamoto, H.; Tsuchida, K.; Kashihara, T.; Kobayashi, K.; Harada, K.; Takahashi, K.; et al. Dose escalation of external beam radiotherapy for high-risk prostate cancer—Impact of multiple high-risk factor. *Asian J. Urol.* **2019**, *6*, 192–199. [CrossRef]
16. Wattson, D.A.; Chen, M.H.; Moran, B.J.; Dosoretz, D.E.; Braccioforte, M.H.; Salenius, S.A.; D'Amico, A.V. The number of high-risk factors and the risk of prostate cancer-specific mortality after brachytherapy: Implications for treatment selection. *Int. J. Radiat. Oncol. Biol. Phys.* **2012**, *82*, e773–e779. [CrossRef]
17. Rodrigues, G.; Lukka, H.; Warde, P.; Brundage, M.; Souhami, L.; Crook, J.; Cury, F.; Catton, C.; Mok, G.; Martin, A.-G.; et al. The prostate cancer risk stratification (ProCaRS) project: Recursive partitioning risk stratification analysis. *Radiother. Oncol.* **2013**, *109*, 204–210. [CrossRef]
18. Fukagai, T.; Namiki, T.S.; Carlile, R.G.; Yoshida, H.; Namiki, M. Comparison of the clinical outcome after hormonal therapy for prostate cancer between Japanese and Caucasian men. *BJU Int.* **2006**, *97*, 1190–1193. [CrossRef]
19. Sabolch, A.; Feng, F.Y.; Daignault-Newton, S.; Halverson, S.; Blas, K.; Phelps, L.; Olson, K.B.; Sandler, H.M.; Hamstra, D.A. Gleason Pattern 5 Is the Greatest Risk Factor for Clinical Failure and Death from Prostate Cancer after Dose-Escalated Radiation Therapy and Hormonal Ablation. *Int. J. Radiat. Oncol. Biol. Phys.* **2011**, *81*, e351–e360. [CrossRef]
20. Tsumura, H.; Ishiyama, H.; Tabata, K.-I.; Katsumata, H.; Kobayashi, M.; Ikeda, M.; Kurosaka, S.; Fujita, T.; Kitano, M.; Satoh, T.; et al. Impact of five-tiered Gleason grade groups on prognostic prediction in clinical stage T3 prostate cancer undergoing high-dose-rate brachytherapy. *Prostate* **2017**, *77*, 1520–1527. [CrossRef]

21. Chin, J.; Rumble, R.B.; Kollmeier, M.; Heath, E.; Efstathiou, J.; Dorff, T.; Berman, B.; Feifer, A.; Jacques, A.; Loblaw, D.A. Brachytherapy for Patients with Prostate Cancer: American Society of Clinical Oncology/Cancer Care Ontario Joint Guideline Update. *J. Clin. Oncol.* **2017**, *35*, 1737–1743. [CrossRef]
22. Viani, G.A.; Stefano, E.J.; Afonso, S.L. Higher-Than-Conventional Radiation Doses in Localized Prostate Cancer Treatment: A Meta-analysis of Randomized, Controlled Trials. *Int. J. Radiat. Oncol.* **2009**, *74*, 1405–1418. [CrossRef] [PubMed]
23. Spratt, D.E.; Zumsteg, Z.S.; Ghadjar, P.; Kollmeier, M.A.; Pei, X.; Cohen, G.; Polkinghorn, W.; Yamada, Y.; Zelefsky, M.J. Comparison of high-dose (86.4 Gy) IMRT vs combined brachytherapy plus IMRT for intermediate-risk prostate cancer. *BJU Int.* **2014**, *114*, 360–367. [CrossRef] [PubMed]
24. Kent, A.R.; Matheson, B.; Millar, J.L. Improved survival for patients with prostate cancer receiving high-dose-rate brachytherapy boost to EBRT compared with EBRT alone. *Brachytherapy* **2019**, *18*, 313–321. [CrossRef] [PubMed]
25. Wedde, T.B.; Småstuen, M.C.; Brabrand, S.; Fosså, S.D.; Kaasa, S.; Tafjord, G.; Russnes, K.M.; Hellebust, T.P.; Lilleby, W. Ten-year survival after High-Dose-Rate Brachytherapy combined with External Beam Radiation Therapy in high-risk prostate cancer: A comparison with the Norwegian SPCG-7 cohort. *Radiother. Oncol.* **2019**, *132*, 211–217. [CrossRef]
26. Kishan, A.U.; Cook, R.R.; Ciezki, J.P.; Ross, A.E.; Pomerantz, M.M.; Nguyen, P.L.; Shaikh, T.; Tran, P.T.; Sandler, K.A.; Stock, R.G.; et al. Radical Prostatectomy, External Beam Radiotherapy, or External Beam Radiotherapy with Brachytherapy Boost and Disease Progression and Mortality in Patients with Gleason Score 9–10 Prostate Cancer. *JAMA* **2018**, *319*, 896–905. [CrossRef]
27. Perera, M.; Papa, N.; Roberts, M.; Williams, M.; Udovicich, C.; Vela, I.; Christidis, D.; Bolton, D.; Hofman, M.S.; Lawrentschuk, N.; et al. Gallium-68 Prostate-specific Membrane Antigen Positron Emission Tomography in Advanced Prostate Cancer—Updated Diagnostic Utility, Sensitivity, Specificity, and Distribution of Prostate-specific Membrane Antigen-avid Lesions: A Systematic Review and Meta-analysis. *Eur. Urol.* **2020**, *77*, 403–417. [CrossRef] [PubMed]
28. Komura, K.; Sweeney, C.J.; Inamoto, T.; Ibuki, N.; Azuma, H.; Kantoff, P.W. Current treatment strategies for advanced prostate cancer. *Int. J. Urol.* **2018**, *25*, 220–231. [CrossRef]

cancers

MDPI

Review

Epithelial-to-Mesenchymal Transition-Related Markers in Prostate Cancer: From Bench to Bedside

Samantha Gogola [1], Michael Rejzer [1], Hisham F. Bahmad [2,*], Wassim Abou-Kheir [3], Yumna Omarzai [2,4] and Robert Poppiti [2,4]

[1] Herbert Wertheim College of Medicine, Florida International University, Miami, FL 33199, USA; sgogo002@med.fiu.edu (S.G.); mrejz001@med.fiu.edu (M.R.)

[2] The Arkadi M. Rywlin M.D. Department of Pathology and Laboratory Medicine, Mount Sinai Medical Center, Miami Beach, FL 33140, USA; yumna.omarzai@msmc.com (Y.O.); robert.poppiti@msmc.com (R.P.)

[3] Department of Anatomy, Cell Biology and Physiological Sciences, Faculty of Medicine, American University of Beirut, Beirut 1107, Lebanon; wa12@aub.edu.lb

[4] Department of Pathology, Herbert Wertheim College of Medicine, Florida International University, Miami, FL 33199, USA

* Correspondence: hfbahmad@gmail.com or hisham.bahmad@msmc.com; Tel.: +1-305-674-2277

Simple Summary: Prostate cancer (PCa) is the second most frequent type of cancer in men worldwide. Treatment options for early-stage PCa include external beam radiation therapy, brachytherapy, radical prostatectomy, active surveillance, or a combination of these. In most patients, however, PCa eventually progresses to castration-resistant prostate cancer (CRPC). Transition of PCa from an androgen-dependent to androgen-independent state is not yet fully understood, but epithelial-to-non-epithelial ("mesenchymal") transition (EMT) plays a crucial role in this process. In this review, we provide a synopsis of the transcriptional factors and signaling pathways involved in EMT, besides the diagnostic and prognostic biomarkers that have been identified in this process.

Abstract: Prostate cancer (PCa) is the second most frequent type of cancer in men worldwide, with 288,300 new cases and 34,700 deaths estimated in the United States in 2023. Treatment options for early-stage disease include external beam radiation therapy, brachytherapy, radical prostatectomy, active surveillance, or a combination of these. In advanced cases, androgen-deprivation therapy (ADT) is considered the first-line therapy; however, PCa in most patients eventually progresses to castration-resistant prostate cancer (CRPC) despite ADT. Nonetheless, the transition from androgen-dependent to androgen-independent tumors is not yet fully understood. The physiological processes of epithelial-to-non-epithelial ("mesenchymal") transition (EMT) and mesenchymal-to-epithelial transition (MET) are essential for normal embryonic development; however, they have also been linked to higher tumor grade, metastatic progression, and treatment resistance. Due to this association, EMT and MET have been identified as important targets for novel cancer therapies, including CRPC. Here, we discuss the transcriptional factors and signaling pathways involved in EMT, in addition to the diagnostic and prognostic biomarkers that have been identified in these processes. We also tackle the various studies that have been conducted from bench to bedside and the current landscape of EMT-targeted therapies.

Keywords: prostate cancer; epithelial-to-mesenchymal transition; mesenchymal-to-epithelial transition; EMT; MET; biomarkers; targeted therapy; review

Citation: Gogola, S.; Rejzer, M.; Bahmad, H.F.; Abou-Kheir, W.; Omarzai, Y.; Poppiti, R. Epithelial-to-Mesenchymal Transition-Related Markers in Prostate Cancer: From Bench to Bedside. *Cancers* **2023**, *15*, 2309. https://doi.org/10.3390/cancers15082309

Academic Editor: Kouji Izumi

Received: 23 March 2023
Revised: 7 April 2023
Accepted: 11 April 2023
Published: 14 April 2023

1. Introduction

Prostate cancer (PCa) is the second most frequent type of cancer in men worldwide, with 288,300 new cases and 34,700 deaths estimated in the United States in 2023 [1–3]. Mortality rates for PCa have decreased in recent years with the use of prostate-specific antigen (PSA) testing; however, there remains a significant disease burden [4,5]. The most common type of PCa is adenocarcinoma, which is graded using the Gleason scoring system [2]. This system is based on the architectural growth patterns of the tumor, with Gleason pattern 1 showing discrete, well-formed small round glands and Gleason pattern 5 showing sheets of tumor cells or individual cells with no gland formation [6,7]. The International Society of Urologic Pathology (ISUP) has recently introduced the Grade Group system, which provides more accurate stratification than the Gleason score alone [8].

Treatment options for early-stage PCa include external beam radiation therapy, brachytherapy, radical prostatectomy, active surveillance, or a combination of these [2]. In more advanced cases, androgen-deprivation therapy (ADT) is considered the first-line therapy, given that PCa cells rely on the androgen receptor (AR) for growth and survival [2,9,10]. Despite these interventions, PCa in many patients eventually progresses to castration-resistant prostate cancer (CRPC), marking the transition from an androgen-dependent to an androgen-independent state. This process is not fully understood; however, continuous AR signaling, *AR* gene amplification, mutations, ligand-independent activation, coregulators, and cancer stem cell (CSC) recruitment are thought to be involved [9,11–17].

2. EMT and MET as Targets for Therapy

In general, epithelial cells exhibit a tight-junction, tightly packed morphology, while non-epithelial ("mesenchymal") cells are characterized by loose packing and increased motility [18,19]. The physiological processes of epithelial-to-non-epithelial ("mesenchymal") transition (EMT) and mesenchymal–epithelial transition (MET) play essential roles in normal embryonic development [20]. Early on, EMT has been linked to the initial generation of the three germ layers from pluripotent stem cells [21]. Subsequently, EMT leads epithelial cells to acquire non-epithelial (mesenchymal) characteristics, as noted by the loss of E-cadherin and the gain of vimentin and N-cadherin [21–23]. This enables cells to disengage from tight junctions and gain mobility to migrate to other tissues [19]. MET complements this process by orchestrating the formation of organized structures once the EMT-induced cells have arrived at their proper location [21]. Beyond embryology, EMT has been shown to also be involved in the migratory processes implicated in wound healing, tissue regeneration, and organ fibrosis [19].

In malignancy, the processes of EMT and MET are often dysregulated to promote cancer progression. Each has been linked to the induction of CSCs capable of generating new tissue [17,21,24], as well as the promotion of enhanced mobility, tissue invasion, and therapy resistance [25]. Because of these factors, EMT and MET have been identified as important targets for novel cancer therapies, including CRPC (Figure 1).

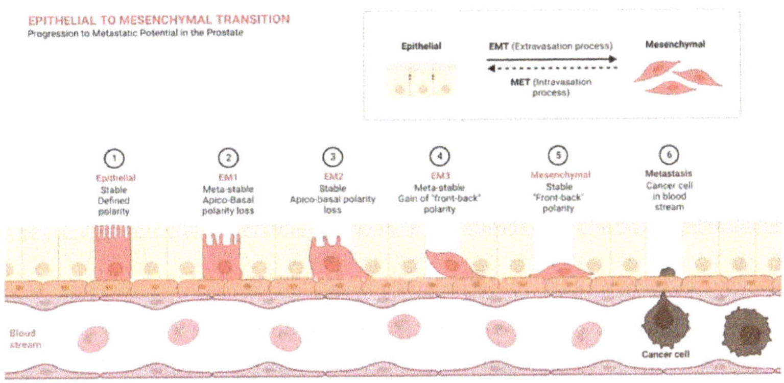

Figure 1. Mechanism of action of EMT in the prostate cell. The progression to metastatic cancer involves the loss of stable apico-basal epithelial cell polarity, the gain of front–back polarity, and eventual metastasis to the bloodstream. Created with BioRender.com (accessed on 11 March 2023).

3. Epithelial-To-Mesenchymal Transition in Cancer Progression

3.1. EMT Initiation

EMT in cancer cells has been implicated in tumor initiation, malignant transformation, CSC survival, metastasis, and treatment resistance [26]. These associations are primarily due to the sequential loss of epithelial characteristics, such as E-cadherin expression that maintains cell–cell interactions, in favor of a non-epithelial ("mesenchymal") phenotype capable of tissue invasion. The initiation of EMT involves a variety of factors intrinsic to the tumor microenvironment (TME), including growth factors and cytokines, hypoxia, and interactions with the extracellular matrix (ECM) [17].

Some of the best-characterized growth factors and cytokines involved in EMT induction include transforming growth factor beta (TGF-β), hepatocyte growth factor (HGF), fibroblast growth factor (FGF), epidermal growth factor (EGF), and platelet-derived growth factor (PDGF). TGF-β is the most studied of these factors, with a variety of tumor mutations leading to augmented expression and EMT activation, primarily through *SMAD*-mediated signaling [27]. Elevated HGF expression has been observed in cancer-associated fibroblasts of the colon, breast, pancreas, and prostate [28]. Enhanced expression of FGF has been connected to an increase in the expression of non-epithelial markers, such as vimentin and FSP-1, as well as the promotion of metalloproteases (MMPs) and cytoskeletal rearrangements [29,30]. EGF overexpression plays a prominent role in various cancers including the breast, prostate, cervix, and head and neck via PI3K/Akt signaling [31]. Excessive PDGF expression has been observed in cancers of the prostate, lung, kidney, ovary, brain, and pancreas and is involved with multiple important EMT pathways, including PI3K/Akt, Notch, and others [32].

Hypoxia commonly occurs in the microenvironment of solid tumors due to overcrowding and impaired diffusion, leading to the inhibition of prolyl hydroxylases and a resultant upregulation of hypoxia-inducible factors (HIFs). With regards to EMT induction, HIF-1-alpha is of particular interest and has been associated with TGF-β signaling, as well as the SMAD, Ras/MEK/ERK, and PI3K/Akt signaling pathways [33]. This hypoxia-driven mechanism has been observed in many different cancers, including breast, ovarian, lung, prostate, and pancreatic cancers, among others [33].

The ECM maintains proper tissue segregation and is a major regulator of intracellular signaling cascades. As such, cancer progression relies heavily on manipulating the ECM, a role for which EMT is particularly well suited. EMT utilizes a dynamic composition of integrins to connect with certain aspects of the ECM, such as type I collagen, which is well known to be augmented in a variety of cancers [34]. The interaction with a2b1 integrin has been investigated and correlated with EMT induction in breast, lung, and pancreatic cancers via NF-kB, JNK, and TGF-β pathway activation [35–38]. Additionally, this action has been observed to directly suppress E-cadherin and indirectly induce N-cadherin, an important early transition in EMT [38]. As EMT progresses, the transitioning cell expands secretion of type 1 collagen and fibronectin, enhancing integrin activation and producing a network by which the transitioning cell can utilize lamellipodia and filopodia for migration [39]. This enhanced mobility is complemented by the induction of various MMPs that cleave type IV collagen in the basal lamina and disrupt epithelial cell junctions, both of which facilitate cell invasion [40]. Furthermore, MMPs have demonstrated an ability to directly induce EMT progression, as evidenced by MMP-3 enhancement of the transcription factor SNAI1 in lung cancer [41].

3.2. EMT Transcription Factors

The cellular alterations seen with EMT result from changes in gene expression that are primarily driven by EMT-regulating transcription factors (EMT-TFs). EMT-TFs are themselves induced through a variety of direct and indirect signaling pathways upregulated in cancer cells. A large number of EMT-TFs have been identified; however, the most well-studied families are SNAIL, TWIST, and zinc-finger E-box-binding homeobox (ZEB) [42].

The SNAIL family of EMT-TFs includes SNAI1 (Snail), SNAI2 (Slug), and SNAI3 (Smuc); however, SNAI3 is a poor EMT-inducer [43,44]. They are most notable for accumulating in the cell nucleus and binding the *CDH1* promoter to suppress the transcription of its encoded protein, E-cadherin [45]. SNAIL expression is regulated through multiple signaling pathways, including receptor tyrosine kinases (RTKs), TGF-β, Notch, Wnt, and others, as well as post-translational modifications [44]. Enhanced SNAIL expression has been correlated with a higher tumor grade and metastatic potential in breast, ovarian, and hepatocellular carcinomas [46–48]. Furthermore, this propensity for EMT-induced metastasis has been shown to involve immunosuppression, with SNAIL-knockdown leading to inhibited tumor growth and metastasis from significant elevations in tumor-infiltrating and systemic immune responses [49].

The TWIST family of EMT-TFs includes TWIST1 and TWIST2. TWIST1 has been shown to directly bind the E-cadherin promoter to repress its expression as well as bind the E-box cis-element in the N-cadherin gene to enhance its expression [50,51]. Additionally, TWIST1 can bind the SNAI2 promoter to enhance SNAIL-mediated EMT induction [52]. TWIST expression is regulated through multiple signaling pathways, including RTKs, TGF-β, Notch, Wnt, TNF-alpha, HIF-1-alpha, and others, as well as post-translational modifications [53]. Enhanced TWIST expression has been observed in many cancers, including breast, bladder, gastric, hepatocellular carcinoma, and others, and is associated with higher tumor grade, metastasis, and therapeutic resistance [50].

The ZEB family of EMT-TFs includes ZEB1 and ZEB2. Both have been shown to bind E-box regions around the *CDH1* promoter to suppress the expression of E-cadherin [54]. ZEB1 has also been shown to repress transcription of the epithelial cell polarity genes *HUGL2, Crumbs3*, and *PATJ* [55]. ZEB expression is regulated through multiple signaling pathways, including RTKs, TGF-β, Notch, Wnt, and others, as well as post-translational modifications [56]. Enhanced ZEB expression has been observed in many cancers, including prostate, bladder, brain, breast, cervical, colon, and others, and is associated with a higher tumor grade, metastasis, and therapeutic resistance [56].

3.3. EMT Signaling Pathways

3.3.1. TGF-β Signaling

TGF-β signaling is a well-known pathway of EMT induction. Its ligands include isoforms from either the TGF-β or bone morphogenic protein (BMP) families, with TGF-β-1, BMP2, and BMP4 being particularly associated with EMT [57–59]. Ligand initially binds to one of two types of serine and threonine kinase receptors, type I receptors, of which there are seven, or type II receptors, of which there are five [60]. Binding leads to the formation of a TGF-β heterotetrameric receptor complex with type II receptors trans-phosphorylating the type I receptors, activating their kinase activity [60]. This induces various signaling cascades, most notably involving SMAD2 and SMAD3, which oligomerize with SMAD4 for nuclear localization [60]. Inside the nucleus, the SMAD complex binds regulatory elements that induce the expression of various EMT genes, including SNAI1/2, TWIST1/2, and ZEB1/2 [61]. TGF-β signaling can also utilize SMAD-independent pathways, including PI3K/Akt and Ras/MEK/ERK [60]. Activated Akt2 has been shown to enhance the translation of the EMT-inducers DAB2 and ILE1, as well as SNAI1 [62–64]. Additionally, MEK/ERK stimulation plays a demonstrated role in the delocalization of zonula occludens and E-cadherin from epithelial cell junctions, driving EMT progression [65].

3.3.2. Receptor Tyrosine Kinase Signaling

Receptor tyrosine kinase (RTK) signaling includes a broad range of pathways initiated by a variety of ligands implicated in EMT, including HGF, FGF, PDGF, EGF, and insulin-like growth factor (IGF). In short, ligand binding to RTKs leads to receptor dimerization and trans-phosphorylation of intracellular domains, initiating additional signaling cascades via Ras, PI3K, FAK, Src, and TAK [66]. Of note, there is a good amount of overlap with the SMAD-independent pathways described with TGF-β signaling, particularly with regards to the Ras/MEK/ERK and PI3K/Akt cascades [67]. Beyond what was previously described, IGF-1 and HGF have been shown to utilize ERK signaling to enhance ZEB1 in PCa cells and SNAI1/2 expression in hepatocellular carcinoma cells, respectively [68,69]. PDGF operates through the PI3K/Akt pathway to augment the transcription of *CDH2*, leading to increases in N-cadherin [70]. *FAK* activation plays an essential role in upregulating *SNAIL* and *TWIST* transcription as well as downregulating E-cadherin expression and promoting its internalization [71]. Increased Src expression has been demonstrated in CRPC and correlated with a greater prevalence of distant metastases [72,73]. Src-suppression in breast carcinoma cells demonstrated an increase in E-cadherin and a decrease in vimentin, reducing the apparent metastatic potential [74]. Similarly, elevations in Src expression showed downregulation of E-cadherin with an apparent increase in pancreatic ductal carcinoma invasiveness [75].

3.3.3. Wnt Signaling

Wnt signaling is activated by the binding of the Wnt ligand to a Frizzled receptor and a lipoprotein receptor-related protein (LRP) [76]. This allows GSK-3-beta to phosphorylate LRP, which recruits Dishevelled and Axin to the plasma membrane, allowing beta-catenin to translocate to the nucleus [76]. Intranuclear beta-catenin is able to form a complex with LEF-1 that leads to the inhibition of *CDH1* transcription, suppressing E-cadherin production [77]. Beta-catenin has also been shown to directly induce SNAI1 and SNAI2 expression in a number of cancers, as well as promote TWIST expression in mammary epithelial cells [78–80].

3.3.4. Notch Signaling

Notch signaling involves an intercellular interaction between the extracellular domain of the Notch receptor and its cell surface ligands, Delta and Jagged [81]. This stimulates proteolytic cleavage of the Notch receptor intracellular domain by ADAM-MMPs and gamma-secretase, allowing for translocation to the nucleus [81]. Once in the nucleus, the cleaved Notch receptor is able to activate the expression of various genes implicated in EMT, including NF-kB, Akt, and p21, as well as directly promote SNAIL expression [82–84]. Furthermore, Notch signaling is capable of inducing HIF-1-alpha release, leading to the upregulation of LOX and subsequent stabilization of SNAI1 [85]. Furthermore, the inhibition of Notch signaling in lung adenocarcinoma has demonstrated reductions in tumor invasiveness and EMT progression [86].

3.3.5. Hedgehog Signaling

Hedgehog (Hh) signaling is mediated through the binding of Hh ligands to PTCH receptors, resulting in the internalization and degradation of the Hh-PTCH complex [87]. This releases the inhibition on Smoothened, which initiates an intracellular cascade that activates the Gli family of transcription factors [87]. Gli1 has been shown to promote the transcription of SNAI1 and has been implicated in promoting EMT-mediated invasion of ileal neuroendocrine tumors [88,89]. Hh signaling is notable for being highly involved in crosstalk with other pathways that promote EMT. Hh induction of TGF-β-1 signaling has been correlated with increased motility and invasiveness in gastric cancer [90]. Hh enhancement of JAG2 expression has been shown to augment the Notch pathway [91]. Furthermore, the inhibition of Hh signaling in pancreatic cancer cells has demonstrated the impairment of EMT-mediated disease progression [92].

4. Studies on EMT in Prostate Cancer

Different studies have elaborated on the role of androgens, signaling pathways, epigenetic alterations, TME, and CSCs in PCa pathogenesis. First, androgens play a critical role in the development of PCa. Specifically, AR is considered a key mediator of PCa growth, including the induction of cell cycle progression, inhibition of apoptosis, and activation of angiogenesis. Second, various signaling pathways are implicated in PCa development and progression. Those include the TGF-β, RTK, WNT, Notch, and Hedgehog signaling pathways. These pathways promote PCa growth by inducing EMT and promoting PCa stemness properties. Third, epigenetic and TME alterations also contribute to PCa development and progression.

4.1. *In Vitro and In Vivo Studies*

4.1.1. EMT Surface Markers

Vimentin is an important cell surface marker of mesenchymal cells and, as such, can be utilized to identify the occurrence of EMT. Studies have found increased co-expression of cytokeratin 8 and vimentin in androgen-independent CRP [16,93]. A follow-up study conducted by the same group sought to determine whether an increase in these biomarkers was associated with worse clinical outcomes [94]. A total of 122 samples from patients with PCa were evaluated, and it was found that these markers were associated with a higher Gleason score. This study also confirmed that the degree of EMT progression is predictive of PSA failure regardless of the Gleason score, pathological state, or surgical margins [94].

4.1.2. EMT Transcription Markers

Evidence indicates that tumors may originate from CSCs that express ZEB1 in prostatic basal stem cells, triggering the induction of EMT with stem cell traits, immune evasion, and epigenomic reprogramming [95]. Basal cells exhibit intrinsic stem-like and neurogenic properties, characterized by genes that are enriched in advanced, anaplastic, castration-resistant, and metastatic PCa [95]. Single-cell RNA-sequencing analysis holds promise for uncovering detailed transcriptomic signatures that can help uncover the lineage contribution to CSCs and their association with PCa progression, drug resistance, and metastasis [95].

In metastatic CRPC (mCRPC), epigenetic reprogramming, especially through polycomb repression, is thought to underlie lineage plasticity [96]. The polycomb repressive complex plays a crucial role in regulating EMT, with Hsp90 acting through EZH2 to reverse its function, leading to tumor growth and tissue invasion [96]. EZH2 also promotes neuroendocrine differentiation through histone methylation at H3 lysine 27, with this differentiation being a significant marker of certain PCa cell lines [96]. Furthermore, polycomb regulation modulates stem cell functions.

In a study utilizing Pten knockout mice, Rb1 loss was found to be a significant driver of lineage plasticity in a Pten loss-induced prostate adenocarcinoma model, as evidenced by an increase in EMT and stemness [97]. Transcriptomic profiling revealed that this phenotype was mediated by *SOX2* and *EZH2*, both of which are epigenetic reprogramming factors. Additional studies have demonstrated a strong link between *TP53*, *RB1*, lineage plasticity, and epigenetic changes that contribute to CRPC [97].

EMT represents a mechanism by which cancer cells can acquire resistance to therapy, including resistance to chemotherapy, radiotherapy, increased drug efflux, and evasion of apoptosis [98]. Importantly, Snail has been shown to prevent treatment-induced apoptosis by interfering with Tp53 or Pten [98]. Two studies utilizing mouse models demonstrated that primary and secondary tumor cells gain therapy resistance through an EMT-dependent mechanism [93,98].

4.1.3. Tumor Microenvironment

The crosstalk between epithelial tumor cells of PCa and surrounding stroma within the tumor microenvironment plays a crucial role in the progression of the disease into its advanced stages and eventual metastasis. Some of the key players within the stroma include mesenchymal stem/progenitor cells, stromal-derived mediators of inflammation, regulators of angiogenesis, connective tissue growth factors, wingless homologs (Wnts), and integrins [17]. A study by Zhou et al. referred to the mechanism of neuroendocrine differentiation that occurs in parallel with castration resistance development in advanced PCa [99]. In addition, it is noteworthy mentioning that the TME evolves in parallel with the PCa clones, where the ECM and vasculature architecture is altered, recruiting specialized tumor-supporting cells that favor tumor spread and colonization at distant sites, particularly the bones where a premetastatic niche is orchestrated [100].

An early study investigating the creation of the TME in PCa highlighted the essential role of cancer-associated fibroblasts (CAFs) [101]. CAFs were found to acquire stemness and an EMT phenotype after interacting with cancer-induced macrophages in the TME. This induction event was subsequently correlated with increased PCa metastasis [101].

A study by Bezzi and colleagues showed that different genetically engineered mouse models with homozygous Pten loss exhibited varied immune compositions in the TME [102]. They demonstrated that the loss of Zbtb7a along with Pten resulted in higher CXCL5 expression, while the loss of Tp53 along with Pten led to increased CLCL17 expression, potentially attracting myeloid cells to the TME through distinct mechanisms [102].

A study conducted by Su and colleagues demonstrated that PRC1 drives the metastasis of certain PCa subtypes through the regulation of CCL2 expression [103]. In the TME, CCL2 was shown to promote PCa self-renewal, angiogenesis, and immune system suppression. They also found that PRC1 combined with immune checkpoint blockade effectively suppresses metastasis in PCa-induced mice, suggesting that CCL2 expression could serve as a biomarker for response to therapy [103]. A separate study found that the inactivation of AR reduces a transcriptional repressor of CCL2, which mediates EMT of prostate tumor cells [93].

4.1.4. TGF-β Signaling

TGF-β is a well-known EMT-inducer via alternative splicing of CD44, forming an isoform capable of migration, invasion, and tumor initiation. An in vitro study using human PCa cells treated with TGF-β showed a decrease in E-cadherin and an increase in N-cadherin, among other EMT and CSC markers [104]. The same study also performed in vitro and in vivo investigations that showed that CD44 promoted PCa cell migration, invasion, and tumor initiation [104].

4.1.5. RTK Signaling

Through both in vivo and in vitro studies, Bluemn and colleagues evaluated the inevitable shift to CRPC through androgen independence [105]. While they observed FGF to be markedly overexpressed in CRPC, the expression of the FGF receptor (FGFR), an RTK, was also found to have increased expression [105,106]. The enhanced activity of these specific RTKs was associated with ligand-independent activation of AR transcription in these models [106]. Another study that used xenograft growth demonstrated that PCa expression of IL6 is capable of activating a specific type of CAF that induces EMT invasiveness and stemness [107]. These findings suggest IL6 and FGF as potential biomarkers.

4.1.6. WNT Signaling

A study performed by Acevedo and colleagues identified FGF-receptor-mediated EMT in PCa progression that utilized SOX9 and Wnt signaling [108]. It was found that, in inducible FGFR1 prostate mouse models, activation with chemical inducers of dimerization led to highly synchronous, stepwise progression to adenocarcinoma linked to EMT [108].

A previous study demonstrated that the loss of *PTEN* can initiate EMT [109]. Another study found that restoring *PTEN* in breast cancer prevented EMT and stemness through the downregulation of Abelson interactor 1 (*Abi1*) [110]. Abi1 is an adapter protein that uses Wnt signaling to regulate the progression of epithelial plasticity in PCa [109].

4.1.7. Notch Signaling

One study has implicated the Notch pathway as an EMT promoter in PCa, with recent research describing it as an important player through activation of the estrogen receptor through the use of castrated mice [111]. The estrogen receptor alpha is expressed in the basal cell layers of the normal prostate and has key roles in coordinating stem cells for prostate development [111]. It was also found that EZH2 was recruited by estrogen receptors and facilitated the binding of these receptors to the Notch promoter [111].

4.1.8. Hedgehog Signaling

A study performed by Ishii and colleagues determined that the Shh-inhibitor vismodegib prevented EMT in CRPC cells, resulting in decreased tumor growth in mice when compared to controls. It was also shown to inhibit cancer cell proliferation via enhanced apoptosis [112].

4.1.9. PI3K/AKT Signaling

Contactin1 (Cntn-1) is an immunoglobulin superfamily cell adhesion neuronal membrane glycoprotein that promotes metastasis through EMT [113]. Cntn-1 downregulation has been shown to decrease PI3K/Akt signaling activity, an important pathway for EMT propagation [114]. This signaling pathway promotes EMT in PCa through the upregulation of EMT-inducing transcription factors and the activation of downstream effectors, such as mTOR and GSK-3β [115]. Activation of the PI3K/AKT pathway upregulates EMT-inducing transcription factors, such as *Snail, Slug,* and *ZEB1*, which in turn repress the expression of epithelial markers, such as E-cadherin, and induce the expression of mesenchymal markers, such as N-cadherin, vimentin, and fibronectin [94]. This results in a loss of cell–cell adhesion and an increase in cell motility and invasiveness.

Normal prostatic epithelium in rodents is composed of basal, secretory luminal, and neuroendocrine cells, with stem cells identified in both basal and luminal lineages [116]. One study suggested that PCa tumors may arise from CSCs with Pten/Akt signaling dysregulation, resulting in a heterogenous population of cells similar to those present in the normal prostatic epithelium [116].

4.1.10. Integration of the Different Signaling Pathways in PCa Progression

The various signaling pathways mentioned above collectively play a role in the progression of PCa. The TGF-β pathway induces EMT via alternative splicing of *CD44*, leading to increased migration, invasion, and tumor initiation. Likewise, *RTK* signaling, specifically *FGF* and *FGFR*, is overexpressed in CRPC, leading to ligand-independent activation of *AR* transcription and increased invasiveness and stemness. The *WNT* signaling pathway is also implicated in EMT, where the loss of *PTEN* initiates this process and promotes stemness through the regulation of *Abi1*. The Notch pathway also promotes EMT, with estrogen receptors and *EZH2* recruiting to the Notch promoter to activate EMT. The interplay between the different pathways highlights their involvement in PCa progression.

4.2. Translational and Clinical Studies

Transcriptional analysis has identified distinct gene signatures associated with various EMT intermediate states, which have facilitated the identification of EMT transcriptional promoter genes that could serve as biomarkers [117]. The analysis of PCa has revealed that epithelial plasticity is directly correlated with poor clinical prognosis [118]. Notably, recent research by Stylianou and colleagues found that EMT biomarkers were enriched in PCa patients who had undergone ADT, which selects for wide-scale transcriptional changes in ADT-resistant tumor cells [118]. *SNAI1* was found to be the primary driver of EMT in their PCa model, with subsequent targeting of *SNAIL* leading to reduced mesenchymal drivers, such as ZEB1, and the re-expression of epithelial markers, such as E-cadherin [119]. Additionally, the loss of *SNAI2* led to a better response to ADT [119]. It was also found that the Wnt pathway Wnt5a/Fzd2 was found to increase EMT markers and predict PCa aggressiveness, while Abi1 controlled epithelial plasticity downstream of the Wnt receptor Fzd2 [109].

A study by Jedroszka and colleagues divided patients into groups based on their expression levels of AR, ESR1, and ESR2 [120]. It was found that in those under the age of 50, there was a completely different expression of EMT genes than in those over the age of 50 [120]. After the investigation of 43 genes involved in EMT, it was found that those under 50 overexpressed *CTNNB1*, *CDH1*, *SMAD2*, *SMAD3*, *TCF3*, and *LEF1*, while those over 50 overexpressed Snail1 and underexpressed *KRT5*, *KRT19*, *OCLN*, *CDH2*, and *MUC1* [120]. The difference in gene expression also predicted the presence of a more aggressive, invasive phenotype in those under 50, regardless of the Gleason score [120]. The reasons for the change in gene expression observed are not fully understood. However, it has been suggested that age-related changes in the hormonal milieu, especially the decrease in androgen levels, may contribute to this phenomenon. Additionally, aging is associated with various epigenetic changes, including alterations in DNA methylation, histone modifications, and non-coding RNA expression, which can impact gene expression. Further research is needed to fully elucidate the mechanisms underlying the age-related differences in EMT gene expression in PCa.

In a study by He and colleagues, single-cell analysis of advanced PCa patients treated with ADT revealed the co-expression of multiple AR isoforms, with resistance to therapy associated with upregulation of EMT and TGF-β gene signatures [121]. The study also found a subset of patient tumors with high expression of dysfunctional cytotoxic CD8+ T cell markers, indicating a potential impact of EMT on immune responses in CRPC [121].

5. Potential Biomarkers of Interest for Targeted Therapy

Based on the known pathways involved in EMT and prior in vitro, in vivo, translational, and clinical studies, many biomarkers have been identified as potential targets for EMT-targeted therapy in PCa. For EMT-driver targeting, the genes for TGF-β, PRC1/2, SNAI1/2, FGF, CNTN1, and BRD4, as well as the transcription factors SOX2, EZH2, and HSP90, have been proposed. For EMT-effector targeting, the genes for ZEB1/2, TWIST1/2, EZH2, Kaiso, ABI1, and CDH1/2, as well as the transcription factors ZEB1, LSD1, and PRC1/2, have been proposed. Due to the crucial role each of these factors plays in regulating the EMT process, inhibiting their expression may be a way of reversing the EMT process and preventing the activation of these pathways. For EMT-stemness targeting, the genes for SOX2 and PRC1/2 have been proposed. The immune targets of IL6, CCL2, and CXCL5 have also been identified as potential targets. Two important biomarkers involved in the cell cycle that have been identified are Tp53 and Rb1. Furthermore, many of these identified biomarkers play roles in various EMT signaling pathways, including RTK, TGF-β, NF-kB, Wnt, PI3K/Akt, PPAR, and Notch. Therefore, inhibitors of these pathways may also have investigational importance. Levels of E-cadherin, vimentin, and N-cadherin may also be useful markers of EMT and MET conversion.

6. Clinical Trials

A number of clinical trials investigating the aforementioned biomarkers were listed on https://clinicaltrials.gov/ (accessed on 15 February 2023). For the purposes of this review, only those clinical trials with specific targeted therapies for the listed biomarkers or those using vimentin and/or N-cadherin as a marker of decreased EMT were included for further analysis, as seen in Table 1.

Analysis of these trials revealed many investigational therapies of interest. Clinical trial *NCT02452008* is recruiting for a study involving LY2157299, a TGF-β receptor inhibitor. Clinical trial *NCT05413421* is recruiting for a study involving ORIC-944, a highly selective, allosteric, small-molecule inhibitor of PRC2 (Figure 2). Dovitinib, an RTK inhibitor with unique inhibitory effects on FGF, underwent investigation in clinical trials *NCT01741116*, *NCT01994590*, and *NCT02065323*. Various EZH2 inhibitors, including CPI-1205, PF-06821497, and Tazverik, are being studied in clinical trials *NCT03480646*, *NCT03460977*, *NCT05567679*, and *NCT04179864*, all of which are currently recruiting. Completed studies involving HSP90 inhibitors AT13387 and STA-9090 were conducted in clinical trials *NCT01685268* and *NCT01270880*. *NCT02140996*, which investigated the Ad-sig-hMUC-1/ecdCD40L vector vaccine meant to disrupt E-cadherin, currently has an unknown status and was last updated in 2016. JBI-802, an LSD1/HDAC6 inhibitor, is being studied in clinical trial *NCT05268666*, which is currently recruiting. *NCT00433446*, *NCT00385827*, and *NCT00401765* have finished studies involving CNTO-328, an anti-IL6 chimeric monoclonal antibody. *NCT00992186* has been completed and involved Carlumab, an anti-CCL2 therapy (Figure 3).

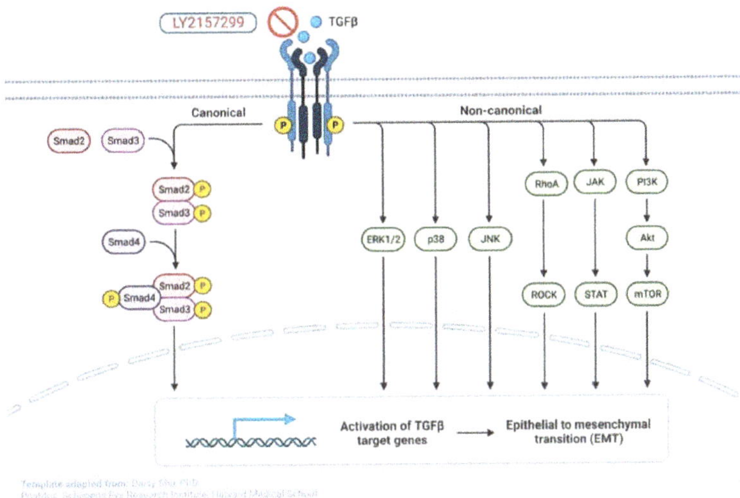

Figure 2. Mechanism of action of the TGF-β inhibitor LY2157299. As shown, inhibition of TGF-β causes downstream inhibition effects on SMAD, ERK1/2, p38, JNK, RhoA/ROCK, JAK/STAT, and PI3K/Akt/mTOR, leading to decreased activation of TGF-β target genes, and a decrease in EMT. Created with BioRender.com (accessed on 11 March 2023).

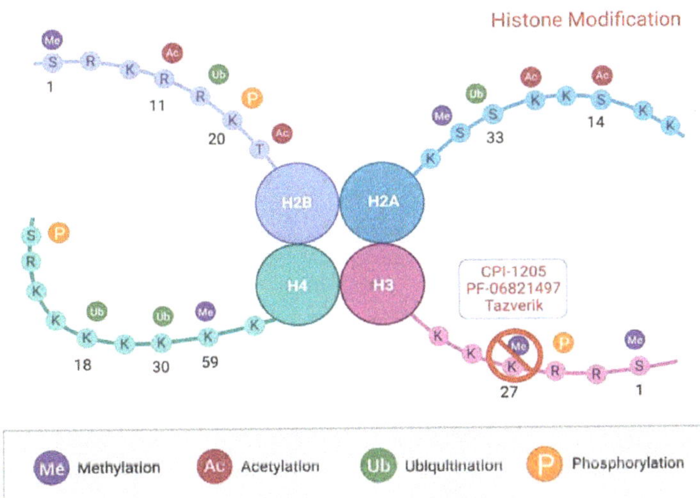

Figure 3. Mechanism of action of the EZH2 inhibitors CPI-1205, PF-06821497, and Tazverik. EZH2 is an enzyme responsible for methylation of histone H3 at lysine 27. Created with BioRender.com (accessed on 11 March 2023).

Table 1. List of clinical trials involving the EMT biomarkers of interest with investigational therapies targeting those biomarkers (https://clinicaltrials.gov/, accessed on 15 February 2023).

Target	NCT Number	Phase	Status	Outcome of Interest
TGF-β	*NCT02452008*	2	Recruiting	Compare the progression-free survival of those with mCRPC who are treated with enzalutamide alone vs. enzalutamide plus LY2157299, a TGF-β receptor inhibitor.
PRC2	*NCT05413421*	1	Recruiting	Establish a phase 2 dose and/or MTD of ORIC-944, a potent, highly selective, allosteric, orally bioavailable, small molecule inhibitor of PRC2.
FGF	*NCT01741116*	2	Completed	Evaluate the efficacy and safety of Dovitinib, an RTK inhibitor with unique inhibitory effects on FGF. No results posted.
	NCT01994590	2	Terminated	Evaluate the safety of adding Dovitinib to abiraterone acetate and prednisone in those with mCRPC. Terminated due to sponsor no longer supplying study drug.
	NCT02065323	2	Withdrawn	Evaluate if adding Dovitinib to ADT will prolong time to disease progression in those with mCRPC receiving ADT for the first time. Withdrawn due to budgeting considerations and time length to development.
EZH2	*NCT03480646*	1, 2	Active, not recruiting	Determine the dose-limiting toxicities in those with mCRPC receiving CPI-1205, a small molecule inhibitor of EZH2.
	NCT03460977	1	Recruiting	Evaluate the safety and efficacy of PF-06821497, an EZH2 inhibitor, in those with CRPC.
	NCT05567679	1	Not yet recruiting	Evaluate if the underlying prostate cancer tumor is more sensitive to the patient's immune system after receiving radical prostatectomy following preoperative treatment with Tazverik, an EZH2 inhibitor.
	NCT04179864	1, 2	Recruiting	Determine the safety and efficacy of combining Tazverik with either enzalutamide or abiraterone/prednisone in those with CRPC who have not received chemotherapy.
HSP90	*NCT01685268*	1, 2	Completed	Determine the safety and antitumor activity of AT13387, an HSP90 inhibitor, either alone or in combination with abiraterone. No results posted.
	NCT01270880	2	Completed	Evaluate the progression-free survival of those receiving STA-9090, an HSP90 inhibitor, with mCRPC refractory to docetaxel. At 6 months, all 18 participants had disease progression.
CDH1	*NCT02140996*	1	Unknown	Assessment of safety and dose level of Ad-sig-hMUC-1/ecdCD40L vector vaccine meant to disrupt e-cadherin. Last status update in 2016 listed it as recruiting.
LSD1	*NCT05268666*	1, 2	Recruiting	Assessment of the MTD and efficacy of JBI-802, an LSD1/HDAC6 inhibitor.
IL6	*NCT00433446*	2	Completed	Determine PSA response to CNTO-328, an anti-IL6 chimeric monoclonal antibody, in those with mCRPC. 3.8% of participants had a reduction in PSA of at least 50%.
	NCT00385827	2	Terminated	Determine the number of participants with adverse events and the progression-free survival in those receiving CNTO-328 for mCRPC. Terminated after determination of a lack of efficacy.
	NCT00401765	1	Completed	Determine the safety and efficacy of CNTO-328 in combination with docetaxel in those with mCRPC. No results posted.
CCL2	*NCT00992186*	2	Completed	Determine the safety and efficacy of Carlumab, an anti-CCL2 therapy, in those with mCRPC. Of 41 participants, 0 had a composite response as measured by: a change in skeletal lesions, extra-skeletal lesions, or PSA.
N-Cadherin and Vimentin	*NCT01990196*	2	Active, not recruiting	Measure vimentin and N-cadherin expression following radical prostatectomy and treatment with degarelix, enzalutamide, trametinib, or dasatinib, which are capable of SRC and/or MEK inhibition of tyrosine kinase.
	NCT02204943	2	Completed	Measure changes in biomarkers of epithelial plasticity such as N-cadherin and vimentin following bone targeting radium-223 in those with mCRPC. No results posted.
	NCT00887640	2	Terminated	Measure percent change in N-cadherin expression at baseline and at 8 weeks following treatment with Temsirolimus in those with mCRPC refractory to treatment.

Abbreviations: ADT: androgen deprivation therapy; CCL2: monocyte chemoattractant protein-1; CDH1: cadherin-1; EZH2: enhancer of zeste homolog 2; FGF: fibroblast growth factor; HSP90: heat shock protein 90; IL6: interleukin-6; LSD1: lysine-specific demethylase 1; mCRPC: metastatic castration-resistant prostate cancer; MEK: mitogen-activated protein kinase kinase; MTD: maximum tolerated dose; NCT: national clinical trial; PRC2: polycomb repressive complex 2; PSA: prostate-specific antigen; RTK: receptor tyrosine kinase; SRC: proto-oncogene tyrosine-protein kinase; TGF-β: transforming growth factor beta.

Of the twenty clinical trials included, seven have been completed, with only three of those having available results. In clinical trial *NCT01270880*, the progression-free survival of individuals with mCRPC who had previously received docetaxel and were treated with STA-9090 was investigated. At the conclusion of phase II, all participants experienced disease progression. In clinical trial *NCT00433446*, the proportion of participants with a PSA response to CNTO-328 was studied, and it was found that only 3.8% of participants experienced a decrease in PSA of at least 50% from baseline. Finally, clinical trial *NCT00992186* evaluated the safety and efficacy of Carlumab, and it was determined that none of the participants experienced any form of composite response at the end of the trial.

There are currently no clinical trials listed that involve therapies specifically targeting PRC1, SNAI1/2, CNTN1, BRD4, SOX2, ZEB1/2, TWIST1/2, Kaiso, ABI1, CXCL5, Tp53, or Rb1.

7. Conclusions and Future Directions

The association of EMT with the progression of cancer grading, metastasis, and therapeutic resistance has been of great investigational importance in recent years. Identifying relevant biomarkers for EMT is essential for the development of therapeutic interventions, particularly in heavily treatment-resistant diseases such as CRPC, where EMT promotes invasion and CSC survival. While there are currently many known biomarkers for EMT, more are being identified with the help of transcriptional analysis. The majority of the analyses performed on the clinical utility of these targets have been through in vivo or in vitro studies, with few being conducted through translational applications.

Of the targets identified in this review, only a small minority of those found on clinicaltrials.gov included investigational therapies. While there were twenty clinical trials found on TGF-β, PRC2, FGF, EZH2, HSP90, CDH1, LSD1, IL6, CCL2, N-cadherin, and vimentin, only seven have been completed at this time, with three of these having posted results. To date, the outcomes of these completed trials do not support EMT biomarker-targeted therapy as an effective means of treatment for PCa, which is surprising given the strength and breadth of investigations assessing EMT involvement in cancer progression. The trial examining STA-9090, an HSP90 inhibitor, showed that all participants had disease progression. The trial involving CNTO-328, an anti-IL6 chimeric monoclonal antibody, concluded that only 3.8% of participants experienced a significant decrease in PSA. Lastly, the trial looking at Carlumab, an anti-CCL2 therapy, indicated that none of the participants experienced a significant response to treatment. Given these disappointing outcomes, the results of the remaining 17 clinical trials are of great importance in guiding the future application of EMT biomarker therapy in clinical practice. Additionally, the results of clinical trials comprising targeted therapies of PRC1, SNAI1/2, CNTN1, BRD4, Sox2, ZEB1/2, TWIST1/2, Kaiso, ABI1, CXCL5, TP53, and RB1 are increasingly important. Finally, since none of the studies found on clinicaltrials.gov implicated the specific application of these therapies for the investigation of EMT, future studies involving these factors should be expected.

Author Contributions: Conceptualization, H.F.B.; methodology, S.G. and M.R.; validation, H.F.B.; data curation, S.G., M.R. and H.F.B.; writing—original draft preparation, S.G. and M.R.; writing—review and editing, H.F.B., W.A.-K., Y.O. and R.P.; visualization, H.F.B.; supervision, R.P.; project administration, H.F.B.; funding acquisition, H.F.B. All authors have read and agreed to the published version of the manuscript.

Funding: This research received no external funding.

Institutional Review Board Statement: Not applicable.

Informed Consent Statement: Not applicable.

Data Availability Statement: Not applicable.

Acknowledgments: Figures were created with BioRender.com (accessed on 11 March 2023).

Conflicts of Interest: The authors declare no conflict of interest. The funders had no role in the design of the study; in the collection, analyses, or interpretation of data; in the writing of the manuscript, or in the decision to publish the results.

References

1. Global Burden of Disease Cancer Collaboration. Global, Regional, and National Cancer Incidence, Mortality, Years of Life Lost, Years Lived with Disability, and Disability-Adjusted Life-years for 32 Cancer Groups, 1990 to 2015: A Systematic Analysis for the Global Burden of Disease Study. *JAMA Oncol.* **2017**, *3*, 524–548. [CrossRef]
2. Gogola, S.; Rejzer, M.; Bahmad, H.F.; Alloush, F.; Omarzai, Y.; Poppiti, R. Anti-Cancer Stem-Cell-Targeted Therapies in Prostate Cancer. *Cancers* **2023**, *15*, 1621. [CrossRef]
3. Siegel, R.L.; Miller, K.D.; Wagle, N.S.; Jemal, A. Cancer statistics, 2023. *CA Cancer J. Clin.* **2023**, *73*, 17–48. [CrossRef]
4. Butler, S.S.; Muralidhar, V.; Zhao, S.G.; Sanford, N.N.; Franco, I.; Fullerton, Z.H.; Chavez, J.; D'Amico, A.V.; Feng, F.Y.; Rebbeck, T.R.; et al. Prostate cancer incidence across stage, NCCN risk groups, and age before and after USPSTF Grade D recommendations against prostate-specific antigen screening in 2012. *Cancer* **2020**, *126*, 717–724. [CrossRef]
5. Ilic, D.; Djulbegovic, M.; Jung, J.H.; Hwang, E.C.; Zhou, Q.; Cleves, A.; Agoritsas, T.; Dahm, P. Prostate cancer screening with prostate-specific antigen (PSA) test: A systematic review and meta-analysis. *BMJ* **2018**, *362*, k3519. [CrossRef]
6. Epstein, J.I. An update of the Gleason grading system. *J. Urol.* **2010**, *183*, 433–440. [CrossRef]
7. Gleason, D.F.; Mellinger, G.T. Prediction of prognosis for prostatic adenocarcinoma by combined histological grading and clinical staging. *J. Urol.* **1974**, *111*, 58–64. [CrossRef]
8. Epstein, J.I.; Zelefsky, M.J.; Sjoberg, D.D.; Nelson, J.B.; Egevad, L.; Magi-Galluzzi, C.; Vickers, A.J.; Parwani, A.V.; Reuter, V.E.; Fine, S.W.; et al. A Contemporary Prostate Cancer Grading System: A Validated Alternative to the Gleason Score. *Eur. Urol.* **2016**, *69*, 428–435. [CrossRef]
9. Debes, J.D.; Tindall, D.J. Mechanisms of androgen-refractory prostate cancer. *N. Engl. J. Med.* **2004**, *351*, 1488–1490. [CrossRef]
10. Cornford, P.; van den Bergh, R.C.N.; Briers, E.; van den Broeck, T.; Cumberbatch, M.G.; de Santis, M.; Fanti, S.; Fossati, N.; Gandaglia, G.; Gillessen, S.; et al. EAU-EANM-ESTRO-ESUR-SIOG Guidelines on Prostate Cancer. Part II-2020 Update: Treatment of Relapsing and Metastatic Prostate Cancer. *Eur. Urol.* **2021**, *79*, 263–282. [CrossRef]
11. Pienta, K.J.; Bradley, D. Mechanisms underlying the development of androgen-independent prostate cancer. *Clin. Cancer Res.* **2006**, *12*, 1665–1671. [CrossRef]
12. Feldman, B.J.; Feldman, D. The development of androgen-independent prostate cancer. *Nat. Rev. Cancer* **2001**, *1*, 34–45. [CrossRef]
13. Nelson, W.G.; de Marzo, A.M.; Isaacs, W.B. Prostate cancer. *N. Engl. J. Med.* **2003**, *349*, 366–381. [CrossRef]
14. Shah, R.B.; Mehra, R.; Chinnaiyan, A.M.; Shen, R.; Ghosh, D.; Zhou, M.; Macvicar, G.R.; Varambally, S.; Harwood, J.; Bismar, T.A.; et al. Androgen-independent prostate cancer is a heterogeneous group of diseases: Lessons from a rapid autopsy program. *Cancer Res.* **2004**, *64*, 9209–9216. [CrossRef]
15. Bahmad, H.F.; Demus, T.; Moubarak, M.M.; Daher, D.; Alvarez Moreno, J.C.; Polit, F.; Lopez, O.; Merhe, A.; Abou-Kheir, W.; Nieder, A.M.; et al. Overcoming Drug Resistance in Advanced Prostate Cancer by Drug Repurposing. *Med. Sci.* **2022**, *10*, 15. [CrossRef]
16. Bahmad, H.F.; Cheaito, K.; Chalhoub, R.M.; Hadadeh, O.; Monzer, A.; Ballout, F.; El-Hajj, A.; Mukherji, D.; Liu, Y.N.; Daoud, G.; et al. Sphere-Formation Assay: Three-Dimensional in vitro Culturing of Prostate Cancer Stem/Progenitor Sphere-Forming Cells. *Front. Oncol.* **2018**, *8*, 347. [CrossRef]
17. Bahmad, H.F.; Jalloul, M.; Azar, J.; Moubarak, M.M.; Samad, T.A.; Mukherji, D.; Al-Sayegh, M.; Abou-Kheir, W. Tumor Microenvironment in Prostate Cancer: Toward Identification of Novel Molecular Biomarkers for Diagnosis, Prognosis, and Therapy Development. *Front. Genet.* **2021**, *12*, 652747. [CrossRef]
18. Martin-Belmonte, F.; Mostov, K. Regulation of cell polarity during epithelial morphogenesis. *Curr. Opin. Cell Biol.* **2008**, *20*, 227–234. [CrossRef]
19. Bryant, D.M.; Mostov, K.E. From cells to organs: Building polarized tissue. *Nat. Rev. Mol. Cell Biol.* **2008**, *9*, 887–901. [CrossRef]
20. Barriere, G.; Fici, P.; Gallerani, G.; Fabbri, F.; Rigaud, M. Epithelial Mesenchymal Transition: A double-edged sword. *Clin. Transl. Med.* **2015**, *4*, 14. [CrossRef]
21. Lamouille, S.; Xu, J.; Derynck, R. Molecular mechanisms of epithelial-mesenchymal transition. *Nat. Rev. Mol. Cell Biol.* **2014**, *15*, 178–196. [CrossRef]
22. Eastham, A.M.; Spencer, H.; Soncin, F.; Ritson, S.; Merry, C.L.; Stern, P.L.; Ward, C.M. Epithelial-mesenchymal transition events during human embryonic stem cell differentiation. *Cancer Res.* **2007**, *67*, 11254–11262. [CrossRef]
23. Ullmann, U.; In't Veld, P.; Gilles, C.; Sermon, K.; de Rycke, M.; van de Velde, H.; van Steirteghem, A.; Liebaers, I. Epithelial-mesenchymal transition process in human embryonic stem cells cultured in feeder-free conditions. *Mol. Hum. Reprod.* **2007**, *13*, 21–32. [CrossRef]
24. Azar, J.; Bahmad, H.F.; Daher, D.; Moubarak, M.M.; Hadadeh, O.; Monzer, A.; Al Bitar, S.; Jamal, M.; Al-Sayegh, M.; Abou-Kheir, W. The Use of Stem Cell-Derived Organoids in Disease Modeling: An Update. *Int. J. Mol. Sci.* **2021**, *22*, 47667. [CrossRef]

25. Papaccio, F.; della Corte, C.M.; Viscardi, G.; di Liello, R.; Esposito, G.; Sparano, F.; Ciardiello, F.; Morgillo, F. HGF/MET and the Immune System: Relevance for Cancer Immunotherapy. *Int. J. Mol. Sci.* **2018**, *19*, 113595. [CrossRef]
26. Chaves, L.P.; Melo, C.M.; Saggioro, F.P.; Reis, R.B.D.; Squire, J.A. Epithelial-Mesenchymal Transition Signaling and Prostate Cancer Stem Cells: Emerging Biomarkers and Opportunities for Precision Therapeutics. *Genes* **2021**, *12*, 1900. [CrossRef]
27. Katz, L.H.; Li, Y.; Chen, J.S.; Muñoz, N.M.; Majumdar, A.; Chen, J.; Mishra, L. Targeting TGF-β signaling in cancer. *Expert Opin. Ther. Targets* **2013**, *17*, 743–760. [CrossRef]
28. Owusu, B.Y.; Galemmo, R.; Janetka, J.; Klampfer, L. Hepatocyte Growth Factor, a Key Tumor-Promoting Factor in the Tumor Microenvironment. *Cancers* **2017**, *9*, 40035. [CrossRef]
29. Strutz, F.; Zeisberg, M.; Ziyadeh, F.N.; Yang, C.Q.; Kalluri, R.; Müller, G.A.; Neilson, E.G. Role of basic fibroblast growth factor-2 in epithelial-mesenchymal transformation. *Kidney Int.* **2002**, *61*, 1714–1728. [CrossRef]
30. Lee, J.G.; Kay, E.P. Cross-talk among Rho GTPases acting downstream of PI 3-kinase induces mesenchymal transformation of corneal endothelial cells mediated by FGF-2. *Invest. Ophthalmol. Vis. Sci.* **2006**, *47*, 2358–2368. [CrossRef]
31. Kim, J.; Kong, J.; Chang, H.; Kim, H.; Kim, A. EGF induces epithelial-mesenchymal transition through phospho-Smad2/3-Snail signaling pathway in breast cancer cells. *Oncotarget* **2016**, *7*, 85021–85032. [CrossRef]
32. Wu, Q.; Hou, X.; Xia, J.; Qian, X.; Miele, L.; Sarkar, F.H.; Wang, Z. Emerging roles of PDGF-D in EMT progression during tumorigenesis. *Cancer Treat. Rev.* **2013**, *39*, 640–646. [CrossRef]
33. Tam, S.Y.; Wu, V.W.C.; Law, H.K.W. Hypoxia-Induced Epithelial-Mesenchymal Transition in Cancers: HIF-1α and Beyond. *Front. Oncol.* **2020**, *10*, 486. [CrossRef]
34. Nissen, N.I.; Karsdal, M.; Willumsen, N. Collagens and Cancer associated fibroblasts in the reactive stroma and its relation to Cancer biology. *J. Exp. Clin. Cancer Res.* **2019**, *38*, 115. [CrossRef]
35. Vallés, A.M.; Boyer, B.; Tarone, G.; Thiery, J.P. Alpha 2 beta 1 integrin is required for the collagen and FGF-1 induced cell dispersion in a rat bladder carcinoma cell line. *Cell Adhes. Commun.* **1996**, *4*, 187–199. [CrossRef]
36. Garamszegi, N.; Garamszegi, S.P.; Samavarchi-Tehrani, P.; Walford, E.; Schneiderbauer, M.M.; Wrana, J.L.; Scully, S.P. Extracellular matrix-induced transforming growth factor-beta receptor signaling dynamics. *Oncogene* **2010**, *29*, 2368–2380. [CrossRef]
37. Medici, D.; Nawshad, A. Type I collagen promotes epithelial-mesenchymal transition through ILK-dependent activation of NF-kappaB and LEF-1. *Matrix Biol.* **2010**, *29*, 161–165. [CrossRef]
38. Koenig, A.; Mueller, C.; Hasel, C.; Adler, G.; Menke, A. Collagen type I induces disruption of E-cadherin-mediated cell-cell contacts and promotes proliferation of pancreatic carcinoma cells. *Cancer Res.* **2006**, *66*, 4662–4671. [CrossRef]
39. Oyanagi, J.; Ogawa, T.; Sato, H.; Higashi, S.; Miyazaki, K. Epithelial-mesenchymal transition stimulates human cancer cells to extend microtubule-based invasive protrusions and suppresses cell growth in collagen gel. *PLoS ONE* **2012**, *7*, e53209. [CrossRef]
40. Nisticò, P.; Bissell, M.J.; Radisky, D.C. Epithelial-mesenchymal transition: General principles and pathological relevance with special emphasis on the role of matrix metalloproteinases. *Cold Spring Harb. Perspect. Biol.* **2012**, *4*, 11908. [CrossRef]
41. Stallings-Mann, M.L.; Waldmann, J.; Zhang, Y.; Miller, E.; Gauthier, M.L.; Visscher, D.W.; Downey, G.P.; Radisky, E.S.; Fields, A.P.; Radisky, D.C. Matrix metalloproteinase induction of Rac1b, a key effector of lung cancer progression. *Sci. Transl. Med.* **2012**, *4*, 142ra195. [CrossRef] [PubMed]
42. Stemmler, M.P.; Eccles, R.L.; Brabletz, S.; Brabletz, T. Non-redundant functions of EMT transcription factors. *Nat. Cell Biol.* **2019**, *21*, 102–112. [CrossRef] [PubMed]
43. Gras, B.; Jacqueroud, L.; Wierinckx, A.; Lamblot, C.; Fauvet, F.; Lachuer, J.; Puisieux, A.; Ansieau, S. Snail family members unequally trigger EMT and thereby differ in their ability to promote the neoplastic transformation of mammary epithelial cells. *PLoS ONE* **2014**, *9*, e92254. [CrossRef]
44. Wang, Y.; Shi, J.; Chai, K.; Ying, X.; Zhou, B.P. The Role of Snail in EMT and Tumorigenesis. *Curr. Cancer Drug Targets* **2013**, *13*, 963–972. [CrossRef]
45. Batlle, E.; Sancho, E.; Francí, C.; Domínguez, D.; Monfar, M.; Baulida, J.; García de Herreros, A. The transcription factor snail is a repressor of E-cadherin gene expression in epithelial tumour cells. *Nat. Cell Biol.* **2000**, *2*, 84–89. [CrossRef]
46. Olmeda, D.; Moreno-Bueno, G.; Flores, J.M.; Fabra, A.; Portillo, F.; Cano, A. SNAI1 is required for tumor growth and lymph node metastasis of human breast carcinoma MDA-MB-231 cells. *Cancer Res.* **2007**, *67*, 11721–11731. [CrossRef]
47. Jin, H.; Yu, Y.; Zhang, T.; Zhou, X.; Zhou, J.; Jia, L.; Wu, Y.; Zhou, B.P.; Feng, Y. Snail is critical for tumor growth and metastasis of ovarian carcinoma. *Int. J. Cancer* **2010**, *126*, 2102–2111. [CrossRef]
48. Min, A.L.; Choi, J.Y.; Woo, H.Y.; Kim, J.D.; Kwon, J.H.; Bae, S.H.; Yoon, S.K.; Shin, S.H.; Chung, Y.J.; Jung, C.K. High expression of Snail mRNA in blood from hepatocellular carcinoma patients with extra-hepatic metastasis. *Clin. Exp. Metastasis* **2009**, *26*, 759–767. [CrossRef]
49. Kudo-Saito, C.; Shirako, H.; Takeuchi, T.; Kawakami, Y. Cancer metastasis is accelerated through immunosuppression during Snail-induced EMT of cancer cells. *Cancer Cell* **2009**, *15*, 195–206. [CrossRef]
50. Vesuna, F.; van Diest, P.; Chen, J.H.; Raman, V. Twist is a transcriptional repressor of E-cadherin gene expression in breast cancer. *Biochem. Biophys. Res. Commun.* **2008**, *367*, 235–241. [CrossRef]
51. Alexander, N.R.; Tran, N.L.; Rekapally, H.; Summers, C.E.; Glackin, C.; Heimark, R.L. N-cadherin gene expression in prostate carcinoma is modulated by integrin-dependent nuclear translocation of Twist1. *Cancer Res.* **2006**, *66*, 3365–3369. [CrossRef] [PubMed]

52. Casas, E.; Kim, J.; Bendesky, A.; Ohno-Machado, L.; Wolfe, C.J.; Yang, J. Snail2 is an essential mediator of Twist1-induced epithelial mesenchymal transition and metastasis. *Cancer Res.* **2011**, *71*, 245–254. [CrossRef] [PubMed]
53. Zhao, Z.; Rahman, M.A.; Chen, Z.G.; Shin, D.M. Multiple biological functions of Twist1 in various cancers. *Oncotarget* **2017**, *8*, 20380–20393. [CrossRef] [PubMed]
54. Eger, A.; Aigner, K.; Sonderegger, S.; Dampier, B.; Oehler, S.; Schreiber, M.; Berx, G.; Cano, A.; Beug, H.; Foisner, R. DeltaEF1 is a transcriptional repressor of E-cadherin and regulates epithelial plasticity in breast cancer cells. *Oncogene* **2005**, *24*, 2375–2385. [CrossRef] [PubMed]
55. Aigner, K.; Dampier, B.; Descovich, L.; Mikula, M.; Sultan, A.; Schreiber, M.; Mikulits, W.; Brabletz, T.; Strand, D.; Obrist, P.; et al. The transcription factor ZEB1 (deltaEF1) promotes tumour cell dedifferentiation by repressing master regulators of epithelial polarity. *Oncogene* **2007**, *26*, 6979–6988. [CrossRef] [PubMed]
56. Perez-Oquendo, M.; Gibbons, D.L. Regulation of ZEB1 Function and Molecular Associations in Tumor Progression and Metastasis. *Cancers* **2022**, *14*, 1864. [CrossRef] [PubMed]
57. Pang, M.F.; Georgoudaki, A.M.; Lambut, L.; Johansson, J.; Tabor, V.; Hagikura, K.; Jin, Y.; Jansson, M.; Alexander, J.S.; Nelson, C.M.; et al. TGF-β1-induced EMT promotes targeted migration of breast cancer cells through the lymphatic system by the activation of CCR7/CCL21-mediated chemotaxis. *Oncogene* **2016**, *35*, 748–760. [CrossRef]
58. Kang, M.H.; Kang, H.N.; Kim, J.L.; Kim, J.S.; Oh, S.C.; Yoo, Y.A. Inhibition of PI3 kinase/Akt pathway is required for BMP2-induced EMT and invasion. *Oncol. Rep.* **2009**, *22*, 525–534. [CrossRef]
59. Deng, G.; Chen, Y.; Guo, C.; Yin, L.; Han, Y.; Li, Y.; Fu, Y.; Cai, C.; Shen, H.; Zeng, S. BMP4 promotes the metastasis of gastric cancer by inducing epithelial-mesenchymal transition via ID1. *J. Cell Sci.* **2020**, *133*, jcs237222. [CrossRef]
60. Huang, F.; Chen, Y.G. Regulation of TGF-β receptor activity. *Cell Biosci.* **2012**, *2*, 9. [CrossRef]
61. Garg, M. Epithelial-mesenchymal transition—Activating transcription factors—Multifunctional regulators in cancer. *World J. Stem Cells* **2013**, *5*, 188–195. [CrossRef] [PubMed]
62. Irie, H.Y.; Pearline, R.V.; Grueneberg, D.; Hsia, M.; Ravichandran, P.; Kothari, N.; Natesan, S.; Brugge, J.S. Distinct roles of Akt1 and Akt2 in regulating cell migration and epithelial-mesenchymal transition. *J. Cell Biol.* **2005**, *171*, 1023–1034. [CrossRef] [PubMed]
63. Chaudhury, A.; Hussey, G.S.; Ray, P.S.; Jin, G.; Fox, P.L.; Howe, P.H. TGF-beta-mediated phosphorylation of hnRNP E1 induces EMT via transcript-selective translational induction of Dab2 and ILEI. *Nat. Cell Biol.* **2010**, *12*, 286–293. [CrossRef] [PubMed]
64. Zhou, B.P.; Deng, J.; Xia, W.; Xu, J.; Li, Y.M.; Gunduz, M.; Hung, M.C. Dual regulation of Snail by GSK-3beta-mediated phosphorylation in control of epithelial-mesenchymal transition. *Nat. Cell Biol.* **2004**, *6*, 931–940. [CrossRef]
65. Xie, L.; Law, B.K.; Chytil, A.M.; Brown, K.A.; Aakre, M.E.; Moses, H.L. Activation of the Erk pathway is required for TGF-beta1-induced EMT in vitro. *Neoplasia* **2004**, *6*, 603–610. [CrossRef]
66. Du, Z.; Lovly, C.M. Mechanisms of receptor tyrosine kinase activation in cancer. *Mol. Cancer* **2018**, *17*, 58. [CrossRef]
67. Guo, X.; Wang, X.F. Signaling cross-talk between TGF-beta/BMP and other pathways. *Cell Res.* **2009**, *19*, 71–88. [CrossRef]
68. Graham, T.R.; Zhau, H.E.; Odero-Marah, V.A.; Osunkoya, A.O.; Kimbro, K.S.; Tighiouart, M.; Liu, T.; Simons, J.W.; O'Regan, R.M. Insulin-like growth factor-I-dependent up-regulation of ZEB1 drives epithelial-to-mesenchymal transition in human prostate cancer cells. *Cancer Res.* **2008**, *68*, 2479–2488. [CrossRef]
69. Grotegut, S.; von Schweinitz, D.; Christofori, G.; Lehembre, F. Hepatocyte growth factor induces cell scattering through MAPK/Egr-1-mediated upregulation of Snail. *Embo. J.* **2006**, *25*, 3534–3545. [CrossRef]
70. Yang, X.; Chrisman, H.; Weijer, C.J. PDGF signalling controls the migration of mesoderm cells during chick gastrulation by regulating N-cadherin expression. *Development* **2008**, *135*, 3521–3530. [CrossRef]
71. Chuang, H.H.; Zhen, Y.Y.; Tsai, Y.C.; Chuang, C.H.; Hsiao, M.; Huang, M.S.; Yang, C.J. FAK in Cancer: From Mechanisms to Therapeutic Strategies. *Int. J. Mol. Sci.* **2022**, *23*, 31726. [CrossRef] [PubMed]
72. Drake, J.M.; Graham, N.A.; Stoyanova, T.; Sedghi, A.; Goldstein, A.S.; Cai, H.; Smith, D.A.; Zhang, H.; Komisopoulou, E.; Huang, J.; et al. Oncogene-specific activation of tyrosine kinase networks during prostate cancer progression. *Proc. Natl. Acad. Sci. USA* **2012**, *109*, 1643–1648. [CrossRef] [PubMed]
73. Tatarov, O.; Mitchell, T.J.; Seywright, M.; Leung, H.Y.; Brunton, V.G.; Edwards, J. SRC family kinase activity is up-regulated in hormone-refractory prostate cancer. *Clin. Cancer Res.* **2009**, *15*, 3540–3549. [CrossRef] [PubMed]
74. Liu, X.; Feng, R. Inhibition of epithelial to mesenchymal transition in metastatic breast carcinoma cells by c-Src suppression. *Acta Biochim. Biophys. Sin.* **2010**, *42*, 496–501. [CrossRef] [PubMed]
75. Nagathihalli, N.S.; Merchant, N.B. Src-mediated regulation of E-cadherin and EMT in pancreatic cancer. *Front. Biosci.* **2012**, *17*, 2059–2069. [CrossRef]
76. Patel, S.; Alam, A.; Pant, R.; Chattopadhyay, S. Wnt Signaling and Its Significance Within the Tumor Microenvironment: Novel Therapeutic Insights. *Front. Immunol.* **2019**, *10*, 2872. [CrossRef]
77. Kim, K.; Lu, Z.; Hay, E.D. Direct evidence for a role of beta-catenin/LEF-1 signaling pathway in induction of EMT. *Cell Biol. Int.* **2002**, *26*, 463–476. [CrossRef]
78. Zucchini-Pascal, N.; Peyre, L.; Rahmani, R. Crosstalk between beta-catenin and snail in the induction of epithelial to mesenchymal transition in hepatocarcinoma: Role of the ERK1/2 pathway. *Int. J. Mol. Sci.* **2013**, *14*, 20768–20792. [CrossRef]

79. Wu, Z.Q.; Li, X.Y.; Hu, C.Y.; Ford, M.; Kleer, C.G.; Weiss, S.J. Canonical Wnt signaling regulates Slug activity and links epithelial-mesenchymal transition with epigenetic Breast Cancer 1, Early Onset (BRCA1) repression. *Proc. Natl. Acad. Sci. USA* **2012**, *109*, 16654–16659. [CrossRef]
80. Howe, L.R.; Watanabe, O.; Leonard, J.; Brown, A.M. Twist is up-regulated in response to Wnt1 and inhibits mouse mammary cell differentiation. *Cancer Res.* **2003**, *63*, 1906–1913.
81. Bray, S.J. Notch signalling: A simple pathway becomes complex. *Nat. Rev. Mol. Cell Biol.* **2006**, *7*, 678–689. [CrossRef] [PubMed]
82. Guo, D.; Ye, J.; Dai, J.; Li, L.; Chen, F.; Ma, D.; Ji, C. Notch-1 regulates Akt signaling pathway and the expression of cell cycle regulatory proteins cyclin D1, CDK2 and p21 in T-ALL cell lines. *Leuk. Res.* **2009**, *33*, 678–685. [CrossRef] [PubMed]
83. Maniati, E.; Bossard, M.; Cook, N.; Candido, J.B.; Emami-Shahri, N.; Nedospasov, S.A.; Balkwill, F.R.; Tuveson, D.A.; Hagemann, T. Crosstalk between the canonical NF-κB and Notch signaling pathways inhibits Pparγ expression and promotes pancreatic cancer progression in mice. *J. Clin. Invest.* **2011**, *121*, 4685–4699. [CrossRef] [PubMed]
84. Leong, K.G.; Niessen, K.; Kulic, I.; Raouf, A.; Eaves, C.; Pollet, I.; Karsan, A. Jagged1-mediated Notch activation induces epithelial-to-mesenchymal transition through Slug-induced repression of E-cadherin. *J. Exp. Med.* **2007**, *204*, 2935–2948. [CrossRef] [PubMed]
85. Sahlgren, C.; Gustafsson, M.V.; Jin, S.; Poellinger, L.; Lendahl, U. Notch signaling mediates hypoxia-induced tumor cell migration and invasion. *Proc. Natl. Acad. Sci. USA* **2008**, *105*, 6392–6397. [CrossRef]
86. Xie, M.; Zhang, L.; He, C.S.; Xu, F.; Liu, J.L.; Hu, Z.H.; Zhao, L.P.; Tian, Y. Activation of Notch-1 enhances epithelial-mesenchymal transition in gefitinib-acquired resistant lung cancer cells. *J. Cell. Biochem.* **2012**, *113*, 1501–1513. [CrossRef]
87. Sari, I.N.; Phi, L.T.H.; Jun, N.; Wijaya, Y.T.; Lee, S.; Kwon, H.Y. Hedgehog Signaling in Cancer: A Prospective Therapeutic Target for Eradicating Cancer Stem Cells. *Cells* **2018**, *7*, 110208. [CrossRef]
88. Fendrich, V.; Waldmann, J.; Esni, F.; Ramaswamy, A.; Mullendore, M.; Buchholz, M.; Maitra, A.; Feldmann, G. Snail and Sonic Hedgehog activation in neuroendocrine tumors of the ileum. *Endocr. Relat. Cancer* **2007**, *14*, 865–874. [CrossRef]
89. Li, X.; Deng, W.; Nail, C.D.; Bailey, S.K.; Kraus, M.H.; Ruppert, J.M.; Lobo-Ruppert, S.M. Snail induction is an early response to Gli1 that determines the efficiency of epithelial transformation. *Oncogene* **2006**, *25*, 609–621. [CrossRef]
90. Yoo, Y.A.; Kang, M.H.; Kim, J.S.; Oh, S.C. Sonic hedgehog signaling promotes motility and invasiveness of gastric cancer cells through TGF-beta-mediated activation of the ALK5-Smad 3 pathway. *Carcinogenesis* **2008**, *29*, 480–490. [CrossRef]
91. Xia, R.; Xu, M.; Yang, J.; Ma, X. The role of Hedgehog and Notch signaling pathway in cancer. *Mol. Biomed.* **2022**, *3*, 44. [CrossRef] [PubMed]
92. Wang, F.; Ma, L.; Zhang, Z.; Liu, X.; Gao, H.; Zhuang, Y.; Yang, P.; Kornmann, M.; Tian, X.; Yang, Y. Hedgehog Signaling Regulates Epithelial-Mesenchymal Transition in Pancreatic Cancer Stem-Like Cells. *J. Cancer* **2016**, *7*, 408–417. [CrossRef] [PubMed]
93. Tsai, Y.C.; Chen, W.Y.; Abou-Kheir, W.; Zeng, T.; Yin, J.J.; Bahmad, H.; Lee, Y.C.; Liu, Y.N. Androgen deprivation therapy-induced epithelial-mesenchymal transition of prostate cancer through downregulating SPDEF and activating CCL2. *Biochim. Biophys. Acta Mol. Basis. Dis.* **2018**, *1864*, 1717–1727. [CrossRef]
94. Cheaito, K.A.; Bahmad, H.F.; Hadadeh, O.; Saleh, E.; Dagher, C.; Hammoud, M.S.; Shahait, M.; Mrad, Z.A.; Nassif, S.; Tawil, A.; et al. EMT Markers in Locally-Advanced Prostate Cancer: Predicting Recurrence? *Front. Oncol.* **2019**, *9*, 131. [CrossRef] [PubMed]
95. Wang, X.; Xu, H.; Cheng, C.; Ji, Z.; Zhao, H.; Sheng, Y.; Li, X.; Wang, J.; Shu, Y.; He, Y.; et al. Identification of a Zeb1 expressing basal stem cell subpopulation in the prostate. *Nat. Commun.* **2020**, *11*, 706. [CrossRef] [PubMed]
96. Nolan, K.D.; Franco, O.E.; Hance, M.W.; Hayward, S.W.; Isaacs, J.S. Tumor-secreted Hsp90 subverts polycomb function to drive prostate tumor growth and invasion. *J. Biol. Chem.* **2015**, *290*, 8271–8282. [CrossRef] [PubMed]
97. Ku, S.Y.; Rosario, S.; Wang, Y.; Mu, P.; Seshadri, M.; Goodrich, Z.W.; Goodrich, M.M.; Labbé, D.P.; Gomez, E.C.; Wang, J.; et al. Rb1 and Trp53 cooperate to suppress prostate cancer lineage plasticity, metastasis, and antiandrogen resistance. *Science* **2017**, *355*, 78–83. [CrossRef]
98. Huang, Y.; Hong, W.; Wei, X. The molecular mechanisms and therapeutic strategies of EMT in tumor progression and metastasis. *J. Hematol. Oncol.* **2022**, *15*, 129. [CrossRef]
99. Zhou, H.; He, Q.; Li, C.; Alsharafi, B.L.M.; Deng, L.; Long, Z.; Gan, Y. Focus on the tumor microenvironment: A seedbed for neuroendocrine prostate cancer. *Front. Cell Dev. Biol.* **2022**, *10*, 955669. [CrossRef]
100. Kang, J.; la Manna, F.; Bonollo, F.; Sampson, N.; Alberts, I.L.; Mingels, C.; Afshar-Oromieh, A.; Thalmann, G.N.; Karkampouna, S. Tumor microenvironment mechanisms and bone metastatic disease progression of prostate cancer. *Cancer Lett.* **2022**, *530*, 156–169. [CrossRef]
101. Comito, G.; Giannoni, E.; Segura, C.P.; Barcellos-de-Souza, P.; Raspollini, M.R.; Baroni, G.; Lanciotti, M.; Serni, S.; Chiarugi, P. Cancer-associated fibroblasts and M2-polarized macrophages synergize during prostate carcinoma progression. *Oncogene* **2014**, *33*, 2423–2431. [CrossRef] [PubMed]
102. Bezzi, M.; Seitzer, N.; Ishikawa, T.; Reschke, M.; Chen, M.; Wang, G.; Mitchell, C.; Ng, C.; Katon, J.; Lunardi, A.; et al. Diverse genetic-driven immune landscapes dictate tumor progression through distinct mechanisms. *Nat. Med.* **2018**, *24*, 165–175. [CrossRef] [PubMed]
103. Su, W.; Han, H.H.; Wang, Y.; Zhang, B.; Zhou, B.; Cheng, Y.; Rumandla, A.; Gurrapu, S.; Chakraborty, G.; Su, J.; et al. The Polycomb Repressor Complex 1 Drives Double-Negative Prostate Cancer Metastasis by Coordinating Stemness and Immune Suppression. *Cancer Cell* **2019**, *36*, 139–155.e110. [CrossRef] [PubMed]

104. Chen, Q.; Gu, M.; Cai, Z.K.; Zhao, H.; Sun, S.C.; Liu, C.; Zhan, M.; Chen, Y.B.; Wang, Z. TGF-β1 promotes epithelial-to-mesenchymal transition and stemness of prostate cancer cells by inducing PCBP1 degradation and alternative splicing of CD44. *Cell Mol. Life Sci.* **2021**, *78*, 949–962. [CrossRef] [PubMed]
105. Bluemn, E.G.; Coleman, I.M.; Lucas, J.M.; Coleman, R.T.; Hernandez-Lopez, S.; Tharakan, R.; Bianchi-Frias, D.; Dumpit, R.F.; Kaipainen, A.; Corella, A.N.; et al. Androgen Receptor Pathway-Independent Prostate Cancer Is Sustained through FGF Signaling. *Cancer Cell* **2017**, *32*, 474.e476–489.e476. [CrossRef] [PubMed]
106. Gregory, C.W.; Whang, Y.E.; McCall, W.; Fei, X.; Liu, Y.; Ponguta, L.A.; French, F.S.; Wilson, E.M.; Earp, H.S., 3rd. Heregulin-induced activation of HER2 and HER3 increases androgen receptor transactivation and CWR-R1 human recurrent prostate cancer cell growth. *Clin. Cancer Res.* **2005**, *11*, 1704–1712. [CrossRef]
107. Giannoni, E.; Bianchini, F.; Masieri, L.; Serni, S.; Torre, E.; Calorini, L.; Chiarugi, P. Reciprocal activation of prostate cancer cells and cancer-associated fibroblasts stimulates epithelial-mesenchymal transition and cancer stemness. *Cancer Res.* **2010**, *70*, 6945–6956. [CrossRef]
108. Acevedo, V.D.; Gangula, R.D.; Freeman, K.W.; Li, R.; Zhang, Y.; Wang, F.; Ayala, G.E.; Peterson, L.E.; Ittmann, M.; Spencer, D.M. Inducible FGFR-1 activation leads to irreversible prostate adenocarcinoma and an epithelial-to-mesenchymal transition. *Cancer Cell* **2007**, *12*, 559–571. [CrossRef]
109. Nath, D.; Li, X.; Mondragon, C.; Post, D.; Chen, M.; White, J.R.; Hryniewicz-Jankowska, A.; Caza, T.; Kuznetsov, V.A.; Hehnly, H.; et al. Abi1 loss drives prostate tumorigenesis through activation of EMT and non-canonical WNT signaling. *Cell Commun. Signal* **2019**, *17*, 120. [CrossRef]
110. Qi, Y.; Liu, J.; Chao, J.; Scheuerman, M.P.; Rahimi, S.A.; Lee, L.Y.; Li, S. PTEN suppresses epithelial-mesenchymal transition and cancer stem cell activity by downregulating Abi1. *Sci. Rep.* **2020**, *10*, 12685. [CrossRef]
111. Shen, Y.; Cao, J.; Liang, Z.; Lin, Q.; Wang, J.; Yang, X.; Zhang, R.; Zong, J.; Du, X.; Peng, Y.; et al. Estrogen receptor α-NOTCH1 axis enhances basal stem-like cells and epithelial-mesenchymal transition phenotypes in prostate cancer. *Cell Commun. Signal* **2019**, *17*, 50. [CrossRef] [PubMed]
112. Ishii, A.; Shigemura, K.; Kitagawa, K.; Sung, S.Y.; Chen, K.C.; Yi-Te, C.; Liu, M.C.; Fujisawa, M. Anti-tumor Effect of Hedgehog Signaling Inhibitor, Vismodegib, on Castration-resistant Prostate Cancer. *Anticancer Res.* **2020**, *40*, 5107–5114. [CrossRef] [PubMed]
113. Liang, Y.; Ma, C.; Li, F.; Nie, G.; Zhang, H. The Role of Contactin 1 in Cancers: What We Know So Far. *Front. Oncol.* **2020**, *10*, 574208. [CrossRef] [PubMed]
114. Chen, B.; Zhang, Y.; Li, C.; Xu, P.; Gao, Y.; Xu, Y. CNTN-1 promotes docetaxel resistance and epithelial-to-mesenchymal transition via the PI3K/Akt signaling pathway in prostate cancer. *Arch. Med. Sci.* **2021**, *17*, 152–165. [CrossRef] [PubMed]
115. Khan, M.I.; Hamid, A.; Adhami, V.M.; Lall, R.K.; Mukhtar, H. Role of epithelial mesenchymal transition in prostate tumorigenesis. *Curr. Pharm. Des.* **2015**, *21*, 1240–1248. [CrossRef]
116. Xin, L.; Lawson, D.A.; Witte, O.N. The Sca-1 cell surface marker enriches for a prostate-regenerating cell subpopulation that can initiate prostate tumorigenesis. *Proc. Natl. Acad. Sci. USA* **2005**, *102*, 6942–6947. [CrossRef]
117. Vasaikar, S.V.; Deshmukh, A.P.; den Hollander, P.; Addanki, S.; Kuburich, N.A.; Kudaravalli, S.; Joseph, R.; Chang, J.T.; Soundararajan, R.; Mani, S.A. EMTome: A resource for pan-cancer analysis of epithelial-mesenchymal transition genes and signatures. *Br. J. Cancer* **2021**, *124*, 259–269. [CrossRef]
118. Stylianou, N.; Lehman, M.L.; Wang, C.; Fard, A.T.; Rockstroh, A.; Fazli, L.; Jovanovic, L.; Ward, M.; Sadowski, M.C.; Kashyap, A.S.; et al. A molecular portrait of epithelial-mesenchymal plasticity in prostate cancer associated with clinical outcome. *Oncogene* **2019**, *38*, 913–934. [CrossRef]
119. Cmero, M.; Kurganovs, N.J.; Stuchbery, R.; McCoy, P.; Grima, C.; Ngyuen, A.; Chow, K.; Mangiola, S.; Macintyre, G.; Howard, N.; et al. Loss of SNAI2 in Prostate Cancer Correlates With Clinical Response to Androgen Deprivation Therapy. *JCO Precis. Oncol.* **2021**, *5*, 337. [CrossRef]
120. Jędroszka, D.; Orzechowska, M.; Hamouz, R.; Górniak, K.; Bednarek, A.K. Markers of epithelial-to-mesenchymal transition reflect tumor biology according to patient age and Gleason score in prostate cancer. *PLoS ONE* **2017**, *12*, e0188842. [CrossRef]
121. He, M.X.; Cuoco, M.S.; Crowdis, J.; Bosma-Moody, A.; Zhang, Z.; Bi, K.; Kanodia, A.; Su, M.J.; Ku, S.Y.; Garcia, M.M.; et al. Transcriptional mediators of treatment resistance in lethal prostate cancer. *Nat. Med.* **2021**, *27*, 426–433. [CrossRef] [PubMed]

cancers

MDPI

Review

Androgen Deprivation Therapy in High-Risk Localized and Locally Advanced Prostate Cancer

Hiroaki Iwamoto [1], Kouji Izumi [1,*], Tomoyuki Makino [1,2] and Atsushi Mizokami [1]

1 Department of Integrative Cancer Therapy and Urology, Kanazawa University Graduate School of Medical Science, 13-1 Takara-Machi, Kanazawa 920-8640, Ishikawa, Japan; iwamoto-h@med.kanazawa-u.ac.jp (H.I.); mackeeen511@gmail.com (T.M.); mizokami@staff.kanazawa-u.ac.jp (A.M.)

2 Department of Urology, Ishikawa Prefectural Central Hospital, Kanazawa 920-8530, Ishikawa, Japan

* Correspondence: kouji1974@staff.kanazawa-u.ac.jp; Tel.: +81-76-265-2393; Fax: +81-76-234-4263

Simple Summary: Androgen deprivation therapy alone is commonly performed for metastatic prostate cancer but is generally not recommended for the treatment of high-risk localized or locally advanced prostate cancer. In this article, we will discuss the position, indications, and future possibilities of ADT for high-risk localized or locally advanced prostate cancer.

Abstract: The recommended treatment for high-risk localized or locally advanced prostate cancer is radical prostatectomy plus extended pelvic lymph node dissection or radiation therapy plus long-term androgen deprivation therapy. However, some patients are treated with androgen deprivation therapy alone for various reasons. In this review, we will discuss the position, indications, complications, and future prospects of androgen deprivation therapy for high-risk localized and locally advanced prostate cancer.

Keywords: prostate cancer; androgen deprivation therapy; high-risk; localized; locally advanced

Citation: Iwamoto, H.; Izumi, K.; Makino, T.; Mizokami, A. Androgen Deprivation Therapy in High-Risk Localized and Locally Advanced Prostate Cancer. *Cancers* **2022**, *14*, 1803. https://doi.org/10.3390/cancers14071803

Academic Editor: Kentaro Inamura

Received: 25 January 2022
Accepted: 30 March 2022
Published: 1 April 2022

Publisher's Note: MDPI stays neutral with regard to jurisdictional claims in published maps and institutional affiliations.

1. Introduction

Prostate cancer (PC) is the most common cancer in men and the leading cause of cancer-related deaths in developed countries [1,2]. Most PC deaths are caused by metastatic disease [3]. Approximately 10% of new PC cases are diagnosed with distant metastasis [4–6]. The development and dissemination of prostate-specific antigen (PSA) screening have contributed to early PC detection, which in turn has reduced PC-related mortality [7–10]. However, approximately 15% of newly diagnosed PCs are high-risk PCs [11]. While localized PC generally has a good prognosis, high-risk PC has a significantly worse prognosis than low- and intermediate-risk PC, with a 15-year PC-specific mortality rate of 22–38% [11–13]. Guidelines differ slightly in their definition of high-risk PC, including locally advanced PC (Table 1). In the D'Amico risk classification, the European Association of Urology (EAU) guidelines, and European Society for Medical Oncology (ESMO) guidelines, patients are classified as high-risk if they meet clinical stage T2c or a PSA level of ≥20 ng/mL or Gleason score of 8–10, while the National Comprehensive Cancer Network (NCCN) guidelines classify patients as high-risk at clinical stage T3 or higher [14–17]. The EAU guidelines classify locally advanced PC at clinical stage T3 or higher or clinical stage N1, and the NCCN guidelines classify very high-risk at clinical stage T3b or higher or primary Gleason pattern 5 or >4 cores with grade group 4 or 5 [15,16]. Briefly, patients with clinical stage T2c, a PSA level of ≥20 ng/mL, or a Gleason score of 8–10 are considered to have high-risk PC. Although each guideline differs slightly, radical prostatectomy (RP) + extended pelvic lymph node dissection (ePLND) or radiation therapy (RT) + long-term androgen deprivation therapy (ADT) is recommended for the treatment of high-risk or locally advanced PC, and ADT alone is currently indicated in a few cases [15–17]. However, ADT has been used aggressively for localized PC in Japan. According to data from 10,280

PC patients diagnosed in Japan in 2004, 41% of non-metastatic castration-sensitive prostate cancer (nmCSPC) patients received ADT as initial treatment [5]. In this review, we provide an overview of ADT therapy, including the position and future possibilities of ADT alone in high-risk or locally advanced PC. Herein, ADT is defined as including gonadotropin-releasing hormone (GnRH) agonist alone, GnRH agonist alone, anti-androgenic agent alone, and combined androgen blockade (CAB) therapy.

Table 1. Definition of high-risk prostate cancer.

	Risk	Clinical Stage		Initial PSA		Gleason Score			References
D'Amico et al.	High	≥T2c	or	>20 ng/mL	or	≥8			[14]
NCCN 2021	High	T3a	or	>20 ng/mL	or	Grade Group 4 or Grade Group 5			[15]
	Very high	T3b/T4	or		or	Primary Gleason pattern 5 or > 4 cores with Grade Group 4 or 5	or	2 or 3 high-risk features	
EAU 2020	High	T2c	or	>20 ng/mL	or	≥8			[16]
	Locally advanced	T3/T4 or N1	and	Any	and	Any			
ESMO 2020	High	≥T2c	or	>20 ng/mL	or	≥8			[17]

PSA = Prostate specific antigen; NCCN = National Comprehensive Cancer Network; EAU = European Association of Urology; ESMO = European Society for Medical Oncology.

2. ADT

2.1. History of ADT

After Huggins and Hodges reported the efficacy of castration therapy, ADT became the gold standard for advanced PC [18]. Surgical castration had been the only method of castration, but Schally and Guillemin elucidated the structure of GnRH, which led to the development of GnRH agonists, and medical castration became possible [19]. Studies have reported the efficacy and tolerability of GnRH agonists as a first-line treatment for advanced PC and concluded that the survival rate, disease progression, and time to treatment failure are comparable between GnRH agonist therapy and orchiectomy [20–23]. Surgical castration is a simple and cost-effective outpatient procedure, while the advantage of medical castration is the avoidance of surgery [20–24]. In recent years, the rate of surgical castration has been reported to be less than 9% [24]. Although castration reduces serum testosterone levels by approximately 90%, 20–40% of dihydrotestosterone (DHT) remains in human PC tissue [25–27]. As this residual androgen may cause inadequate treatment of PC or relapse, CAB therapy, which combines ADT with an antiandrogen drug, has been proposed [28–30]. Recently, GnRH antagonists are developed. GnRH agonists have been reported to result in a transient increase in testosterone levels that occurs early in the administration, which is called a testosterone surge that can cause urinary tract obstruction and spinal cord compression [31–33]. GnRH antagonists do not cause testosterone surges, and testosterone levels reach castration levels early, so they may be particularly useful in patients with symptomatic metastatic PC [34]. In addition, ADT has made progress with the development of the new androgen receptor signaling-targeted agent (ARSTs), such as enzalutamide, abiraterone acetate, apalutamide, and darolutamide [35–38]. The effects of ADT are generally not permanent and eventually lead to castration-resistant PC (CRPC) [6]. The treatment for CRPC includes alternative ADT [39], ARST [35–38], and chemotherapy such as docetaxel [40,41] and cabazitaxel [42,43].

ADT is effective in improving patients' quality of life by reducing bone pain, pathological fractures, spinal cord compression, and ureteral obstruction, which are symptoms specific to advanced PC, such as bone metastases or local enlargement of PC [18,44,45]. However, ADT has various adverse effects, such as hot flashes [46–50], sexual dysfunction [46,49–52], breast enlargement [48,49,53,54], depression [49,55], dementia [56–61], osteoporosis [62–66], obesity [46,67], diabetes [68–73], and cardiovascular (CV) toxicity [68,74–80].

Dementia, osteoporosis, and CV toxicity are important side effects of ADT in older patients. We summarize these AEs for older patients with PC in the next section.

2.2. ADT for High-Risk Localized and Locally Advanced PC

Various guidelines do not recommend ADT alone as an initial treatment for high-risk or locally advanced PC [15–17]. However, in clinical practice, some patients, especially older ones, are treated with ADT alone as the initial therapy. In the USA, the use of GnRH agonists has increased since the 1990s [81], and as of 2009, 22% of patients with localized PC aged >66 years were being treated with ADT alone [82]. In Japan, approximately 30% of patients with localized PC were treated with ADT alone [5]. As shown in Tables 2 and 3, many studies have reported on the efficacy of ADT alone for localized PC, but worldwide, there are more negative reports.

Table 2. Negative data of ADT for high-risk localized and locally advanced prostate cancer.

Study	Study Specification	Patient Characteristics	Size	Findings	References
Merglen et al. (2007)	retrospective cohort study	Patients with localized PC treated with either total prostatectomy, radiation therapy, watchful waiting, hormone therapy, or other treatment	844	Patients who received ADT alone already had an increased risk of PCSM at 5 years (HR 3.5, 95% CI 1.4–8.7)	[83]
Lee et al. (2018)	retrospective study	Patients diagnosed with localized PC who underwent ADT or treatment-free follow-up	340	In clinically unfavorable localized intermediate- and high-risk PC, initiation of ADT within 12 months of diagnosis was not associated with improved 5-year all-cause mortality or PCSM compared with patients who received no conservative treatment	[84]
Lu-Yao et al. (2008)	retrospective cohort study	Patients diagnosed with localized PC who underwent ADT or treatment-free follow-up	19,271	ADT is not associated with improved survival among the majority of elderly men with localized prostate cancer when compared with conservative management	[85]

Table 2. *Cont.*

Study	Study Specification	Patient Characteristics	Size	Findings	References
Potosky et al. (2014)	retrospective cohort study	Newly diagnosed patients with localized PC	15,170	ADT was associated with neither a risk of all-cause mortality (HR 1.04, 95% CI 0.97–1.11) nor PCSM (HR 1.03, 95% CI 0.89–1.19).	[86]
Lu-Yao et al. (2014)	retrospective cohort study	Patients aged 66 years or older with localized PC who did not receive curative treatment	66,717	ADT is not associated with improved long-term overall or disease-specific survival for men with localized PC.	[87]
Sammon et al. (2015)	retrospective cohort study	Newly diagnosed patients with locally advanced or localized PC	46,376	There was an increased risk of all-cause mortality in the ADT group compared to the observation group (HR 1.37, 95% CI 1.20–1.56)	[82]

ADT = Androgen deprivation therapy; PC = Prostate cancer; PCSM = Prostate cancer specific mortality; HR = Hazard ratio; CI = Confidence interval.

Table 3. Positive data of ADT for high-risk localized and locally advanced prostate cancer.

Study	Study Specification	Patient Characteristics	Size	Findings	References
Labrie et al. (2002)	prospective study	Patients with newly diagnosed locally advanced or localized PC who have undergone CAB	57	In patients with stage T2–T3 cancer who continued CAB for more than 6.5 years and discontinued treatment there were only two cases of PSA elevation. Long-term continuous CAB was suggested to be a possibility for long-term control or cure of localized PC	[88]
Akaza et al. (2006)	prospective cohort study	Patients with newly diagnosed locally advanced or localized PC who have undergone ADT	151	In men with localized or locally advanced PC, primary ADT inhibited PC progression and resulted in a life expectancy similar to that of the normal population	[89]
Kawakami et al. (2006)	retrospective cohort study	Newly diagnosed localized PC patients with or without ADT	7044	The use of ADT therapy appeared to control disease in the majority of patients who received it, at least for an intermediate period	[90]
Akaza et al. (2010)	retrospective cohort study	Patients with newly diagnosed locally advanced or localized PC who have undergone ADT	15,461	ADT resulted in a long-term survival rate comparable to the general population	[91]

Table 3. *Cont.*

Study	Study Specification	Patient Characteristics	Size	Findings	References
Matsumoto et al. (2014)	retrospective cohort study	Patients with newly diagnosed locally PC at intermediate to high risk who have undergone ADT	410	When prostate cancer with no capsular invasion and a GS of less than 8 was treated with ADT, the expected survival rate was similar to that of the general population	[92]
Studer et al. (2014)	randomized controlled trial	PC patients without distant metastasis treated with immediate or delayed ADT	985	Deferred ADT was inferior to immediate ADT in terms of overall survival (HR 1.21; 95% CI 1.05–1.39)	[93]
Nguyen et al. (2011)	meta-analysis of randomized controlled trial	Patients diagnosed with PC	4141	ADT was associated with lower PCSM (443/2527 vs. 552/2278 events; RR, 0.69; 95% CI, 0.56–0.84; $p < 0.001$) and lower all-cause mortality (1140/2527 vs. 1213/2278 events; RR, 0.86; 95% CI 0.80–0.93; $p < 0.001$)	[80]

ADT = Androgen deprivation therapy; PC = Prostate cancer; CAB = Combined androgen blockade; PSA = Prostate specific antigen; GS = Gleason score; HR = Hazard ratio; PCSM = Prostate cancer specific mortality; CI = Confidence interval; RR = Relative risk.

2.2.1. Negative Data of ADT for High-Risk Localized and Locally Advanced PC

A cohort study of 844 patients with localized PC who underwent total prostatectomy, RT, watchful waiting, ADT, or other treatment, with data collected from the Geneva Cancer Registry, revealed that patients who received hormone therapy alone had increased PC-specific mortality at 5 years [83].

A retrospective cohort study of 340 patients diagnosed with localized PC and followed up with ADT or no treatment at a single center in Singapore found no improvement in 5-year all-cause mortality or PC-specific mortality (PCSM) when ADT was initiated within 12 months of diagnosis [84].

A retrospective cohort study comparing 7867 patients who were newly diagnosed with localized PC and received ADT with 11,404 patients who did not receive ADT was selected from the population-based Surveillance, Epidemiology, and End Results (SEER) program database and linked Medicare files. The study showed that ADT was not associated with improved survival for the majority of older men compared with conservative management [85].

A retrospective study of 15,170 patients with newly diagnosed clinically localized PC who were not receiving curative treatment was conducted using data from three integrated healthcare delivery systems within the HMO Cancer Research Network in the USA. The results showed that ADT was not associated with either overall or PCSM risk. However, ADT predominantly reduced the risk of all-cause mortality only in a subgroup of men at high-risk for cancer progression [86].

A retrospective cohort study of 66,717 patients aged ≥66 years with localized PC who did not receive curative treatment, from the National Cancer Institute's SEER program and Medicare data, found that primary ADT was not associated with improved long-term overall survival (OS) or disease-specific survival at 15 years [87].

In a retrospective cohort study of 46,376 patients newly diagnosed with locally advanced or localized PC from the National Cancer Institute's SEER program and Medicare data and not treated with curative intent, ADT was associated with decreased survival compared with observation management [82].

As shown above, many large cohort studies have rejected the efficacy of ADT for localized PC. However, some studies have shown the efficacy of ADT in localized PC.

2.2.2. Positive Data of ADT for High-Risk Localized and Locally Advanced PC

In a previous study, 57 patients with newly diagnosed locally advanced or localized PC who discontinued long-term CAB therapy were followed for at least 5 years. Among 20 patients with stage T2 to T3 cancer who discontinued continuous CAB therapy after 6.5 years, two cases of PSA elevations occurred, with a 90% non-failure rate. This study suggested that long-term and continuous CAB was associated with the possibility of long-term control or cure of localized PC [88].

In a prospective cohort study of 151 patients with newly diagnosed locally advanced or localized PC who underwent ADT from 104 sites in Japan, ADT reduced PC progression, resulting in a life expectancy similar to that of the normal population [89].

A retrospective study of data from The Cancer of the Prostate Strategic Urologic Research Endeavor (CaPSURE) in the USA compared 993 patients with newly diagnosed localized PC who received ADT with 6051 patients who did not receive ADT. The results revealed that ADT use controlled the disease in the majority of patients with PC at an intermediate period of 5 years [90].

In an analysis of the Japan Study Group of Prostate Cancer (J-CaP) surveillance study of 15,461 patients with locally advanced or localized PC in Japan, ADT resulted in long-term survival rates similar to that in the general population [91].

In a report of 410 patients with intermediate- to high-risk localized PC treated with ADT alone from five centers in Japan, the expected survival rate was similar to that of the general population in the absence of capsular invasion and with a Gleason score of $\geq$8 [92].

In the European Organization for Research and Treatment of Cancer (EORTC) trial 30891, a randomized, prospective study compared 492 patients with PC without distant metastases who received immediate ADT with 493 patients who received delayed ADT. The results indicated that the delayed ADT group had a significantly inferior OS rate to the immediate ADT group [93].

In a pooled analysis of a randomized trial of 4141 patients with unfavorable-risk PC, ADT use was associated with a decreased risk of PCSM and all-cause mortality [80].

As described above, most of the studies demonstrating the efficacy of ADT for localized PC were reported from Japan. However, there have been reports of racial differences in the efficacy of ADT for localized PC.

2.2.3. Differences in the Efficacy of ADT by Race

A retrospective study of 165 patients with PC who underwent ADT at The Queen's Medical Center in Honolulu compared 59 Caucasian men (CM) and 105 Japanese American men (JAM) [94]. Although no significant difference was found in the patient background, JAMs who received ADT had a better prognosis than CMs in terms of both overall and cause-specific survival (p = 0.001 and 0.036, respectively). The multivariate analysis also revealed that race was one of the significant prognostic factors (p = 0.03).

A retrospective study compared data from a total of 15,513 patients with PC who received ADT from the CaPSURE database in the USA and the J-CaP database in Japan [95]. Men who underwent ADT at J-CaP (n = 13,880) were older and had higher risk of disease than men who underwent ADT at CaPSURE (n = 1633) and had a higher rate of CAB (66.9% vs. 46.4%). The multivariate regression showed that the sub-hazard ratio for PCSM was 0.52 (95% confidence interval 0.40–0.68) for J-CaP versus CaPSURE, and the adjusted PCSM for men receiving ADT in Japan was less than half that of men in the USA.

Although further large-scale prospective studies are awaited, Asians, including Japanese, may be expected to benefit more from ADT than Caucasians.

2.2.4. Position of ADT in High-Risk Localized and Locally Advanced PC

The efficacy of RP and RT for localized PC has been recognized [96–98]. A randomized clinical trial (RCT) reported that improved survival with long-term ADT plus RT for patients with locally advanced PC has led to the recommendation of combined RT and ADT for high-risk cases [99,100]. RP was not recommended for patients with high-risk PC; however, recent reports have led to a reevaluation. In a meta-analysis including 118,830 patients and comparing the prognosis of RP and RT for localized PC, the prognosis was significantly better with RP, even in the high-risk group [101]. In a retrospective study of 42,765 patients with high-risk PC, the RP group had a significantly better prognosis than the RT plus ADT group [102]. Based on the above, RP plus ePLND or RT plus ADT is recommended for the treatment of high-risk or locally advanced PC [15–17]. However, RP is not recommended for patients with an expected life expectancy of $\leq$5 years, and ADT alone may be an option [15]. Older patients are more likely to have several comorbidities and should be aware of adverse events (AEs) from ADT.

2.3. *Evidence of ARST for Castration-Sensitive Prostate Cancer*

In recent years, evidence of ARST for castration-sensitive prostate cancer (CSPC) has been accumulating. In the ARCHES trial, in which 1150 patients with metastatic CSPC (mCSPC) were randomized 1:1 to enzalutamide plus ADT or placebo plus ADT, the enzalutamide plus ADT group had significantly longer radiographic progression-free survival than the placebo group (not reached vs. 19.0 months, $p < 0.001$, HR = 0.39) [103]. In the ENZAMET study, in which 1125 patients with mCSPC were randomized to enzalutamide plus ADT or non-steroidal antiandrogen plus ADT, both groups did not reach the median OS; however, the enzalutamide plus ADT group had a significantly longer OS [104]. In the LATITUDE trial, in which 1199 patients with mCSPC were randomized to abiraterone acetate plus prednisone (n = 597) or placebo (n = 602), the abiraterone acetate plus prednisone group had significantly prolonged OS compared with the placebo group (53.3 vs. 36.5 months, $p < 0.0001$, HR = 0.66) [105]. In the TITAN trial, in which 1052 patients with mCSPC were randomized 1:1 to apalutamide plus ADT or placebo plus ADT, the apalutamide plus ADT group had a significantly longer OS than the placebo group (not reached vs. 52.2 months, $p < 0.0001$, HR = 0.65) [106].

As mentioned above, ARST for mCSPC is effective. However, evidence on ARST for nmCSPC is limited. In the STAMPEDE trial, which randomized 1974 patients with high-risk nmCSPC to ARST plus ADT (n = 986) or ADT (n = 988), both groups did not reach the median OS; however, the ARST plus ADT group had a significantly longer OS ($p < 0.0001$, HR = 0. 60) [107]. Of the 1974 patients in this study, 774 (39%) had positive lymph nodes and 1684 (85%) received concomitant RT.

There are no reports of ARST being given for nmCSPC rather than in combination with other therapies. At present, ARST for nmCSPC is not recommended.

2.4. *Adverse Effects of ADT in Older Patients*

As discussed in the previous section, there are a variety of AEs in ADT. In particular, dementia, osteoporosis, and CV toxicity are important side effects of ADT in older patients. We summarize these AEs for older patients with PC.

2.4.1. Risk of Developing Dementia Due to ADT in Older Patients

Low testosterone levels are associated with dementia risk in older men [108]. Low testosterone level and ADT have been reported to be associated with elevated levels of beta-amyloid protein, which characterizes Alzheimer's disease [55,109]. As shown in Table 4, the association of ADT with dementia risk was reported in a large cohort study.

Table 4. Risk of ADT-induced dementia in older patients.

Study	Study Specification	Patient Characteristics	Size	Findings	References
Krasnova et al. (2020)	retrospective cohort study	Older patients diagnosed with PC who have received ADT or who have not received ADT	100,414	The risk of dementia was 17% higher and the risk of Alzheimer's disease 23% higher in the group that received ADT	[56]
Jayadevappa et al. (2019)	retrospective cohort study	Older patients diagnosed with PC who have received ADT or who have not received ADT	154,089	Exposure to ADT, compared with no ADT exposure, was associated with a diagnosis of Alzheimer disease (HR 1.14, 95% CI, 1.10–1.18, $p < 0.001$) and dementia (HR 1.20, 95% CI 1.17–1.24, $p < 0.001$)	[57]
Robinson et al. (2019)	retrospective cohort study	Patients with PC and matched prostate-cancer-free controls (Older patients accounted for about 90%)	146,985	In men with prostate cancer, GnRH agonist treatment (HR 1.15, 95% CI 1.07–1.23) and orchiectomy (HR 1.60, 95% CI 1.32–1.93) were associated with an increased risk of dementia, as compared to no treatment in PC-free men	[58]
Liu et al. (2021)	retrospective cohort study	Patients diagnosed with PC who have received ADT or who have not received ADT (Older patients accounted for about 70%)	47,384	There was no statistical difference in the incidence of dementia between the ADT group and the group not receiving ADT (aHR, 1.12, 95% CI 0.87–1.43 in Taiwan, aHR 1.02, 95% CI: 0.85–1.23 in the UK)	[59]
Nead et al. (2017)	meta-analysis	Patients diagnosed with PC who have received ADT or who have not received ADT	50,541	ADT administration was associated with a 47% increase in dementia risk (HR 1.47, 95% CI 1.08–2.00, $p = 0.02$)	[60]
Cui et al. (2021)	meta-analysis	Patients diagnosed with PC who have received ADT or who have not received ADT	776,251	ADT administration was associated with a 21% increase in dementia risk (pooled HR = 1.21, 95% CI 1.13–1.30, $p < 0.001$)	[61]

PC = Prostate cancer; ADT = Androgen deprivation therapy; HR = Hazard ratio; CI = Confidence interval; GnRH = Gonadotropin releasing hormone; aHR = adjusted HR.

A retrospective cohort study of 100,414 older patients with PC, using data from the National Cancer Institute's SEER program and Medicare, noted a 17% higher risk of dementia and 23% higher risk of Alzheimer's disease in the ADT group [56].

A retrospective cohort study of 154,089 older patients with PC using the National Cancer Institute's SEER-Medicare linked database reported a 14% increase in Alzheimer's disease and 20% increase in dementia in the ADT group [57].

Based on data from the Prostate Cancer Database Sweden (PCBaSe Sweden), a retrospective cohort study of 146,985 men (with PC, $n = 25{,}967$; without PC, $n = 121{,}018$) was conducted [58]. Approximately 90% of the patients were older. The GnRH agonist PC group had a 15% increased risk of dementia compared with controls without PC.

However, a retrospective cohort study of 47,384 patients with PC from the National Health Insurance database in Taiwan and the Health Improvement Network in the United Kingdom (UK) showed contradictory results [59]. Approximately 70% of the patients were older. The incidence of dementia in the ADT group was 2.74 per 1000 person-years compared with 3.03 per 1000 person-years in the non-ADT group in Taiwan and 2.81 per 1000 person-years compared with 2.79 per 1000 person-years in the UK, with no significant difference between the ADT and non-ADT groups.

Two meta-analyses have examined the relationship between ADT and dementia risk. The first meta-analysis, including 50,541 patients with PC, showed a 47% increased risk of dementia in the ADT group [60]. The second meta-analysis, which included 339,400 cases treated with ADT and 436,851 controls, found a 21% increased risk of dementia in the ADT group [61].

Although some negative results were observed, the results of retrospective studies have suggested that ADT is causally associated with an increased risk of dementia. Further evidence from prospective studies is needed. The risk of dementia should be considered when providing ADT older patients with PC. Special consideration should be given to the risk of dementia in men at high-risk for cognitive decline.

2.4.2. Risk of ADT-Induced Dementia in Older Patients

ADT causes deficiencies in testosterone and estrogen. Furthermore, it has been reported to decrease bone density by increasing bone turnover and resorption [110,111].

As shown in Table 5, several large retrospective cohort studies have investigated the increased risk of osteoporosis and fracture with ADT.

Table 5. Risk of developing osteoporosis due to ADT in older patients.

Study	Study Specification	Patient Characteristics	Size	Findings	References
Smith et al. (2005)	retrospective cohort study	Older patients diagnosed with PC who have received ADT or who have not received ADT	11,661	The rate of any clinical fracture was 7.88 per 100 person-years at risk in men receiving a GnRH agonist compared with 6.51 per 100 person-years in matched controls (RR 1.21, 95% CI, 1.14–1.29, $p = 0.001$)	[62]
Alibhai et al. (2010)	retrospective cohort study	Older patients diagnosed with PC who have received ADT or who have not received ADT	38,158	ADT was associated with an increased risk of fragility fracture (HR 1.65, 95% CI 1.53–1.78) and any fracture (HR 1.46, 95% CI 1.39–1.54)	[63]
Shahinian et al. (2005)	retrospective cohort study	Older patients diagnosed with PC who have received ADT or who have not received ADT	50,613	In patients who received ADT as primary treatment, the RR of any fracture was 1.44 (95% CI 1.33–1.56)	[64]
Beebe-Dimer et al. (2012)	retrospective cohort study	Older patients diagnosed with PC who have received ADT or who have not received ADT	80,844	ADT was associated with an increased rate of fracture in both non-metastatic patients (aHR 1.34, 95% CI 1.29–1.39) and metastatic patients (aHR 1.51, 95% CI 1.36–1.67)	[65]

Table 5. *Cont.*

Study	Study Specification	Patient Characteristics	Size	Findings	References
Kim et al. (2019)	meta-analysis of prospective cohort study	Patients diagnosed with PC who have received ADT or who have not received ADT	533	Statistically significant decreases of BMD change relative to the control group were observed in the ADT treatment group in the lumbar spine (95% CI −6.72 to −0.47, $p = 0.02$), femoral neck (95% CI −4.73 to −1.48, $p = 0.0002$), and total hip (95% CI −2.99 to −0.19, $p = 0.03$)	[66]

PC = Prostate cancer; ADT = Androgen deprivation therapy; GnRH = Gonadotropin releasing hormone; RR = Relative risk; HR = Hazard ratio; CI = Confidence interval; aHR = adjusted HR; BMD = Bone mineral density; MD = Mineral density.

In a retrospective cohort study of 11,661 older patients with PC using medical claims data from a 5% national random sample of Medicare beneficiaries, the risk of fracture was 21% higher in the ADT group [62].

In a retrospective cohort study of 38,158 older patients with PC using linked administrative databases in Ontario, Canada, the risk of fracture was 46% higher in the ADT group [63].

Two large backward-looking cohort studies used the US National Cancer Institute's SEER program and Medicare databases [64,65]. In the first retrospective cohort study of 50,613 older patients with PC between 1992 and 1997, the risk of fracture was 44% higher in the ADT group [64]. In the second retrospective cohort study of 80,844 older patients with PC between 1996 and 2003, the risk of fracture was 34% higher in the group of patients with non-metastatic PC who received ADT [65].

No large prospective studies have been performed to date, but a meta-analysis of a few cases was conducted. A meta-analysis of a prospective cohort study including 533 patients with PC found that bone mineral density (BMD) was significantly decreased in the ADT group [66].

Despite the paucity of prospective studies, previous ones have consistently shown that ADT reduces bone density and increases the risk of fracture. When ADT is performed in older patients, care must be taken to avoid fractures.

2.4.3. Risk of CV Toxicity Due to ADT in Older Patients

In a retrospective cohort study of 73,196 older patients with localized PC using the SEER database, Keating et al. first showed in 2006 that GnRH agonist use significantly increased the risk of developing coronary artery disease, myocardial infarction, and sudden cardiac death [74].

Since then, various studies have investigated the association between ADT and CV risk events in patients with PC (Table 6).

Table 6. Risk of cardiovascular toxicity due to ADT in older patients.

Study	Study Specification	Patient Characteristics	Size	Findings	References
Keating et al. (2006)	retrospective cohort study	Older patients with localized PC	73,196	GnRH agonist use was associated with increased risk of coronary heart disease (aHR 1.16, $p < 0.001$), myocardial infarction (adjusted HR 1.11, $p = 0.03$), and sudden cardiac death (aHR 1.16, $p = 0.004$)	[74]
Keating et al. (2010)	retrospective cohort study	Patients diagnosed with local or regional PC (older patients accounted for about 60%)	37,443	The group of patients who received ADT was significantly more likely to have coronary artery disease (aHR 1.19, 95% CI = 1.10–1.28), myocardial infarction (aHR 1.28, 95% CI = 1.08–1.52), sudden cardiac death (aHR 1.35, 95% CI = 1.18–1.54), and stroke (aHR 1.22, 95% CI = 1.10–1.36) were increased	[68]
O'Farrell et al. (2015)	retrospective cohort study	Patients with PC and matched PC-free controls (older patients accounted for about 90%)	229,147	CVD risk was increased in men on GnRH agonists compared with the comparison cohort (HR 1.21, 95% CI 1.18–1.25)	[75]
O'Farrell et al. (2016)	retrospective cohort study	Patients with PC and matched PC-free controls (older patients accounted for about 90%)	233,193	GnRH agonist users and surgically castrated men had a higher risk of thromboembolic disease than the comparison cohort: HR 1.67, 95% CI 1.40–1.98 and HR 1.61, 95% CI 1.15–2.28, respectively	[76]
Zhao et al. (2014)	meta-analysis of retrospective cohort study	Patients diagnosed with PC who have received ADT or who have not received ADT	295,407	CVD was related to GnRH (HR 1.19, 95% CI 1.04–1.36, $p < 0.001$) and GnRH plus oral antiandrogen (HR 1.46, 95% CI 1.03–2.08, $p = 0.04$). ADT was associated with cardiovascular mortality (HR 1.17, 95% CI 1.04–1.32, $p = 0.01$)	[77]
Meng et al. (2016)	meta-analysis of retrospective cohort study	Patients diagnosed with PC who have received ADT or who have not received ADT	160,485	The incidence of stroke in ADT users was 12% higher than control groups, (HR 1.12, 95% CI 0.95–1.32, $p = 0.16$)	[78]
Alibhai et al. (2009)	retrospective cohort study	Older patients diagnosed with prostate cancer who received ADT or who were not diagnosed with prostate cancer who did not receive ADT	38,158	ADT use was not associated with AMI (HR 0.91, 95% CI 0.84–1.00) or sudden cardiac death (HR 0.96, 95% CI 0.83–1.10)	[79]

PC = Prostate cancer; GnRH = Gonadotropin releasing hormone; HR = Hazard ratio; aHR = adjusted HR; CI = Confidence interval; ADT = Androgen deprivation therapy; CVD = cardiovascular disease; CAB = Combined androgen blockade.

In a retrospective cohort study of 37,443 patients (older patients accounted for a 60%) with local or regional PC diagnosed by the Veterans Healthcare Administration, CV toxicity was significantly higher in the ADT group [68].

Two large retrospective cohort studies using PCBaSe Sweden have reported CV toxicity [75,76]: (i) A retrospective cohort study of 41,362 patients with PC and 187,785 age-matched controls without PC. Older patients accounted for 90% of the study population. The risk of ischemic heart disease was 21% higher in the group using GnRH agonists [75]. (ii) Another retrospective cohort study of 42,263 patients with PC and 190,930 age-matched controls without PC. Older patients accounted for about 90% of the study population. The risk of thromboembolism was 67% higher in the group using GnRH agonists and 61% higher in the group that underwent surgical castration [76].

Several meta-analyses have also been conducted. A meta-analysis of retrospective cohort studies included 129,802 patients with PC who underwent ADT and 165,605 PC patients who did not undergo ADT. The results showed that the risk of CV disease (CVD) was 19% higher in the group using GnRH agonists than in the control group, and 46% higher in the CAB group. The risk of CV mortality was 17% higher in the ADT group [77].

A meta-analysis of both RCTs and observational studies included 74,538 patients with PC who received ADT and 85,947 patients without PC who did not receive ADT. The results showed 12% higher incidence of stroke in the ADT group than in the control group [78].

As mentioned above, many studies have shown that ADT increases the CV risk in patients with PC. However, some reports show no increased risk. A retrospective cohort study of 38,158 older patients with PC using linked administrative data at the Institute for Clinical Evaluative Sciences in Ontario, Canada, found no increased risk of acute myocardial infarction or sudden cardiac death in the ADT group [79].

Large cohort studies and meta-analyses have consistently reported an increased CV risk with ADT, and this complication should be considered with caution when providing ADT in older patients.

2.5. ADT in the Older

Results of retrospective studies have suggested that ADT alone may be indicated for high-risk localized and locally advanced PC in Asians, especially Japanese [58,59]. ADT alone is also an option for older patients with high-risk localized and locally advanced PC, regardless of ethnicity [15].

However, when ADT is used in older patients, side effects such as dementia, osteoporosis, and CV toxicity should be addressed. A meta-analysis of people aged ≥65 years revealed that patients with dementia had a significantly increased mortality risk compared with controls (odds ratio (OR) 2.63, 95% CI 2.17–3.21) [112].

The Lancet Commission on dementia prevention, intervention, and care identified 12 risk factors (low education, hypertension, hearing impairment, smoking, obesity, depression, physical inactivity, diabetes, infrequent social contact, alcoholism, head injury, and air pollution) for dementia that can be improved [113]. Improving these risk factors when administering ADT to older patients may help reduce the risk of developing dementia.

Fractures can be life-threatening in older patients receiving ADT. However, bisphosphonates and human monoclonal antibody (denosumab) can reduce the rate of bone loss in patients on ADT [114].

Moreover, a meta-analysis of 1824 patients with osteoporosis from 20 RCTs showed that kinesiology significantly improved BMD at the lumbar spine and femoral neck [115]. These preventive measures can reduce the risk of osteoporosis development in older patients, and ADT can be performed relatively safely.

CV toxicity is a life-threatening complication for older patients. A joint scientific statement in 2010 (American Heart Association, American Cancer Society, American Urological Association) has recommended assessment of CV profile before ADT initiation [116].

Metabolic syndrome (MetS) has been pointed out as a mechanism of CV toxicity caused by ADT [117]. Because testosterone maintains lean body mass, ADT-induced gonadal hypofunction was suggested to contribute to MetS development [118]. MetS is a collection of metabolic abnormalities including hypertension, central obesity, insulin resistance, and atherosclerotic dyslipidemia, and is considered an important CV risk factor [119]. A recent meta-analysis indicated that MetS doubles the CVD risk and increases all-cause mortality by 1.5 times [120].

Weight control is an important factor in MetS prevention [121]. For obese patients, a weight loss of 5–10 kg, even if not to normal weight, was shown to be effective in improving MetS and CV risk and increasing life expectancy [122]. Furthermore, losing at least 5% of body weight can lead to short-term improvements in insulin resistance, MetS, and related risk factors. In addition, a certain degree of aerobic exercise and physical activity has been found to contribute to CV risk reduction [123] and is recommended by the World Health Organization (WHO) 2020 guidelines on physical activity and sedentary behavior [124].

PDE5 inhibitors are gaining attention as agents to prevent increased CV risk [125]. A meta-analysis of randomized, placebo-controlled trials indicated that PDE5 inhibitors had anti-remodeling properties and improved cardiac inotropism with a good safety profile [126]. However, at this time, no studies have examined the efficacy of PDE5 inhibitors in reducing CV risk in patients with PC receiving GnRH agonists.

GnRH antagonists may also contribute to CV risk reduction. In a pooled analysis of six phase III prospective trials of 2328 patients with PC, patients using GnRH antagonists had a 56% reduction in cardiac events compared with patients using GnRH agonists [127].

A recent multinational randomized phase III trial reported that GnRH antagonist therapy, compared with a GnRH agonist, reduced adverse CV events by 54% in a total of 930 patients with advanced PC (GnRH agonist group, n = 308; GnRH antagonist group, n = 622) [128].

An RCT that investigated CVD-related mortality after treatment of advanced PC with atherosclerotic CVD with GnRH agonist or GnRH antagonist is currently underway and its results are awaited [129].

Further large-scale prospective studies are awaited, but administration of a GnRH antagonist rather than a GnRH agonist may prevent increased CV risk.

Other drugs besides ADT, such as angiogenesis inhibitors and immune checkpoint inhibitors, have also been reported, and future studies are awaited [130].

3. Conclusions

ADT alone for high-risk localized and locally advanced PC, while useful, is not generally first-line therapy. However, ADT may be a useful option for Asians, including Japanese and older patients, with measures to prevent adverse effects. We look forward to further research on racial differences in the efficacy of ADT and progress in countermeasures against adverse effects.

Author Contributions: K.I. had full access to all the data and takes responsibility for the integrity and the accuracy of its content. Study concept and design, K.I.; drafting of the manuscript, H.I. and K.I.; critical revision of the manuscript, T.M.; supervision, A.M. All authors have read and agreed to the published version of the manuscript.

Funding: This research received no external funding.

Conflicts of Interest: The authors declare no conflict of interest.

References

1. Siegel, R.L.; Miller, K.D.; Fuchs, H.E.; Jemal, A. Cancer Statistics, 2021. *CA Cancer J. Clin.* **2021**, *71*, 7–33. [CrossRef] [PubMed]
2. Sung, H.; Ferlay, J.; Siegel, R.L.; Laversanne, M.; Soerjomataram, I.; Jemal, A.; Bray, F. Global Cancer statistics 2020: GLOBOCAN Estimates of Incidence and Mortality Worldwide for 36 Cancers in 185 Countries. *CA Cancer J. Clin.* **2021**, *71*, 209–249. [CrossRef] [PubMed]
3. DeSantis, C.E.; Lin, C.C.; Mariotto, A.B.; Siegel, R.L.; Stein, K.D.; Kramer, J.L.; Alteri, R.; Robbins, A.S.; Jemal, A. Cancer Treatment and Survivorship Statistics, 2014. *CA Cancer J. Clin.* **2014**, *64*, 252–271. [CrossRef] [PubMed]

4. Cetin, K.; Beebe-Dimmer, J.L.; Fryzek, J.P.; Markus, R.; Carducci, M.A. Recent Time Trends in the Epidemiology of stage IV Prostate Cancer in the United States: Analysis of Data from the Surveillance, Epidemiology, and End Results Program. *Urology* **2010**, *75*, 1396–1404. [CrossRef] [PubMed]
5. Fujimoto, H.; Nakanishi, H.; Miki, T.; Kubota, Y.; Takahashi, S.; Suzuki, K.; Kanayama, H.O.; Mikami, K.; Homma, Y. Oncological Outcomes of the Prostate Cancer Patients Registered in 2004: Report from the Cancer Registration Committee of the JUA. *Int. J. Urol.* **2011**, *18*, 876–881. [CrossRef]
6. Iwamoto, H.; Izumi, K.; Shimada, T.; Kano, H.; Kadomoto, S.; Makino, T.; Naito, R.; Yaegashi, H.; Shigehara, K.; Kadono, Y.; et al. Androgen Receptor Signaling-Targeted Therapy and Taxane Chemotherapy Induce Visceral Metastasis in Castration-Resistant Prostate Cancer. *Prostate* **2021**, *81*, 72–80. [CrossRef]
7. Byers, T.; Barrera, E.; Fontham, E.T.; Newman, L.A.; Runowicz, C.D.; Sener, S.F.; Thun, M.J.; Winborn, S.; Wender, R.C.; American Cancer Society Incidence and Mortality Ends Committee. A Midpoint Assessment of the American Cancer Society Challenge Goal to Halve the U.S. Cancer Mortality Rates between the Years 1990 and 2015. *Cancer* **2006**, *107*, 396–405. [CrossRef]
8. Schröder, F.H.; Hugosson, J.; Roobol, M.J.; Tammela, T.L.; Ciatto, S.; Nelen, V.; Kwiatkowski, M.; Lujan, M.; Lilja, H.; Zappa, M.; et al. Prostate-Cancer Mortality at 11 Years of Follow-Up. *N. Engl. J. Med.* **2012**, *366*, 981–990. [CrossRef]
9. Catalona, W.J. Prostate Cancer Screening. *Med. Clin. N. Am.* **2018**, *102*, 199–214. [CrossRef]
10. Welch, H.G.; Albertsen, P.C. Reconsidering Prostate Cancer Mortality—The Future of PSA Screening. *N. Engl. J. Med.* **2020**, *382*, 1557–1563. [CrossRef]
11. Cooperberg, M.R.; Broering, J.M.; Carroll, P.R. Time Trends and Local Variation in Primary Treatment of Localized Prostate Cancer. *J. Clin. Oncol.* **2010**, *28*, 1117–1123. [CrossRef] [PubMed]
12. Eggener, S.E.; Scardino, P.T.; Walsh, P.C.; Han, M.; Partin, A.W.; Trock, B.J.; Feng, Z.; Wood, D.P.; Eastham, J.A.; Yossepowitch, O.; et al. Predicting 15-Year Prostate Cancer Specific Mortality After Radical Prostatectomy. *J. Urol.* **2011**, *185*, 869–875. [CrossRef] [PubMed]
13. Rider, J.R.; Sandin, F.; Andrén, O.; Wiklund, P.; Hugosson, J.; Stattin, P. Long-Term Outcomes Among Noncuratively Treated Men According to Prostate Cancer Risk Category in a Nationwide, Population-Based Study. *Eur. Urol.* **2013**, *63*, 88–96. [CrossRef] [PubMed]
14. D'Amico, A.V.; Whittington, R.; Malkowicz, S.B.; Schultz, D.; Blank, K.; Broderick, G.A.; Tomaszewski, J.E.; Renshaw, A.A.; Kaplan, I.; Beard, C.J.; et al. Biochemical Outcome After Radical Prostatectomy, External Beam Radiation Therapy, or Interstitial Radiation Therapy for Clinically Localized Prostate Cancer. *JAMA* **1998**, *280*, 969–974. [CrossRef]
15. National Comprehensive Cancer Network. NCCN Clinical Practice Guidelines in Oncology. *Prostate Cancer* **2021**, *2*, 185–197.
16. Mottet, N.; van den Bergh, R.C.N.; Briers, E.; Van den Broeck, T.; Cumberbatch, M.G.; De Santis, M.; Fanti, S.; Fossati, N.; Gandaglia, G.; Gillessen, S.; et al. EAU-EANM-ESTRO-ESUR-SIOG Guidelines on Prostate Cancer-2020 Update. Part 1: Screening, Diagnosis, and Local Treatment with Curative Intent. *Eur. Urol.* **2021**, *79*, 243–262. [CrossRef]
17. Parker, C.; Castro, E.; Fizazi, K.; Heidenreich, A.; Ost, P.; Procopio, G.; Tombal, B.; Gillessen, S.; ESMO Guidelines Committee. Prostate Cancer: ESMO Clinical Practice Guidelines for Diagnosis, Treatment and Follow-Up. *Ann. Oncol.* **2020**, *31*, 1119–1134. [CrossRef]
18. Huggins, C.; Hodges, C.V. Studies on Prostatic Cancer: I. The Effect of Castration, of Estrogen and of Androgen Injection on Serum Phosphatases in Metastatic Carcinoma of the Prostate. *J. Urol.* **2002**, *168*, 9–12. [CrossRef]
19. Schally, A.V.; Arimura, A.; Kastin, A.J.; Matsuo, H.; Baba, Y.; Redding, T.W.; Nair, R.M.; Debeljuk, L.; White, W.F. Gonadotropin-Releasing Hormone: One Polypeptide Regulates Secretion of Luteinizing and Follicle-Stimulating Hormones. *Science* **1971**, *173*, 1036–1038. [CrossRef]
20. Bennett, C.L.; Tosteson, T.D.; Schmitt, B.; Weinberg, P.D.; Ernstoff, M.S.; Ross, S.D. Maximum Androgen-Blockade with Medical or Surgical Castration in Advanced Prostate Cancer: A Meta-Analysis of Nine Published Randomized Controlled Trials and 4128 Patients Using Flutamide. *Prostate Cancer Prostatic Dis.* **1999**, *2*, 4–8. [CrossRef]
21. Prostate Cancer Trialists' Collaborative Group. Maximum Androgen Blockade in Advanced Prostate Cancer: An Overview of the Randomised Trials. *Lancet* **2000**, *355*, 1491–1498. [CrossRef]
22. Seidenfeld, J.; Samson, D.J.; Hasselblad, V.; Aronson, N.; Albertsen, P.C.; Bennett, C.L.; Wilt, T.J. Single-Therapy Androgen Suppression in Men with Advanced Prostate Cancer: A Systematic Review and Meta-Analysis. *Ann. Intern. Med.* **2000**, *132*, 566–577. [CrossRef] [PubMed]
23. Samson, D.J.; Seidenfeld, J.; Schmitt, B.; Hasselblad, V.; Albertsen, P.C.; Bennett, C.L.; Wilt, T.J.; Aronson, N. Systematic Review and Meta-Analysis of Monotherapy Compared with Combined Androgen Blockade for Patients with Advanced Prostate Carcinoma. *Cancer* **2002**, *95*, 361–376. [CrossRef] [PubMed]
24. Garje, R.; Chennamadhavuni, A.; Mott, S.L.; Chambers, I.M.; Gellhaus, P.; Zakharia, Y.; Brown, J.A. Utilization and Outcomes of Surgical Castration in Comparison to Medical Castration in Metastatic Prostate Cancer. *Clin. Genitourin. Cancer* **2020**, *18*, e157–e166. [CrossRef]
25. Labrie, F.; Luu-The, V.; Labrie, C.; Simard, J. DHEA and its transformation into androgens and estrogens in peripheral target tissues: Intracrinology. *Front. Neuroendocrinol.* **2001**, *22*, 185–212. [CrossRef]
26. Mizokami, A.; Koh, E.; Fujita, H.; Maeda, Y.; Egawa, M.; Koshida, K.; Honma, S.; Keller, E.T.; Namiki, M. The Adrenal Androgen Androstenediol Is Present in Prostate Cancer Tissue after Androgen Deprivation Therapy and Activates Mutated Androgen Receptor. *Cancer Res.* **2004**, *64*, 765–771. [CrossRef]

27. Nishiyama, T.; Hashimoto, Y.; Takahashi, K. The Influence of Androgen Deprivation Therapy on Dihydrotestosterone Levels in the Prostatic Tissue of Patients with Prostate Cancer. *Clin. Cancer Res.* **2004**, *10*, 7121–7126. [CrossRef]
28. Labrie, F.; Dupont, A.; Belanger, A.; Cusan, L.; Lacourciere, Y.; Monfette, G.; Laberge, J.G.; Emond, J.P.; Fazekas, A.T.; Raynaud, J.P.; et al. New Hormonal Therapy in Prostatic Carcinoma: Combined Treatment with an LHRH Agonist and an Antiandrogen. *Clin. Investig. Med.* **1982**, *5*, 267–275.
29. Bélanger, A.; Dupont, A.; Labrie, F. Inhibition of Basal and Adrenocorticotropin-Stimulated Plasma Levels of Adrenal Androgens After Treatment with an Antiandrogen in Castrated Patients with Prostatic Cancer. *J. Clin. Endocrinol. Metab.* **1984**, *59*, 422–426. [CrossRef]
30. Labrie, F. Endocrine Therapy for Prostate Cancer. *Endocrinol. Metab. Clin. N. Am.* **1991**, *20*, 845–872. [CrossRef]
31. Van Poppel, H.; Nilsson, S. Testosterone Surge: Rationale for Gonadotropin-Releasing Hormone Blockers? *Urology* **2008**, *71*, 1001–1006. [CrossRef] [PubMed]
32. Sasagawa, I.; Kubota, Y.; Nakada, T.; Suzuki, H.; Hirano, J.; Sugano, O.; Kato, H.; Imamura, A.; Mastushita, K.; Onmura, Y.; et al. Influence of Luteinizing Hormone-Releasing Hormone Analogues on Serum Levels of Prostatic Acid Phosphatase and Prostatic Specific Antigen in Patients with Metastatic Carcinoma of the Prostate. *Int. Urol. Nephrol.* **1998**, *30*, 745–753. [CrossRef] [PubMed]
33. Thompson, I.M.; Zeidman, E.J.; Rodriguez, F.R. Sudden Death Due to Disease Flare with Luteinizing Hormone-Releasing Hormone Agonist Therapy for Carcinoma of the Prostate. *J. Urol.* **1990**, *144*, 1479–1480. [CrossRef]
34. Klotz, L.; Boccon-Gibod, L.; Shore, N.D.; Andreou, C.; Persson, B.E.; Cantor, P.; Jensen, J.K.; Olesen, T.K.; Schröder, F.H. The Efficacy and Safety of Degarelix: A 12-Month, Comparative, Randomized, Open-Label, Parallel-Group phase III Study in Patients with Prostate Cancer. *BJU Int.* **2008**, *102*, 1531–1538. [CrossRef]
35. De Bono, J.S.; Logothetis, C.J.; Molina, A.; Fizazi, K.; North, S.; Chu, L.; Chi, K.N.; Jones, R.J.; Goodman, O.B., Jr.; Saad, F.; et al. Abiraterone and Increased Survival in Metastatic Prostate Cancer. *N. Engl. J. Med.* **2011**, *364*, 1995–2005. [CrossRef]
36. Scher, H.I.; Fizazi, K.; Saad, F.; Taplin, M.E.; Sternberg, C.N.; Miller, K.; de Wit, R.; Mulders, P.; Chi, K.N.; Shore, N.D.; et al. Increased Survival with Enzalutamide in Prostate Cancer After Chemotherapy. *N. Engl. J. Med.* **2012**, *367*, 1187–1197. [CrossRef]
37. Smith, M.R.; Saad, F.; Chowdhury, S.; Oudard, S.; Hadaschik, B.A.; Graff, J.N.; Olmos, D.; Mainwaring, P.N.; Lee, J.Y.; Uemura, H.; et al. Apalutamide Treatment and Metastasis-Free Survival in Prostate Cancer. *N. Engl. J. Med.* **2018**, *378*, 1408–1418. [CrossRef]
38. Fizazi, K.; Shore, N.; Tammela, T.L.; Ulys, A.; Vjaters, E.; Polyakov, S.; Jievaltas, M.; Luz, M.; Alekseev, B.; Kuss, I.; et al. Darolutamide in Nonmetastatic, Castration-Resistant Prostate Cancer. *N. Engl. J. Med.* **2019**, *380*, 1235–1246. [CrossRef]
39. Iwamoto, H.; Kano, H.; Shimada, T.; Naito, R.; Makino, T.; Kadamoto, S.; Yaegashi, H.; Shigehara, K.; Izumi, K.; Kadonoa, Y.; et al. Effectiveness of Vintage Hormone Therapy as Alternative Androgen Deprivation Therapy for Non-Metastatic Castration-Resistant Prostate Cancer. *In Vivo* **2021**, *35*, 1247–1252. [CrossRef]
40. Tannock, I.F.; de Wit, R.; Berry, W.R.; Horti, J.; Pluzanska, A.; Chi, K.N.; Oudard, S.; Théodore, C.; James, N.D.; Turesson, I.; et al. Docetaxel plus Prednisone or Mitoxantrone plus Prednisone for Advanced Prostate Cancer. *N. Engl. J. Med.* **2004**, *351*, 1502–1512. [CrossRef]
41. Shimura, Y.; Suga, Y.; Itai, S.; Iwamoto, H.; Takezawa, Y.; Yaegashi, H.; Izumi, K.; Shimada, T.; Sai, Y.; Matsushita, R.; et al. Comparison of Tolerability Between 2-Weekly and 3-Weekly Docetaxel Regimen in Castration-Resistant Prostate Cancer. *Anticancer Res.* **2020**, *40*, 4291–4297. [CrossRef] [PubMed]
42. De Bono, J.S.; Oudard, S.; Ozguroglu, M.; Hansen, S.; Machiels, J.P.; Kocak, I.; Gravis, G.; Bodrogi, I.; Mackenzie, M.J.; Shen, L.; et al. Prednisone plus Cabazitaxel or Mitoxantrone for Metastatic Castration-Resistant Prostate Cancer Progressing After Docetaxel Treatment: A Randomised Open-Label Trial. *Lancet* **2010**, *376*, 1147–1154. [CrossRef]
43. Iwamoto, H.; Kano, H.; Shimada, T.; Naito, R.; Makino, T.; Kadomoto, S.; Yaegashi, H.; Shigehara, K.; Izumi, K.; Kadono, Y.; et al. Sarcopenia and Visceral Metastasis at Cabazitaxel Initiation Predict Prognosis in Patients with Castration-Resistant Prostate Cancer Receiving Cabazitaxel Chemotherapy. *In Vivo* **2021**, *35*, 1703–1709. [CrossRef] [PubMed]
44. Shahinian, V.B.; Kuo, Y.F.; Freeman, J.L.; Orihuela, E.; Goodwin, J.S. Increasing Use of Gonadotropin-Releasing Hormone Agonists for the Treatment of Localized Prostate Carcinoma. *Cancer* **2005**, *103*, 1615–1624. [CrossRef]
45. The Medical Research Council Prostate Cancer Working Party Investigators Group. Immediate versus deferred treatment for advanced prostatic cancer: Initial results of the Medical Research Council Trial. *Br. J. Urol.* **1997**, *79*, 235–246. [CrossRef] [PubMed]
46. Walker, L.M.; Tran, S.; Robinson, J.W. Luteinizing hormone-releasing hormone agonists: A quick reference for prevalence rates of potential adverse effects. *Clin. Genitourin. Cancer* **2013**, *11*, 375–384. [CrossRef]
47. Holzbeierlein, J.M.; McLaughlin, M.D.; Thrasher, J.B. Complications of androgen deprivation therapy for prostate cancer. *Curr. Opin. Urol.* **2004**, *14*, 177–183. [CrossRef]
48. Kunath, F.; Grobe, H.R.; Rücker, G.; Motschall, E.; Antes, G.; Dahm, P.; Wullich, B.; Meerpohl, J.J. Non-steroidal antiandrogen monotherapy compared with luteinizing hormone-releasing hormone agonists or surgical castration monotherapy for advanced prostate cancer: A Cochrane systematic review. *BJU Int.* **2015**, *116*, 30–36. [CrossRef]
49. Magnan, S.; Zarychanski, R.; Pilote, L.; Bernier, L.; Shemilt, M.; Vigneault, E.; Fradet, V.; Turgeon, A.F. Intermittent vs Continuous Androgen Deprivation Therapy for Prostate Cancer: A Systematic Review and Meta-analysis. *JAMA Oncol.* **2015**, *1*, 1261–1269. [CrossRef] [PubMed]
50. Sciarra, A.; Fasulo, A.; Ciardi, A.; Petrangeli, E.; Gentilucci, A.; Maggi, M.; Innocenzi, M.; Pierella, F.; Gentile, V.; Salciccia, S.; et al. A meta-analysis and systematic review of randomized controlled trials with degarelix versus gonadotropin-releasing hormone agonists for advanced prostate cancer. *Medicine* **2016**, *95*, e3845. [CrossRef]

51. Fowler, F.J., Jr.; McNaughton Collins, M.; Walker Corkery, E.; Elliott, D.B.; Barry, M.J. The impact of androgen deprivation on quality of life after radical prostatectomy for prostate carcinoma. *Cancer* **2002**, *95*, 287–295. [CrossRef] [PubMed]
52. Potosky, A.L.; Knopf, K.; Clegg, L.X.; Albertsen, P.C.; Stanford, J.L.; Hamilton, A.S.; Gilliland, F.D.; Eley, J.W.; Stephenson, R.A.; Hoffman, R.M. Quality-of-life outcomes after primary androgen deprivation therapy: Results from the Prostate Cancer Outcomes Study. *J. Clin. Oncol. Off. J. Am. Soc. Clin. Oncol.* **2001**, *19*, 3750–3757. [CrossRef] [PubMed]
53. Iversen, P.; McLeod, D.G.; See, W.A.; Morris, T.; Armstrong, J.; Wirth, M.P. Antiandrogen monotherapy in patients with localized or locally advanced prostate cancer: Final results from the bicalutamide Early Prostate Cancer programme at a median follow-up of 9.7 years. *BJU Int.* **2010**, *105*, 1074–1081. [CrossRef] [PubMed]
54. Fagerlund, A.; Cormio, L.; Palangi, L.; Lewin, R.; Santanelli di Pompeo, F.; Elander, A.; Selvaggi, G. Gynecomastia in Patients with Prostate Cancer: A Systematic Review. *PLoS ONE* **2015**, *10*, e0136094. [CrossRef] [PubMed]
55. Nead, K.T.; Sinha, S.; Yang, D.D.; Nguyen, P.L. Association of androgen deprivation therapy and depression in the treatment of prostate cancer: A systematic review and meta-analysis. *Urol. Oncol.* **2017**, *35*, 664.e661–664.e669. [CrossRef] [PubMed]
56. Krasnova, A.; Epstein, M.; Marchese, M.; Dickerman, B.A.; Cole, A.P.; Lipsitz, S.R.; Nguyen, P.L.; Kibel, A.S.; Choueiri, T.K.; Basaria, S.; et al. Risk of dementia following androgen deprivation therapy for treatment of prostate cancer. *Prostate Cancer Prostatic Dis.* **2020**, *23*, 410–418. [CrossRef] [PubMed]
57. Jayadevappa, R.; Chhatre, S.; Malkowicz, S.B.; Parikh, R.B.; Guzzo, T.; Wein, A.J. Association Between Androgen Deprivation Therapy Use and Diagnosis of Dementia in Men with Prostate Cancer. *JAMA Netw. Open* **2019**, *2*, e196562. [CrossRef] [PubMed]
58. Robinson, D.; Garmo, H.; Van Hemelrijck, M.; Damber, J.E.; Bratt, O.; Holmberg, L.; Wahlund, L.O.; Stattin, P.; Adolfsson, J. Androgen deprivation therapy for prostate cancer and risk of dementia. *BJU Int.* **2019**, *124*, 87–92. [CrossRef]
59. Liu, J.M.; Shen, C.Y.; Lau, W.C.Y.; Shao, S.C.; Man, K.K.C.; Hsu, R.J.; Wu, C.T.; Lai, E.C. Association between Androgen Deprivation Therapy and Risk of Dementia in Men with Prostate Cancer. *Cancers* **2021**, *13*, 3861. [CrossRef] [PubMed]
60. Nead, K.T.; Sinha, S.; Nguyen, P.L. Androgen deprivation therapy for prostate cancer and dementia risk: A systematic review and meta-analysis. *Prostate Cancer Prostatic Dis.* **2017**, *20*, 259–264. [CrossRef] [PubMed]
61. Cui, H.; Wang, Y.; Li, F.; He, G.; Jiang, Z.; Gang, X.; Wang, G. Quantifying observational evidence for risk of dementia following androgen deprivation therapy for prostate cancer: An updated systematic review and meta-analysis. *Prostate Cancer Prostatic Dis.* **2021**, *24*, 15–23. [CrossRef] [PubMed]
62. Smith, M.R.; Lee, W.C.; Brandman, J.; Wang, Q.; Botteman, M.; Pashos, C.L. Gonadotropin-releasing hormone agonists and fracture risk: A claims-based cohort study of men with nonmetastatic prostate cancer. *J. Clin. Oncol. Off. J. Am. Soc. Clin. Oncol.* **2005**, *23*, 7897–7903. [CrossRef]
63. Alibhai, S.M.; Duong-Hua, M.; Cheung, A.M.; Sutradhar, R.; Warde, P.; Fleshner, N.E.; Paszat, L. Fracture types and risk factors in men with prostate cancer on androgen deprivation therapy: A matched cohort study of 19,079 men. *J. Urol.* **2010**, *184*, 918–923. [CrossRef]
64. Shahinian, V.B.; Kuo, Y.F.; Freeman, J.L.; Goodwin, J.S. Risk of fracture after androgen deprivation for prostate cancer. *N. Engl. J. Med.* **2005**, *352*, 154–164. [CrossRef]
65. Beebe-Dimmer, J.L.; Cetin, K.; Shahinian, V.; Morgenstern, H.; Yee, C.; Schwartz, K.L.; Acquavella, J. Timing of androgen deprivation therapy use and fracture risk among elderly men with prostate cancer in the United States. *Pharmacoepidemiol. Drug Saf.* **2012**, *21*, 70–78. [CrossRef]
66. Kim, D.K.; Lee, J.Y.; Kim, K.J.; Hong, N.; Kim, J.W.; Hah, Y.S.; Koo, K.C.; Kim, J.H.; Cho, K.S. Effect of Androgen-Deprivation Therapy on Bone Mineral Density in Patients with Prostate Cancer: A Systematic Review and Meta-Analysis. *J. Clin. Med.* **2019**, *8*, 113. [CrossRef]
67. Smith, M.R.; Finkelstein, J.S.; McGovern, F.J.; Zietman, A.L.; Fallon, M.A.; Schoenfeld, D.A.; Kantoff, P.W. Changes in body composition during androgen deprivation therapy for prostate cancer. *J. Clin. Endocrinol. Metab.* **2002**, *87*, 599–603. [CrossRef] [PubMed]
68. Keating, N.L.; O'Malley, A.J.; Freedland, S.J.; Smith, M.R. Diabetes and cardiovascular disease during androgen deprivation therapy: Observational study of veterans with prostate cancer. *J. Natl. Cancer Inst.* **2010**, *102*, 39–46. [CrossRef] [PubMed]
69. Braga-Basaria, M.; Dobs, A.S.; Muller, D.C.; Carducci, M.A.; John, M.; Egan, J.; Basaria, S. Metabolic syndrome in men with prostate cancer undergoing long-term androgen-deprivation therapy. *J. Clin. Oncol. Off. J. Am. Soc. Clin. Oncol.* **2006**, *24*, 3979–3983. [CrossRef] [PubMed]
70. Crawley, D.; Garmo, H.; Rudman, S.; Stattin, P.; Haggstrom, C.; Zethelius, B.; Holmberg, L.; Adolfsson, J.; Van Hemelrijck, M. Association between duration and type of androgen deprivation therapy and risk of diabetes in men with prostate cancer. *Int. J. Cancer* **2016**, *139*, 2698–2704. [CrossRef] [PubMed]
71. Smith, M.R.; Lee, H.; Nathan, D.M. Insulin sensitivity during combined androgen blockade for prostate cancer. *J. Clin. Endocrinol. Metab.* **2006**, *91*, 1305–1308. [CrossRef] [PubMed]
72. Bosco, C.; Crawley, D.; Adolfsson, J.; Rudman, S.; Van Hemelrijck, M. Quantifying the evidence for the risk of metabolic syndrome and its components following androgen deprivation therapy for prostate cancer: A meta-analysis. *PLoS ONE* **2015**, *10*, e0117344. [CrossRef] [PubMed]
73. Wang, H.; Sun, X.; Zhao, L.; Chen, X.; Zhao, J. Androgen deprivation therapy is associated with diabetes: Evidence from meta-analysis. *J. Diabetes Investig.* **2016**, *7*, 629–636. [CrossRef] [PubMed]

74. Keating, N.L.; O'Malley, A.J.; Smith, M.R. Diabetes and cardiovascular disease during androgen deprivation therapy for prostate cancer. *J. Clin. Oncol. Off. J. Am. Soc. Clin. Oncol.* **2006**, *24*, 4448–4456. [CrossRef]
75. O'Farrell, S.; Garmo, H.; Holmberg, L.; Adolfsson, J.; Stattin, P.; Van Hemelrijck, M. Risk and timing of cardiovascular disease after androgen-deprivation therapy in men with prostate cancer. *J. Clin. Oncol. Off. J. Am. Soc. Clin. Oncol.* **2015**, *33*, 1243–1251. [CrossRef] [PubMed]
76. O'Farrell, S.; Sandström, K.; Garmo, H.; Stattin, P.; Holmberg, L.; Adolfsson, J.; Van Hemelrijck, M. Risk of thromboembolic disease in men with prostate cancer undergoing androgen deprivation therapy. *BJU Int.* **2016**, *118*, 391–398. [CrossRef] [PubMed]
77. Zhao, J.; Zhu, S.; Sun, L.; Meng, F.; Zhao, L.; Zhao, Y.; Tian, H.; Li, P.; Niu, Y. Androgen deprivation therapy for prostate cancer is associated with cardiovascular morbidity and mortality: A meta-analysis of population-based observational studies. *PLoS ONE* **2014**, *9*, e107516. [CrossRef] [PubMed]
78. Meng, F.; Zhu, S.; Zhao, J.; Vados, L.; Wang, L.; Zhao, Y.; Zhao, D.; Niu, Y. Stroke related to androgen deprivation therapy for prostate cancer: A meta-analysis and systematic review. *BMC Cancer* **2016**, *16*, 180. [CrossRef] [PubMed]
79. Alibhai, S.M.; Duong-Hua, M.; Sutradhar, R.; Fleshner, N.E.; Warde, P.; Cheung, A.M.; Paszat, L.F. Impact of androgen deprivation therapy on cardiovascular disease and diabetes. *J. Clin. Oncol. Off. J. Am. Soc. Clin. Oncol.* **2009**, *27*, 3452–3458. [CrossRef] [PubMed]
80. Nguyen, P.L.; Je, Y.; Schutz, F.A.; Hoffman, K.E.; Hu, J.C.; Parekh, A.; Beckman, J.A.; Choueiri, T.K. Association of androgen deprivation therapy with cardiovascular death in patients with prostate cancer: A meta-analysis of randomized trials. *JAMA* **2011**, *306*, 2359–2366. [CrossRef] [PubMed]
81. Sammon, J.D.; Abdollah, F.; Reznor, G.; Pucheril, D.; Choueiri, T.K.; Hu, J.C.; Kim, S.P.; Schmid, M.; Sood, A.; Sun, M.; et al. Patterns of Declining Use and the Adverse Effect of Primary Androgen Deprivation on All-cause Mortality in Elderly Men with Prostate Cancer. *Eur. Urol.* **2015**, *68*, 32–39. [CrossRef] [PubMed]
82. Merglen, A.; Schmidlin, F.; Fioretta, G.; Verkooijen, H.M.; Rapiti, E.; Zanetti, R.; Miralbell, R.; Bouchardy, C. Short- and long-term mortality with localized prostate cancer. *Arch Intern. Med.* **2007**, *167*, 1944–1950. [CrossRef] [PubMed]
83. Lee, H.J.; Lee, A.; Huang, H.H.; Lau, W.K.O. Primary androgen deprivation therapy as monotherapy in unfavourable intermediate- and high-risk localised prostate cancer: A Singaporean single-centre perspective. *Int. Urol. Nephrol.* **2018**, *50*, 665–673. [CrossRef]
84. Lu-Yao, G.L.; Albertsen, P.C.; Moore, D.F.; Shih, W.; Lin, Y.; DiPaola, R.S.; Yao, S.L. Survival following primary androgen deprivation therapy among men with localized prostate cancer. *JAMA* **2008**, *300*, 173–181. [CrossRef]
85. Potosky, A.L.; Haque, R.; Cassidy-Bushrow, A.E.; Ulcickas Yood, M.; Jiang, M.; Tsai, H.T.; Luta, G.; Keating, N.L.; Smith, M.R.; Van Den Eeden, S.K. Effectiveness of primary androgen-deprivation therapy for clinically localized prostate cancer. *J. Clin. Oncol. Off. J. Am. Soc. Clin. Oncol.* **2014**, *32*, 1324–1330. [CrossRef]
86. Lu-Yao, G.L.; Albertsen, P.C.; Moore, D.F.; Shih, W.; Lin, Y.; DiPaola, R.S.; Yao, S.L. Fifteen-year survival outcomes following primary androgen-deprivation therapy for localized prostate cancer. *JAMA Intern. Med.* **2014**, *174*, 1460–1467. [CrossRef]
87. Labrie, F.; Candas, B.; Gomez, J.L.; Cusan, L. Can combined androgen blockade provide long-term control or possible cure of localized prostate cancer? *Urology* **2002**, *60*, 115–119. [CrossRef]
88. Akaza, H.; Homma, Y.; Usami, M.; Hirao, Y.; Tsushima, T.; Okada, K.; Yokoyama, M.; Ohashi, Y.; Aso, Y. Efficacy of primary hormone therapy for localized or locally advanced prostate cancer: Results of a 10-year follow-up. *BJU Int.* **2006**, *98*, 573–579. [CrossRef]
89. Kawakami, J.; Cowan, J.E.; Elkin, E.P.; Latini, D.M.; DuChane, J.; Carroll, P.R. Androgen-deprivation therapy as primary treatment for localized prostate cancer: Data from Cancer of the Prostate Strategic Urologic Research Endeavor (CaPSURE). *Cancer* **2006**, *106*, 1708–1714. [CrossRef]
90. Akaza, H. Future prospects for luteinizing hormone-releasing hormone analogues in prostate cancer treatment. *Pharmacology* **2010**, *85*, 110–120. [CrossRef]
91. Matsumoto, K.; Hagiwara, M.; Tanaka, N.; Hayakawa, N.; Ishida, M.; Ninomiya, A.; Nakajima, Y.; Nakamura, S. Survival following primary androgen deprivation therapy for localized intermediate- or high-risk prostate cancer: Comparison with the life expectancy of the age-matched normal population. *Med. Oncol.* **2014**, *31*, 979. [CrossRef] [PubMed]
92. Studer, U.E.; Whelan, P.; Wimpissinger, F.; Casselman, J.; de Reijke, T.M.; Knönagel, H.; Loidl, W.; Isorna, S.; Sundaram, S.K.; Collette, L. Differences in time to disease progression do not predict for cancer-specific survival in patients receiving immediate or deferred androgen-deprivation therapy for prostate cancer: Final results of EORTC randomized trial 30891 with 12 years of follow-up. *Eur. Urol.* **2014**, *66*, 829–838. [CrossRef] [PubMed]
93. Fukagai, T.; Namiki, T.S.; Carlile, R.G.; Yoshida, H.; Namiki, M. Comparison of the clinical outcome after hormonal therapy for prostate cancer between Japanese and Caucasian men. *BJU Int.* **2006**, *97*, 1190–1193. [CrossRef]
94. Cooperberg, M.R.; Hinotsu, S.; Namiki, M.; Carroll, P.R.; Akaza, H. Trans-Pacific variation in outcomes for men treated with primary androgen-deprivation therapy (ADT) for prostate cancer. *BJU Int.* **2016**, *117*, 102–109. [CrossRef]
95. Kupelian, P.A.; Elshaikh, M.; Reddy, C.A.; Zippe, C.; Klein, E.A. Comparison of the efficacy of local therapies for localized prostate cancer in the prostate-specific antigen era: A large single-institution experience with radical prostatectomy and external-beam radiotherapy. *J. Clin. Oncol. Off. J. Am. Soc. Clin. Oncol.* **2002**, *20*, 3376–3385. [CrossRef]
96. Bill-Axelson, A.; Holmberg, L.; Filén, F.; Ruutu, M.; Garmo, H.; Busch, C.; Nordling, S.; Häggman, M.; Andersson, S.O.; Bratell, S.; et al. Radical prostatectomy versus watchful waiting in localized prostate cancer: The Scandinavian prostate cancer group-4 randomized trial. *J. Natl. Cancer Inst.* **2008**, *100*, 1144–1154. [CrossRef]

97. Bill-Axelson, A.; Holmberg, L.; Garmo, H.; Rider, J.R.; Taari, K.; Busch, C.; Nordling, S.; Häggman, M.; Andersson, S.O.; Spångberg, A.; et al. Radical prostatectomy or watchful waiting in early prostate cancer. *N. Engl. J. Med.* **2014**, *370*, 932–942. [CrossRef]
98. Bolla, M.; Collette, L.; Blank, L.; Warde, P.; Dubois, J.B.; Mirimanoff, R.O.; Storme, G.; Bernier, J.; Kuten, A.; Sternberg, C.; et al. Long-term results with immediate androgen suppression and external irradiation in patients with locally advanced prostate cancer (an EORTC study): A phase III randomised trial. *Lancet* **2002**, *360*, 103–106. [CrossRef]
99. Roach, M., 3rd; Bae, K.; Speight, J.; Wolkov, H.B.; Rubin, P.; Lee, R.J.; Lawton, C.; Valicenti, R.; Grignon, D.; Pilepich, M.V. Short-term neoadjuvant androgen deprivation therapy and external-beam radiotherapy for locally advanced prostate cancer: Long-term results of RTOG 8610. *J. Clin. Oncol. Off. J. Am. Soc. Clin. Oncol.* **2008**, *26*, 585–591. [CrossRef]
100. Wallis, C.J.D.; Saskin, R.; Choo, R.; Herschorn, S.; Kodama, R.T.; Satkunasivam, R.; Shah, P.S.; Danjoux, C.; Nam, R.K. Surgery Versus Radiotherapy for Clinically-Localized Prostate Cancer: A Systematic Review and Meta-analysis. *Eur. Urol.* **2016**, *70*, 21–30. [CrossRef]
101. Ennis, R.D.; Hu, L.; Ryemon, S.N.; Lin, J.; Mazumdar, M. Brachytherapy-Based Radiotherapy and Radical Prostatectomy Are Associated with Similar Survival in High-Risk Localized Prostate Cancer. *J. Clin. Oncol. Off. J. Am. Soc. Clin. Oncol.* **2018**, *36*, 1192–1198. [CrossRef] [PubMed]
102. Armstrong, A.J.; Szmulewitz, R.Z.; Petrylak, D.P.; Holzbeierlein, J.; Villers, A.; Azad, A.; Alcaraz, A.; Alekseev, B.; Iguchi, T.; Shore, N.D.; et al. ARCHES: A Randomized, Phase III Study of Androgen Deprivation Therapy with Enzalutamide or Placebo in Men with Metastatic Hormone-Sensitive Prostate Cancer. *J. Clin. Oncol. Off. J. Am. Soc. Clin. Oncol.* **2019**, *37*, 2974–2986. [CrossRef] [PubMed]
103. Davis, I.D.; Martin, A.J.; Stockler, M.R.; Begbie, S.; Chi, K.N.; Chowdhury, S.; Coskinas, X.; Frydenberg, M.; Hague, W.E.; Horvath, L.G.; et al. Enzalutamide with Standard First-Line Therapy in Metastatic Prostate Cancer. *N. Engl. J. Med.* **2019**, *381*, 121–131. [CrossRef] [PubMed]
104. Fizazi, K.; Tran, N.; Fein, L.; Matsubara, N.; Rodriguez-Antolin, A.; Alekseev, B.Y.; Özgüroğlu, M.; Ye, D.; Feyerabend, S.; Protheroe, A.; et al. Abiraterone acetate plus prednisone in patients with newly diagnosed high-risk metastatic castration-sensitive prostate cancer (LATITUDE): Final overall survival analysis of a randomised, double-blind, phase 3 trial. *Lancet Oncol.* **2019**, *20*, 686–700. [CrossRef]
105. Chi, K.N.; Chowdhury, S.; Bjartell, A.; Chung, B.H.; Pereira de Santana Gomes, A.J.; Given, R.; Juárez, A.; Merseburger, A.S.; Özgüroğlu, M.; Uemura, H.; et al. Apalutamide in Patients with Metastatic Castration-Sensitive Prostate Cancer: Final Survival Analysis of the Randomized, Double-Blind, Phase III TITAN Study. *J. Clin. Oncol. Off. J. Am. Soc. Clin. Oncol.* **2021**, *39*, 2294–2303. [CrossRef]
106. Attard, G.; Murphy, L.; Clarke, N.W.; Cross, W.; Jones, R.J.; Parker, C.C.; Gillessen, S.; Cook, A.; Brawley, C.; Amos, C.L.; et al. Abiraterone acetate and prednisolone with or without enzalutamide for high-risk non-metastatic prostate cancer: A meta-analysis of primary results from two randomised controlled phase 3 trials of the STAMPEDE platform protocol. *Lancet* **2021**, *399*, 447–460. [CrossRef]
107. Carcaillon, L.; Brailly-Tabard, S.; Ancelin, M.L.; Tzourio, C.; Foubert-Samier, A.; Dartigues, J.F.; Guiochon-Mantel, A.; Scarabin, P.Y. Low testosterone and the risk of dementia in elderly men: Impact of age and education. *Alzheimers Dement.* **2014**, *10*, S306–S314. [CrossRef]
108. Gandy, S.; Almeida, O.P.; Fonte, J.; Lim, D.; Waterrus, A.; Spry, N.; Flicker, L.; Martins, R.N. Chemical andropause and amyloid-beta peptide. *JAMA* **2001**, *285*, 2195–2196. [CrossRef]
109. Manolagas, S.C.; Weinstein, R.S. New Developments in the Pathogenesis and Treatment of Steroid-Induced Osteoporosis. *J. Bone Miner. Res.* **1999**, *14*, 1061–1066. [CrossRef]
110. Riggs, B.L.; Khosla, S.; Melton, L.J., 3rd. Sex Steroids and the Construction and Conservation of the Adult Skeleton. *Endocr. Rev.* **2002**, *23*, 279–302. [CrossRef]
111. Dewey, M.E.; Saz, P. Dementia, Cognitive Impairment and Mortality in Persons Aged 65 and over Living in the Community: A Systematic Review of the Literature. *Int. J. Geriatr. Psychiatry* **2001**, *16*, 751–761. [CrossRef] [PubMed]
112. Livingston, G.; Huntley, J.; Sommerlad, A.; Ames, D.; Ballard, C.; Banerjee, S.; Brayne, C.; Burns, A.; Cohen-Mansfield, J.; Cooper, C.; et al. Dementia Prevention, Intervention, and Care: 2020 Report of the Lancet Commission. *Lancet* **2020**, *396*, 413–446. [CrossRef]
113. Poon, Y.; Pechlivanoglou, P.; Alibhai, S.M.H.; Naimark, D.; Hoch, J.S.; Papadimitropoulos, E.; Hogan, M.E.; Krahn, M. Systematic Review and Network Meta-Analysis on the Relative Efficacy of Osteoporotic Medications: Men with Prostate Cancer on Continuous Androgen-Deprivation Therapy to Reduce Risk of Fragility Fractures. *BJU. Int.* **2018**, *121*, 17–28. [CrossRef] [PubMed]
114. Yan, Y.; Tan, B.; Fu, F.; Chen, Q.; Li, W.; Chen, W.; He, H. Exercise vs Conventional Treatment for Treatment of Primary Osteoporosis: A Systematic Review and Meta-Analysis of Randomized Controlled Trials. *Orthop. Surg.* **2021**, *13*, 1474–1487. [CrossRef] [PubMed]
115. Levine, G.N.; D'Amico, A.V.; Berger, P.; Clark, P.E.; Eckel, R.H.; Keating, N.L.; Milani, R.V.; Sagalowsky, A.I.; Smith, M.R.; Zakai, N.; et al. Androgen-Deprivation Therapy in Prostate Cancer and Cardiovascular Risk: A Science Advisory from the American Heart Association, American Cancer Society, and American Urological Association: Endorsed by the American Society for Radiation Oncology. *CA Cancer J. Clin.* **2010**, *60*, 194–201. [CrossRef]

116. Muniyan, S.; Xi, L.; Datta, K.; Das, A.; Teply, B.A.; Batra, S.K.; Kukreja, R.C. Cardiovascular Risks and Toxicity—The Achilles Heel of Androgen Deprivation Therapy in Prostate Cancer Patients. *Biochim. Biophys. Acta Rev. Cancer* **2020**, *1874*, 188383. [CrossRef]
117. Makhsida, N.; Shah, J.; Yan, G.; Fisch, H.; Shabsigh, R. Hypogonadism and Metabolic Syndrome: Implications for Testosterone Therapy. *J. Urol.* **2005**, *174*, 827–834. [CrossRef]
118. Rochlani, Y.; Pothineni, N.V.; Kovelamudi, S.; Mehta, J.L. Metabolic Syndrome: Pathophysiology, Management, and Modulation by Natural Compounds. *Ther. Adv. Cardiovasc. Dis.* **2017**, *11*, 215–225. [CrossRef]
119. Mottillo, S.; Filion, K.B.; Genest, J.; Joseph, L.; Pilote, L.; Poirier, P.; Rinfret, S.; Schiffrin, E.L.; Eisenberg, M.J. The Metabolic Syndrome and Cardiovascular Risk a Systematic Review and Meta-Analysis. *J. Am. Coll. Cardiol.* **2010**, *56*, 1113–1132. [CrossRef]
120. Grundy, S.M.; Cleeman, J.I.; Daniels, S.R.; Donato, K.A.; Eckel, R.H.; Franklin, B.A.; Gordon, D.J.; Krauss, R.M.; Savage, P.J.; Smith, S.C., Jr.; et al. Diagnosis and Management of the Metabolic Syndrome: An American Heart Association/National Heart, Lung, and Blood Institute Scientific Statement. *Circulation* **2005**, *112*, 2735–2752. [CrossRef]
121. Wing, R.R.; Blair, E.H.; Bononi, P.; Marcus, M.D.; Watanabe, R.; Bergman, R.N. Caloric Restriction Per Se Is a Significant Factor in Improvements in Glycemic Control and Insulin Sensitivity During Weight Loss in Obese NIDDM Patients. *Diabetes Care* **1994**, *17*, 30–36. [CrossRef]
122. Lee, D.C.; Pate, R.R.; Lavie, C.J.; Sui, X.; Church, T.S.; Blair, S.N. Leisure-Time Running Reduces All-Cause and Cardiovascular Mortality Risk. *J. Am. Coll. Cardiol.* **2014**, *64*, 472–481. [CrossRef] [PubMed]
123. Bull, F.C.; Al-Ansari, S.S.; Biddle, S.; Borodulin, K.; Buman, M.P.; Cardon, G.; Carty, C.; Chaput, J.P.; Chastin, S.; Chou, R.; et al. World Health Organization 2020 Guidelines on Physical Activity and Sedentary Behaviour. *Br. J. Sports Med.* **2020**, *54*, 1451–1462. [CrossRef]
124. Das, A.; Durrant, D.; Salloum, F.N.; Xi, L.; Kukreja, R.C. PDE5 Inhibitors as Therapeutics for Heart Disease, Diabetes and Cancer. *Pharmacol. Ther.* **2015**, *147*, 12–21. [CrossRef] [PubMed]
125. Giannetta, E.; Feola, T.; Gianfrilli, D.; Pofi, R.; Dall'Armi, V.; Badagliacca, R.; Barbagallo, F.; Lenzi, A.; Isidori, A.M. Is Chronic Inhibition of Phosphodiesterase type 5 Cardioprotective and Safe? A Meta-Analysis of Randomized Controlled Trials. *BMC Med.* **2014**, *12*, 185. [CrossRef] [PubMed]
126. Albertsen, P.C.; Klotz, L.; Tombal, B.; Grady, J.; Olesen, T.K.; Nilsson, J. Cardiovascular Morbidity Associated with Gonadotropin Releasing Hormone Agonists and an Antagonist. *Eur. Urol.* **2014**, *65*, 565–573. [CrossRef] [PubMed]
127. Shore, N.D.; Saad, F.; Cookson, M.S.; George, D.J.; Saltzstein, D.R.; Tutrone, R.; Akaza, H.; Bossi, A.; van Veenhuyzen, D.F.; Selby, B.; et al. Oral Relugolix for Androgen-Deprivation Therapy in Advanced Prostate Cancer. *N. Engl. J. Med.* **2020**, *382*, 2187–2196. [CrossRef]
128. Melloni, C.; Slovin, S.F.; Blemings, A.; Goodman, S.G.; Evans, C.P.; Nilsson, J.; Bhatt, D.L.; Zubovskiy, K.; Olesen, T.K.; Dugi, K.; et al. Cardiovascular Safety of Degarelix Versus Leuprolide for Advanced Prostate Cancer: The PRONOUNCE Trial Study Design. *JACC Cardiooncol.* **2020**, *2*, 70–81. [CrossRef] [PubMed]
129. Krebs, M.; Solimando, A.G.; Kalogirou, C.; Marquardt, A.; Frank, T.; Sokolakis, I.; Hatzichristodoulou, G.; Kneitz, S.; Bargou, R.; Kübler, H.; et al. miR-221-3p Regulates VEGFR2 Expression in High-Risk Prostate Cancer and Represents an Escape Mechanism from Sunitinib In Vitro. *J. Clin. Med.* **2020**, *9*, 670. [CrossRef]
130. Solimando, A.G.; Kalogirou, C.; Krebs, M. Angiogenesis as Therapeutic Target in Metastatic Prostate Cancer—Narrowing the Gap between Bench and Bedside. *Front. Immunol.* **2022**, *13*, 842038. [CrossRef] [PubMed]

cancers

MDPI

Review

Treatment Strategies for High-Risk Localized and Locally Advanced and Oligometastatic Prostate Cancer

Tomoyuki Makino [1,2], Kouji Izumi [1,*], Hiroaki Iwamoto [1] and Atsushi Mizokami [1]

1 Department of Integrative Cancer Therapy and Urology, Kanazawa University Graduate School of Medical Science, 13-1 Takara-machi, Kanazawa 920-8640, Ishikawa, Japan; mackeeen511@gmail.com (T.M.); iwamoto-h@med.kanazawa-u.ac.jp (H.I.); mizokami@staff.kanazawa-u.ac.jp (A.M.)
2 Department of Urology, Ishikawa Prefectural Central Hospital, Kanazawa 920-8530, Ishikawa, Japan
* Correspondence: kouji1974@staff.kanazawa-u.ac.jp; Tel.: +81-76-265-2393; Fax: +81-76-234-4263

Simple Summary: The definitions of locally advanced and oligometastatic prostate cancer are ambiguous, and there are no standard treatments for these. Although multidisciplinary treatment combining systemic and local treatment may be effective, there are many unresolved issues such as the choice of local treatment, use of new endocrine agents and chemotherapy, and selection of optimal patients. The present article discusses the definitions, diagnoses, and treatment of very high-risk prostate cancer and oligometastatic prostate cancer.

Abstract: Despite the significant advances in the treatment of high-risk prostate cancer, patients with very high-risk features such as being locally advanced (clinical stage T3–4 or minimal nodal involvement), having a high Gleason pattern, or with oligometastasis may still have a poor prognosis despite aggressive treatment. Multidisciplinary treatment with both local and systemic therapies is thought to be effective, however, unfortunately, there is still no standard treatment. However, in recent years, local definitive therapy using a combination of radiotherapy and androgen deprivation is being supported by several randomized clinical trials. This study reviews the current literature with a focus on the definition of very high-risk prostate cancer, the role of modern imaging, and its treatment options.

Keywords: prostate cancer; locally advanced; oligometastasis; very high-risk

Citation: Makino, T.; Izumi, K.; Iwamoto, H.; Mizokami, A. Treatment Strategies for High-Risk Localized and Locally Advanced and Oligometastatic Prostate Cancer. *Cancers* **2021**, *13*, 4470. https://doi.org/10.3390/cancers13174470

Academic Editor: David Wong

Received: 6 August 2021
Accepted: 1 September 2021
Published: 5 September 2021

1. Introduction

With the introduction of prostate cancer (PC) screening, more men are continuously being diagnosed with clinically nonmetastatic PC. However, 17–31% of them have high-risk localized or locally advanced disease requiring curative treatment [1]. In addition, with the development of new imaging techniques, several types of oligometastatic PC which are between locally advanced cancer and widely metastatic cancer are being discovered [2]. Thus, accurate diagnosis will become more important in the future. Recent advancements have also been made in radiotherapy (RT) for PC due to innovations in medical and physical engineering, and excellent long-term results have been reported [3–9]. However, the definitions of locally advanced PC and oligometastatic PC are still ambiguous, and there is no standard treatment for these. Furthermore, no studies directly compare local treatment options such as radical prostatectomy (RP) and RT. Thus, the superiority or inferiority of these treatments is unknown. So far, the standard treatment for oligometastatic PC has been systemic therapy, specifically androgen deprivation therapy (ADT). In recent years, however, the significance of combined local treatment has been discussed, and the results of large-scale clinical trials have been reported with and without combined RT [6,10]. In addition, attempts to further enhance disease control by concomitant metastasis-directed therapy (MDT) have been made [11–13], and radical curing of oligometastatic PC may be expected in the future. The present article reviews the definition, diagnosis, and treatment (especially RT) of locally advanced (focusing on very high-risk PC) and oligometastatic PC, focusing on previous reports.

2. Locally Advanced PC

2.1. Definition

Since D'Amico et al. proposed the risk classification of localized PC, risk stratification has been conducted by various research groups and guidelines. Cases with a high risk of recurrence are defined as "high-risk PC" [14]; however, because of the heterogeneity in prognosis among these cases, they have been further subdivided into "very high-risk PC" [15]. Sphan et al. studied 712 PC patients with prostate-specific antigen (PSA) > 20 ng/mL and found that a combination of additional risk factors (e.g., Gleason score (GS) 8–10, clinical stage (c) T3–4) at presentation were associated with unfavorable histopathology and worse cancer-specific outcomes [16]. Similarly, Walz and Joniau showed that patients with two or more high-risk features (e.g., PSA > 20 ng/mL, GS 8–10, cT3–4) had worse biochemical recurrence-free survival (RFS) and prostate cancer-specific survival (CSS) than those with only one high-risk feature [17,18]. In contrast, the preoperative criteria of the National Comprehensive Cancer Network (NCCN) identifies those with primary Gleason pattern 5 on biopsy or ≥4 cores containing pattern 4 (odds ratio (OR): 3.17; $p < 0.001$) as the high-risk subgroup, who are most likely to experience early (within one year) biochemical recurrence after surgery [19]. In recent years, the NCCN defined very high-risk PC patients as those with cT3b–4 or primary Gleason pattern 5 or >4 cores with grade group ≥ 4 according to the International Society of Urological Pathology [20].

Lymph node involvement was considered as a sign of further metastases indicating poor prognosis. However, low nodal metastatic burden in surgical specimens indicates better outcomes than visceral or bone metastasis. Patients with ≤2 positive lymph nodes treated with RP with extended pelvic lymph node dissection show significantly better CSS outcomes at 15-year follow-up compared to those with ≥2 positive lymph nodes (84% vs. 62%, respectively; $p < 0.001$) [21]. Moreover, patients with a GS < 8 and ≤2 positive lymph nodes had relatively favorable outcomes at 10 years among patients with lymph node metastases treated with RP and extended pelvic lymphadenectomy [22]. These findings suggest that the current staging system of PC does not accurately reflect prognosis and treatment paradigms may need to be reconsidered for better outcomes. Indeed, the recent European Association of Urology (EAU) guidelines state that cN+ patients are categorized as having high-risk locally advanced disease; and that cT3–4 or cN+ (any PSA and any GS) cases can be ultimately managed locally through a multimodal approach [23]. The definitions of very high-risk PC reported so far are shown in Table 1.

Table 1. Definition of very high-risk prostate cancer.

Source (Year)	Definition	Reference
Spahn (2010)	2 high-risk features (PSA > 20 ng/mL, GS 8–10, and cT3–4)	[16]
Walz (2011)		[17]
Sundi (2014)	Primary Gleason pattern 5 or 4 cores containing pattern 4	[19]
Joniau (2015)	GS 8–10 in combination with 1 other high-risk factor (PSA > 20 ng/mL and cT3–4)	[18]
NCCN guidelines (2019v2)	cT3b–4 or primary Gleason pattern 5 or >4 cores with Grade Group 4 or 5	[20]
EAU guidelines (2019)	cT3–4 or cN+, any PSA, any GS	[23]

PSA = Prostate specific antigen; GS = Gleason score; NCCN = National Comprehensive Cancer Network; EAU = European Association of Urology.

2.2. *Diagnosis*

Imaging studies are very important in the diagnosis of locally advanced PC. A cohort study of high-risk PC using multi-parametric magnetic resonance imaging (mpMRI) with a combination of T2-weighted, diffusion-weighted, and dynamic contrast-enhanced images reported an 89% positivity rate of extracapsular invasion and an OR of 10.3 for predicting extracapsular invasion [24]. In addition, a meta-analysis including 17 studies that used mpMRI to detect extracapsular invasion reported a sensitivity of 0.55 (95% confidence interval (CI): 0.43–0.66) and a specificity of 0.87 (95% CI: 0.82–0.91), suggesting the usefulness of mpMRI for diagnosing locally advanced PC [25]. The NCCN, EAU, and American Urological Association guidelines recommend mpMRI for the diagnosis of locally advanced PC [20,23,26], and it is expected to become more widely used in the future.

2.3. *Treatment*

Previously, ADT alone has been the most common treatment for very high-risk PC. Although combining systemic treatment with ADT and local treatment has recently become more common, there is no standardized treatment for the choice of local treatment because it is unknown which is better between RP and RT; no direct comparison studies have been conducted. Recently, RP plus RT and RT plus ADT in patients with T3-4N0-1M0 PC were compared and PC-specific survival rates for patients undergoing RP plus RT and RT plus ADT, respectively, were 88.9% and 74.2% for T3a/bN0-NXM0 disease, 75.7% and 58.6% for T3a/bN1M0 disease, and 72.0% and 60.5% for T4N0–NXM0 disease. [27]. A retrospective analysis was also performed in 2935 elderly (≥65 years) males in the Surveillance Epidemiology and End Results (SEER)-Medicare linked database who underwent external beam RT (EBRT) versus RP for locally advanced PC [28]. EBRT was associated with higher overall and prostate-specific mortality (hazard ratio (HR): 1.41; 95% CI: 1.09–1.82 vs. HR: 2.35; 95% CI: 1.85–2.98, respectively). Although RP-treated patients appeared to have better prognoses than RT-treated ones, these studies are not prospective comparative studies, and the method and dose of irradiation are unknown. Thus, caution should be taken in interpreting these results, and definitive conclusions cannot be drawn.

2.3.1. RP

In most high-risk patients, surgery is performed with the goal of cure. However, for clinical T3b–4 PC, RP can be thought of as "debulking" the primary tumor in order to improve local control. Moltzahn et al. evaluated a multicenter cohort of 266 patients with very high-risk locally advanced PC (cT3b–4) treated surgically. Despite poor pathologic characteristics, the 10-year cancer-specific mortality rate was relatively low (5.6–12.9%) and was influenced by comorbidities and age [29]. In a report based on the SEER database including 1093 patients with cT4 or cN1 PC, the five-year overall survival (OS) of patients treated with RP or combined ADT and RT was significantly better than that of patients treated with ADT alone or without treatment [30]. The long-term outcome of PC patients who underwent RP in a European cohort has also been reported [31]; this assessed the 20-year oncological outcomes of 22,843 patients, of which there were 3230 high-risk and 903 very high-risk patients based on the NCCN classification. High-risk patients had a 20-year biochemical RFS rate of 34.5%, whereas very high-risk patients had the steepest decline in biochemical RFS and did not reach the 20-year follow-up (30.5% at 15 years). The 20-year metastasis-free survival (MFS) of the high- and very high-risk groups were 64.8% and 64.1%, respectively. The 20-year CSS in the high- and very high-risk groups were 69.6% and 60.8%, respectively. In recent years, robot-assisted RP (RARP) has rapidly become popular, and there has been an accumulating number of reports with good results comparable to those of conventional open surgery. In a recent report, the three-year RFS of RARP plus extended pelvic lymph node dissection for locally advanced PC of cT3 or higher was 95.8% [32].

2.3.2. Radiation Therapy

The first large comprehensive study comparing long-term follow-up of risk-stratified patients for each treatment option has been reported [33]. Among them, brachytherapy with EBRT plus ADT, as well as high-dose-rate (HDR) brachytherapy were reported as treatment options with relatively good results for high-risk patients. On the other hand, in a randomized phase 3 trial of 1205 patients with locally advanced PC staged at cT3-4N0/NXM0, cT1–2 + PSA > 40 ng/mL, or cT1–2 + PSA 20–40 ng/mL + GS 8–10, the 10-year OS of patients treated with combined ADT and RT was significantly better than that of patients treated with ADT alone, at 55% and 49%, respectively (HR: 0.70; 95% CI: 0.57–0.85; $p < 0.001$), and the risk of death was reduced by 30% [5]. Furthermore, many large studies have demonstrated that ADT plus RT was more effective than ADT alone [34–37]. The prospective randomized trial RTOG 85-31 evaluated the effectiveness of adjuvant ADT after definitive RT (a total dose of 65–70 Gy including a boost to the prostate) in patients with cT3 and/or regional lymph node involvement and showed the addition of ADT significantly improved 10-year OS (49% vs. 39%, $p = 0.002$) [3,4]. The GETUG 12 trial evaluated the addition of docetaxel and estramustine to adjuvant ADT in RT or RP among patients with high-risk localized PC and showed that the combined group significantly improved the eight-year RFS (62% vs. 50%, $p = 0.017$) [7].

Although local treatment of PC in men with pelvic lymph node metastasis was considered futile, the advantage of combining ADT with RT may be a promising treatment option. Rusthoven et al. reported that additional EBRT for prostate to ADT improved the 10-year estimated CSS (67% and 53%, respectively; $p < 0.001$) in 796 patients with cT1-4N1M0 PC [8]. Evaluation of 3540 patients with clinically lymph node positive PC from the National Cancer Data Base also reported treatment with ADT plus RT was associated with a 50% reduction in five-year all-cause mortality when compared to treatment with ADT alone (HR: 0.5, 95% CI: 0.37–0.67; $p < 0.001$) [9]. Moreover, the duration of ADT was reported to be superior in terms of local control and prognosis with long-term treatment (24–36 months) compared with short-term treatment ($\leq$6 months) [36]. In addition, in the case of very high-risk PC, potential micrometastases may be present, and hormonal therapy is expected to have a therapeutic effect on these. Thus, these findings establish the significance of combined long-term ADT and RT for very high-risk PC.

As for the significance of combining RT and hormonal therapy, there may be additive and synergistic effects due to the possibility of enhanced apoptosis. Zitman et al. reported that Shionogi tumors can be transplanted into mice and that castration may sensitize them to the cell-killing effects of radiation [38]. In addition, Pollack et al. reported that castration and fractionated irradiation significantly amplified the growth retardation effect in rat PC cells [39].

The options of RT have since diversified to include three-dimensional conformal RT (3D-CRT), intensity-modulated RT, volumetric-modulated arc therapy, stereotactic body RT, and brachytherapy, specifically permanent low-dose-rate (LDR) brachytherapy and temporary HDR brachytherapy. However, it is unclear which irradiation method is optimal so far. Although the therapeutic effect differs depending on the irradiation method, an index called the biologically effective dose (BED) is a common indicator for judging the effectiveness, with higher BED indicating more effective treatment. Stone and Stock et al. reported that the risk of PSA recurrence decreases with increasing BED in brachytherapy with or without EBRT treatment [40]. A recent meta-analysis on appropriate irradiation doses for PC by Zaorsky et al. reported that an increase in BED to 200 Gy was associated with increased PC control, however, doses above 200 Gy did not result in additional clinical benefit [41].

The α/β value of PC cells is an index of their responsiveness to irradiation. This was analyzed and reported to be 1.5 Gy, which is much lower than that of normal tumor cells [42,43]. This is lower than the normal tissue α/β value of 3 Gy. Theoretically, this finding suggests that hypofractionated irradiation with an increased dose per line can safely increase the dose to the prostate without increasing the frequency of late adverse events in normal tissues. Although hypofractionated irradiation has been tested in various irradiation methods and its therapeutic results are being reported, there are still few reports for high- and very high-risk PC.

- Three-dimensional conformal radiotherapy

The most widespread method of external irradiation is 3D-CRT. In this method, the irradiation area is adjusted according to the shape of the target affected area, so that normal tissues are, as much as possible, not exposed to radiation. It has been reported that 3D-CRT for high-risk localized or locally advanced PC is associated with excellent tumor control and survival outcomes [44–46]. Zelefsky et al. have shown that the 10-year PSA relapse-free survival outcomes for stage T3a and T3b tumors were 44% and 32%, respectively, whereas the 10-year CSS outcomes for stage T3a and T3b tumors were 88% and 79%, respectively [44].

- Intensity-modulated radiotherapy

Intensity-modulated radiotherapy (IMRT) is an evolved form of 3D-CRT which provides optimal dose distribution to lesions that are close to risk organs or have complex shapes by irradiating these with a radiation beam with spatially and temporally non-uniform intensity from multiple directions. Currently, IMRT is the standard form of EBRT for PC, rather than 3D-CRT, because of its ability to reduce gastrointestinal and genitourinary (GU) toxicities, biochemical recurrence, and mortality [47–49]. In addition, IMRT may also be used to irradiate pelvic lymph nodes in cases of high-risk or locally advanced PC. A well-conducted, non-randomized, propensity-matched retrospective analysis of 42,481 patients in the U.S. National Cancer Database found IMRT to be beneficial in intermediate-risk ($p < 0.001$) and high-risk PC ($p < 0.001$), but not in low-risk PC ($p = 0.54$) [50]. Moreover, the results of high-dose RT (78 Gy in 92.5% of patients) with IMRT for cT3–4 PC showed eight-year RFS, CSS, and OS rates of 53.2% (95% CI: 43.4–62.1%), 96.6% (95% CI: 91.2–98.7%), and 89.1% (95% CI: 81.5–93.7%), respectively, at a median observation period of 97 months without grade 4 or higher side effects [51]. Wilcox et al. reported the mid-term results of modern EBRT, using combined ADT and dose-escalated IMRT (78 Gy) with MRI-computed tomography (CT) fusion and daily image guidance with fiducial markers. High-risk PC patients had five-year biochemical RFS and CSS rates of 91.3% and 97.7%, respectively, and late rectal adverse event rates of 1.6% for grade 2 and 0% for grade 3, after a median follow-up of 59 months [52]. In an analysis of IMRT for T3b PC, Goupy et al. found the five-year risks of biochemical recurrence, clinical recurrence, and cancer-specific death to be 24.8%, 21.7%, and 10.3%, respectively [53]. On the other hand, there have been few trials of the aforementioned hypofractionated irradiation in high-risk PC. In a multicenter phase 3 trial, the Hypofractionated Irradiation for Prostate Cancer (HYPRO) trial, hypofractionated RT (64.6 Gy; 19 fractions of 3–4 Gy, three fractions per week) was compared with conventionally fractionated RT (78 Gy; 39 fractions of 2 Gy, five fractions per week) for the treatment with IMRT of T1b-4N0/NXM0/MX PC, including 74% high-risk PC patients [54]. This study reported that the five-year relapse-free survival was 80.5% (95% CI: 75.7–84.4%) for patients treated with hypofractionation and 77.1% (95% CI: 71.9–81.5%) for those treated with conventional fractionation (adjusted HR: 0.86; 95% CI: 0.63–1.16; log-rank $p = 0.36$). A phase 2 study of hypofractionated IMRT (70 Gy/28 fractions) using image-guided radiation techniques for PC, including high-risk, is currently underway (UMIN000007810), and the report on its results is awaited.

- Volumetric-modulated arc therapy

Volumetric-modulated arc therapy (VMAT) is a new irradiation method, combining conventional IMRT and rotational irradiation technology to shorten the treatment time. This has resulted in a reduction in patient burden as well as a further improvement in irradiation accuracy. Although the clinical use of VMAT is increasing significantly worldwide, most currently published data are limited to planning and feasibility studies [55]. Results relative to toxicity and clinical outcome are emerging, but are still sparse, and there are few reports in PC treatment. One such study by Hegazy et al. reported that the three-year biochemical RFS rates for high-risk PC were 48% at a median follow-up period of 34 months [56]. Therefore, larger trials with longer follow-up periods are needed in the future.

- Stereotactic body radiotherapy

Stereotactic body radiotherapy (SBRT) is an advanced conformal RT technique that allows for ultra-hypofractionation, thereby significantly reducing the overall treatment time [57,58]. Available studies have convincingly shown that SBRT can be performed safely and with excellent results in patients with low- and intermediate-risk PC [59–61]. However, the role of SBRT in patients with high- and very high-risk PC remains unclear, as only a few patients were included in the clinical trials conducted [59]. A recent systematic report showed that biochemical control rates ranged from 82–100% at two years and 56–100% at three years, with only a few studies reporting longer-term follow-up data [62]. Thus, with the currently available evidence, it can be concluded that SBRT with or without pelvic elective nodal irradiation cannot be considered the standard of care in high-risk PC due to a lack of high-level evidence [62].

- LDR and HDR brachytherapy

Brachytherapy is a type of RT in which a sealed radiation source is placed directly into the body [63]. The placement of the radiation source into the prostate can be permanent or temporary. In permanent interstitial brachytherapy, also known as seed brachytherapy, an LDR radioactive source is placed in the prostate and left permanently to gradually release radiation over time. In temporary brachytherapy, a needle or catheter is first placed in the prostate to confirm its exact location, and then a radioactive source is temporarily introduced into the prostate. The radiation is delivered using a HDR device and the actual treatment time lasts a few minutes.

Although LDR brachytherapy is indicated for patients with low-risk PC and low volume intermediate-risk PC, there is a significant risk of extracapsular diffusion that is not included in the high-dose region of seed implantation in high-risk patients [63]. In such cases, brachytherapy may be combined with EBRT to ensure that appropriate targets are treated. The ASCENDE-RT study is a randomized comparison of two methods of dose escalation in the context of combined modality therapy for high- and intermediate-risk PC (NCCN classification) that includes 12 months of ADT and whole pelvic irradiation to 46 Gy compared with ^{125}I brachytherapy and EBRT boost to a total of 78 Gy. This study found that the LDR boost improved PSA control compared to EBRT alone, but at the cost of higher GU late toxicity [64]. In recent years, there has been an expansion of the indications for sealed small source therapy, which allows for high-dose local irradiation, and good results have been reported in high-risk PC patients, especially for trimodal therapy (a combination of LDR brachytherapy, EBRT, and hormonal therapy) [65,66]. Moreover, a phase 3 multicenter randomized controlled trial (UMIN000003992) investigating trimodal therapy (with LDR brachytherapy, EBRT, and hormonal therapy) for high-risk PC is currently underway, and future results are highly anticipated [67].

With respect to radiobiology, the degree of dose increase that can be achieved with HDR brachytherapy may be more effective in killing PC cells when compared to other EBRT techniques and LDR brachytherapy [68]. Thus, the current clinical evidence for equivalent outcomes with either LDR and HDR or HDR brachytherapy having a theoretical advantage was supported by radiobiological models. There are no other prospective randomized comparisons of EBRT and HDR boost, although some single institution reports have demonstrated favorable biochemical control rates for high-risk localized and locally advanced PC [69–74]. Yamazaki et al. have shown the efficacy of dose escalating RT in patients with cT3b–4 PC. The biochemical disease-free rate at five years was 78.9% (95% CI: 69.8–87.9%) in the EBRT and HDR boost group compared to 66.5% (95% CI, 56.1–76.9%) in the conventional EBRT group treated with 70–72 Gy [73]. Moreover, Kasahara et al. reported the outcomes of HDR brachytherapy combined with hypofractionated EBRT in 66 patients classified as very high-risk PC (NCCN classification) [74]. The five-year biochemical failure-free, distant metastasis-free, PC-specific, and OS rates were 88.7%, 89.2%, 98.5%, and 97.0%, respectively. However, all these studies are retrospective, with small cohort sizes and short follow-up periods. Kishan et al. recently reported a retrospective multicenter study analyzing RP, EBRT, and EBRT with a brachytherapy boost (LDR in 262 patients, HDR in 174 patients) in 1809 patients with GS 9–10 PC [75]. The five-year MFS rates were 76% for RP, 76% for EBRT, and 92% for EBRT plus brachytherapy, which was associated with a significantly lower rate of distant metastasis (HR: 0.27 (95% CI: 0.17–0.43) for RP and 0.30 (95% CI: 0.19–0.47) for EBRT). The 7.5-year OS rates were 83% for RP, 82% for EBRT, and 90% for EBRT plus brachytherapy, which was associated with significantly lower all-cause mortality (HR: 0.66 (95% CI: 0.46–0.96) for RP and 0.61 (95% CI: 0.45–0.84) for EBRT). The superiority of brachytherapy boost over both RP and EBRT was clearly shown by these results. Interestingly, EBRT with brachytherapy potentially offers improved local control over EBRT, which may prevent subsequent metastases.

Incidentally, the BED achieved with HDR brachytherapy boost is typically much higher than can be achieved with EBRT alone. At an α/β ratio of 1.5, the BEDs were 200–300 Gy for HDR brachytherapy versus −187 Gy for EBRT monotherapy (80 Gy in 2 Gy fractions) [76]. In contrast, the combination of EBRT at a dose of 45 Gy with a permanent implant of ^{125}I with a D90 (minimal dose received by 90% of the target volume) ≥130 Gy achieved a BED of >220 Gy, using an α/β ratio of 2 [40,77]. Moreover, conventionally fractionated RT with or without dose-escalated and hypofractionated RT reached a BED of 140–200 Gy using an α/β ratio of 1.5 [41]. Thus, from the BED perspective, an HDR boost may be more efficient.

Table 2 shows the results of various treatments for high-risk localized and very high-risk PC that have been reported so far.

Table 2. Summary of the treatment of high-risk localized and very high-risk prostate cancer.

Study	No. of Patients	Eligibility Criteria	Treatment	Median Follow-Up	Outcome	Reference
Radical prostatectomy for patients presenting with locally advanced disease						
Moltzahn	266	cT3b–4, N0 or N1, M0	RP + PLND ± adjuvant ADT and/or RT	9.3 years	10-year CSS 87.1–94.4%	[29]
External beam radiotherapy for patients presenting with locally advanced disease						
RTOG 85-31	977	cT3 or N1 or RP + PSM and/or SVI	RT vs. RT + ADT (lifelong)	11 years	10-year OS 39% vs. 49%, p = 0.002; 10-year CSS 78% vs. 84%, p = 0.005; 10-year MFS 61% vs. 76%, p < 0.0001	[3,4]
Intergroup randomized study	1205	cT3–4, N0/Nx, M0 or cT1–2 with either PSA > 40 ng/mL or PSA 20–40 ng/mL and GS 8–10	ADT (lifelong) vs. ADT + RT	8 years (range, 0–15.2)	10-year OS 49% vs. 55% (HR 0.70, 95% CI 0.57–0.85, p < 0.001); CSS higher in combined treatment (HR 0.46, 95% CI 0.34–0.61, p < 0.001); 10-year PFS 46% vs. 74% (HR 0.31, 95% CI 0.25–0.39)	[5]
STAMPEDE	638/2962	Two of the following are met; cT3–4, GS 8–10, PSA > 40 ng/mL	SOC vs. SOC + ZA vs. SOC + DOC vs. SOC + ZA + DOC	3.6 years (IQR 2.5–5)	5-year OS 55% vs. 57% vs. 63% vs. 60%; SOC + DOC (HR 0.78, 95% CI 0.66–0.93, p = 0.006) and SOC + DOC + ZA (HR 0.82, 95% CI 0.69–0.97, p = 0.022) compared to SOC only, respectively	[6]
GETUG 12	413	cT3–4 or GS 8–10 or PSA > 20 ng/mL or pN1	ADT (3 years) + local treatment + CT (DOC + EMT) vs. ADT + local treatment	8.8 years (IQR 8.1–9.7)	8-year RFS 62% vs. 50% (adjusted HR 0.71, 95% CI 0.54–0.94, p = 0.017)	[7]

Table 2. *Cont.*

Study	No. of Patients	Eligibility Criteria	Treatment	Median Follow-Up	Outcome	Reference
Rusthoven	796	cT1–4, N1, M0	RT vs. no local treatment	5.2 years	10-year OS 45% vs. 29% (HR 0.58, 95% CI 0.48–0.71, $p < 0.001$); 10-year CSS 67% vs. 53% (HR 0.61, 95% CI 0.47–0.80, $p < 0.001$)	[8]
Lin	3540	cN1, M0 or Mx	ADT + RT vs. ADT alone	5.2 years	5-year OS 71.5% vs. 53.2% (HR 0.50, 95% CI 0.37–0.67, $p < 0.001$)	[9]
Various modalities of radiotherapy						
Zelefsky	296	cT3, N0, M0	3D-CRT or IMRT+ ADT (3 months)	8 years (range, 2–16)	10-year RFS T3a/T3b: 44%/32%; 10-year CSS T3a/T3b: 88%/79%	[44]
Mizowaki	120	cT3–4, N0, M0	IMRT + ADT (6 months)	97 months (range, 21–120)	8-year RFS 53.2%; 8-year CSS 96.6%; 8-year OS 89.1%	[51]
Goupy	276	cT3b, N0–1, M0	IMRT + ADT (3 years)	26 months (95% CI, 33–39)	5-year RFS 75.2%; 5-year CSS 89.7%; 5-year OS 78.8%	[53]
Yamazaki	249	cT3b–4, N0, M0	HDR + EBRT vs. HDEBRT vs. Conv EBRT	64 months (range, 13–153)	5-year RFS 78.9% vs. 88.1% vs. 66.5% ($p = 0.0003$)	[73]
Kishan	1809	Gleason score 9–10	RP vs. EBRT vs. EBRT + LDR/HDR	RP, 4.2 years; EBRT 5.1 years; EBRT + LDR/HDR 6.3 years	5-year MFS 76% vs. 76% vs. 92% ($p < 0.001$); 7.5-year OS 83% vs. 82% vs. 90% ($p < 0.05$)	[75]

RP = radical prostatectomy; PLND = pelvic lymph node dissection; ADT = androgen deprivation therapy; RT = radiotherapy; SOC = standard of care; ZA = zoledronic acid; DOC = docetaxel; IQR = inter-quartile range; HR = hazard ratio; CI = confidence interval; OS = overall survival; CSS = cancer-specific survival; MFS = metastasis-free survival; PFS = progression-free survival; RFS = recurrence-free survival; CT = chemotherapy; EMT = estramustine; 3D-CRT = three-dimensional conformal radiation therapy; IMRT = intensity modulated radiation therapy; HDR = high-dose-rate; LDR = low-dose-rate; HD = high dose; Conv = conventional; EBRT = external beam radiotherapy.

3. Oligometastatic PC

3.1. Definition

Oligometastasis is a concept first proposed by Hellman and Weichselbaum in 1995 [78]. It is considered as a metastatic carcinoma that lies between locally advanced carcinoma and widely metastatic carcinoma, and it should be treated separately from both in terms of prognosis and treatment [2]. Although oligometastasis is usually defined as a limited number of clinically detectable metastases, it has no formally established definition. The recently reported definitions of oligometastatic PC are shown in Table 3. There are many definitions of metastatic sites, ranging from bone and lymph nodes to any site, and the number of metastases is often reported to be three to five or less [79–85]. Basically, these disease states are not special biologically and pathologically, but are just in between non-visualized and bulky metastatic disease, and may be treated as early/low metastatic disease.

Table 3. Definition of oligometastatic prostate cancer.

Source	No. of Patients	Number of Metastases	Number of Metastases	Detection	Reference
Tabata	35	5	Bone only; each site < 50% size of vertebral body	Bone scan	[79]
Ahmed	17	5	NS	^{11}C-choline PET–CT, MRI, biopsy, CT	[80]
Berkovic	24	3	Bone or LN	Bone scan, ^{18}F-FDG PET–CT, ^{11}C-choline PET–CT	[81]

Table 3. Cont.

Source	No. of Patients	Number of Metastases	Number of Metastases	Detection	Reference
Schick	50	4	NS	Bone scan, ^{18}F-choline PET–CT, ^{11}C-acetate PET–CT	[82]
Decaestecker	50	3	Bone or LN	^{18}F-FDG PET–CT, ^{18}F-choline PET–CT	[83]
Ost	119	3	Any	^{18}F-FDG PET–CT, ^{18}F-choline PET–CT	[84]

CT = computed tomography; MRI = magnetic resonance imaging; PET = positron emission tomography; FDG = fluorodeoxyglucose; LN = lymph node; NS = not specified.

3.2. Diagnosis

In addition to conventional imaging methods using CT and bone scintigraphy, many reports have used positron emission tomography-CT (PET-CT) using ^{18}F-fluorodeoxyglucose and ^{11}C-choline, as well as whole-body MRI (WB-MRI) for diagnosis. Shen et al. conducted a meta-analysis of the diagnostic performance of bone metastases and reported that choline PET-CT, MRI, and bone scintigraphy had sensitivities of 87%, 95%, and 79%, respectively, and specificities of 97%, 96%, and 82%, respectively [86]. Recently, PET using prostate-specific membrane antigen (PSMA), a type II transmembrane protein highly expressed in PC, as a tracer has been attracting attention as a promising new imaging modality [87,88]. Maurer et al. reported that ^{68}Ga-PMSA-PET had a sensitivity of 66% and a specificity of 99% for the diagnosis of lymph node metastasis [89]. In addition, a meta-analysis including 1309 patients reported that the positivity rates of ^{68}Ga-PSMA-PET for patients with biochemical recurrence were 42%, 58%, 76%, and 95% for PSA categories 0–0.2, 0.2–1, 1–2, and >2 ng/mL, respectively [90]. Thus, PSMA-PET has improved specificity and sensitivity compared to standard imaging (CT, MRI, and bone scintigraphy), and also improves the detection of metastatic disease in biochemically recurrent PC with low serum PSA levels. Therefore, it is expected to reliably diagnose clinical stage, which would lead to early intervention in cases of locally advanced cancer with potential metastasis and in more extensive metastatic cancer, even in oligometastatic PC. This also allows for the accurate detection of metastatic sites in biochemically recurrent cases. Thus, PSMA PET/CT, which has relatively high sensitivity and specificity compared to other imaging modalities, is increasingly being used for staging and defining oligometastatic PC. Although there are currently no randomized data showing better clinical outcomes with the use of PSMA PET/CT for oligometastatic disease, hopefully more patients will be diagnosed at an earlier stage of metastasis due to the higher detection rate. This accuracy in diagnosing metastasis in turn will allow for multidisciplinary treatment combining MDT.

3.3. Treatment

In the past, treatment of oligometastatic PC was discussed only in terms of ADT, which is the cornerstone of systemic treatment. However, in recent years, the significance of combined local treatment has been widely discussed; MDT may be useful in some cases and should be considered as part of multimodal therapy. The following mechanisms have been postulated: suppression of growth factors and immunosuppressive cytokines by eradicating the primary tumor site [91], reduction of circulating tumor cells [92], and promotion of the anticancer immune response by the abscopal effect (i.e., regression of metastases after therapeutic irradiation of the primary tumor site) [93]. However, there is no standardized treatment for the choice of local treatment because the superiority of RT over surgery is unknown due to the lack of direct comparative studies. Although there is no standardized treatment, there have been a few recent reports suggesting the efficacy of local RT. In 2018, a randomized controlled trial, the HORRAD trial, compared ADT with local radiation versus ADT alone for PC complicated by bone metastases [10]. Although the two groups had no significant difference in OS (HR: 0.90; 95% CI: 0.70–1.14; $p = 0.4$), a subanalysis suggested that RT to the prostate improved OS in patients with low tumor volume (<5 bone lesions). In 2018, the STAMPEDE trial investigated ADT ± docetaxel with local irradiation [6]; this was a phase 3 randomized controlled trial in which patients with newly metastatic PC were randomized 1:1 to receive ADT ± docetaxel as standard therapy with or without concomitant RT to the prostate. RT consisted of either daily irradiation (55 Gy/20 doses) for four weeks or weekly irradiation (36 Gy/6 doses) for six weeks. Although survival was significantly prolonged in the standard treatment plus RT group (HR: 0.76, 95% CI: 0.68–0.84; $p < 0.0001$), OS was not prolonged in the standard treatment plus RT group (HR: 0.92, 95% CI: 0.80–1.06; $p = 0.266$). Notably, in the subanalysis by tumor volume, there was a significant difference in OS at three years in the low metastatic volume group (73% in the standard treatment group vs. 81% in the standard treatment plus radiation group; HR: 0.68, 95% CI: 0.52–0.90; $p = 0.007$), whereas combined radiation treatment had no prognostic effect in the high metastatic volume group. In fact, the results of the HORRAD and STAMPEDE trials suggest the usefulness of local irradiation, since the combination of hormonal therapies with local RT was found to prolong prognosis in low metastatic burden [6,10]. However, the options for RT are diversifying, and it is currently unclear which irradiation method is optimal. Radiobiologically, the α/β value of PC is as low as 1.5 Gy, therefore RT for PC is considered to be more effective with higher doses in smaller fractions [42,43]. In summary, the efficacy of HDR brachytherapy, which delivers a high dose per instance of irradiation, has been recognized for the control of the primary disease; however, there are no reports of HDR brachytherapy against PC with oligometastasis.

These results suggest that the combined local irradiation is effective for patients with low metastatic volume. The CHAARTED study defines high metastatic volume as the presence of visceral metastases or ≥4 bone lesions with ≥1 beyond the vertebral bodies and pelvis [94], whereas low metastatic volume is often defined as having <3 bone metastases, which is exactly in line with the definition of oligometastasis. Furthermore, a few randomized controlled trials are currently underway to test the efficacy of local treatment for metastatic PC [95]. The SWOG 1802 trial (NCT01751438) is evaluating the effect of local treatment (external beam radiation or surgery) in addition to systemic treatment for M1 PC, while the g-RAMPP trial (NCT02454543) is evaluating the effect of RP plus extended lymph node dissection in addition to systemic treatment for M1b PC (≤5 bone metastases). These studies are expected to evaluate the efficacy of local treatment, and future results will be interesting.

As for systemic treatment, ADT is the basic treatment for locally advanced PC. Docetaxel and abiraterone, which is a new anti-androgenic agent, are both currently being used upfront, and the choice of these agents is also noteworthy. However, considering that the CHAARTED study, which demonstrated the benefit of early docetaxel administration in patients with untreated metastatic PC, was unable to show the survival benefit of docetaxel uptake in patients with low metastatic volume [94], the use of early chemotherapy or novel ADT for oligometastatic PC should be further investigated.

Treatment of metastases consists of surgical resection or SBRT. The goals may be to control the cancer, slow down further metastasis, and avoid or delay systemic therapy-related toxicity. A systematic review has given an overview of the current evidence for MDT in oligometastatic PC [11]. Local control rates at two years ranged between 76–100%. Progression free survival (PFS), its definition was inconsistent, was reported from 38–100% at one year and 22–83% at two years. The ORIOLE Trial, a randomized phase 2 study comparing observation and MDT, showed a significantly better PFS of MDT than observation (median, not reached vs. 5.8 months; HR: 0.30; 95% CI: 0.11–0.81; $p = 0.002$) [12]. Moreover, an interim analysis of a large prospective trial involving SBRT in oligometastatic PC patients with up to five metastatic sites was reported [13]. The proportion of patients who did not require treatment escalation (e.g., modification of ADT, introduction of chemotherapy, or palliative RT) was 51.7% (95% CI: 44.1–59.3%) at two years after SBRT, and the median survival without treatment escalation over the entire follow-up period was 27.1 months (95% CI: 21.8–29.4 months). In addition, PSA reduction was observed in 75% of patients. Therefore, the SBRT shows very promising potential for the long-term suppression of oligometastatic PC.

4. Conclusions

Although there is still no standard treatment for very high-risk locally advanced or oligometastatic PC, a major shift in treatment strategy is underway, with reports on the benefits of combined local RT with ADT as a cornerstone. On the other hand, RT delivery methods and protocols vary from study to study, which is an issue that remains unresolved. It will be interesting to see the results of currently ongoing large-scale studies in this field which will be reported in the future.

Author Contributions: K.I. had full access to all the data and takes responsibility for the integrity and the accuracy of its content. Study concept and design: K.I. Drafting of the manuscript: T.M. and K.I. Critical revision of the manuscript: H.I. Supervision: A.M. All authors have read and agreed to the published version of the manuscript.

Funding: This research received no external funding.

Conflicts of Interest: The authors declare no conflict of interest.

References

1. Cooperberg, M.R.; Cowan, J.; Broering, J.M.; Carroll, P.R. High-Risk Prostate Cancer in the United States, 1990–2007. *World J. Urol.* **2008**, *26*, 211–218. [CrossRef] [PubMed]
2. Gillessen, S.; Attard, G.; Beer, T.M.; Beltran, H.; Bossi, A.; Bristow, R.; Carver, B.; Castellano, D.; Chung, B.H.; Clarke, N.; et al. Management of Patients with Advanced Prostate Cancer: The Report of the Advanced Prostate Cancer Consensus Conference Apccc 2017. *Eur. Urol.* **2018**, *73*, 178–211. [CrossRef] [PubMed]
3. Lawton, C.A.; Winter, K.; Murray, K.; Machtay, M.; Mesic, J.B.; Hanks, G.E.; Coughlin, C.T.; Pilepich, M.V. Updated Results of the Phase Iii Radiation Therapy Oncology Group (Rtog) Trial 85-31 Evaluating the Potential Benefit of Androgen Suppression Following Standard Radiation Therapy for Unfavorable Prognosis Carcinoma of the Prostate. *Int. J. Radiat. Oncol. Biol. Phys.* **2001**, *49*, 937–946. [CrossRef]
4. Pilepich, M.V.; Winter, K.; Lawton, C.A.; Krisch, R.E.; Wolkov, H.B.; Movsas, B.; Hug, E.B.; Asbell, S.O.; Grignon, D. Androgen Suppression Adjuvant to Definitive Radiotherapy in Prostate Carcinoma—Long-Term Results of Phase III Rtog 85-31. *Int. J. Radiat. Oncol. Biol. Phys.* **2005**, *61*, 1285–1290. [CrossRef] [PubMed]
5. Mason, M.D.; Parulekar, W.R.; Sydes, M.R.; Brundage, M.; Kirkbride, P.; Gospodarowicz, M.; Cowan, R.; Kostashuk, E.C.; Anderson, J.; Swanson, G.; et al. Final Report of the Intergroup Randomized Study of Combined Androgen-Deprivation Therapy Plus Radiotherapy Versus Androgen-Deprivation Therapy Alone in Locally Advanced Prostate Cancer. *J. Clin. Oncol* **2015**, *33*, 2143–2150. [CrossRef]
6. Parker, C.C.; James, N.D.; Brawley, C.D.; Clarke, N.W.; Hoyle, A.P.; Ali, A.; Ritchie, A.W.S.; Attard, G.; Chowdhury, S.; Cross, W.; et al. Radiotherapy to the Primary Tumour for Newly Diagnosed, Metastatic Prostate Cancer (Stampede): A Randomised Controlled Phase 3 Trial. *Lancet* **2018**, *392*, 2353–2366. [CrossRef]
7. Fizazi, K.; Faivre, L.; Lesaunier, F.; Delva, R.; Gravis, G.; Rolland, F.; Priou, F.; Ferrero, J.M.; Houede, N.; Mourey, L.; et al. Androgen Deprivation Therapy Plus Docetaxel and Estramustine Versus Androgen Deprivation Therapy Alone for High-Risk Localised Prostate Cancer (Getug 12): A Phase 3 Randomised Controlled Trial. *Lancet Oncol.* **2015**, *16*, 787–794. [CrossRef]
8. Rusthoven, C.G.; Carlson, J.A.; Waxweiler, T.V.; Raben, D.; Dewitt, P.E.; Crawford, E.D.; Maroni, P.D.; Kavanagh, B.D. The Impact of Definitive Local Therapy for Lymph Node-Positive Prostate Cancer: A Population-Based Study. *Int. J. Radiat. Oncol. Biol. Phys.* **2014**, *88*, 1064–1073. [CrossRef]
9. Lin, C.C.; Gray, P.J.; Jemal, A.; Efstathiou, J.A. Androgen Deprivation with or without Radiation Therapy for Clinically Node-Positive Prostate Cancer. *J. Natl. Cancer Inst.* **2015**, *107*, djv119. [CrossRef]
10. Boevé, L.M.S.; Hulshof, M.C.C.M.; Vis, A.N.; Zwinderman, A.H.; Twisk, J.W.R.; Witjes, W.P.J.; Delaere, K.P.J.; Moorselaar, R.J.A.V.; Verhagen, P.C.M.S.; van Andel, G. Effect on Survival of Androgen Deprivation Therapy Alone Compared to Androgen Deprivation Therapy Combined with Concurrent Radiation Therapy to the Prostate in Patients with Primary Bone Metastatic Prostate Cancer in a Prospective Randomised Clinical Trial: Data from the Horrad Trial. *Eur. Urol.* **2019**, *75*, 410–418.
11. Rogowski, P.; Roach, M., 3rd; Schmidt-Hegemann, N.S.; Trapp, C.; von Bestenbostel, R.; Shi, R.; Buchner, A.; Stief, C.; Belka, C.; Li, M. Radiotherapy of Oligometastatic Prostate Cancer: A Systematic Review. *Radiat. Oncol.* **2021**, *16*, 50. [CrossRef] [PubMed]
12. Phillips, R.; Shi, W.Y.; Deek, M.; Radwan, N.; Lim, S.J.; Antonarakis, E.S.; Rowe, S.P.; Ross, A.E.; Gorin, M.A.; Deville, C.; et al. Outcomes of Observation Vs Stereotactic Ablative Radiation for Oligometastatic Prostate Cancer: The Oriole Phase 2 Randomized Clinical Trial. *JAMA Oncol.* **2020**, *6*, 650–659. [CrossRef]

13. Bowden, P.; See, A.W.; Frydenberg, M.; Haxhimolla, H.; Costello, A.J.; Moon, D.; Ruljancich, P.; Grummet, J.; Crosthwaite, A.; Pranavan, G.; et al. Fractionated Stereotactic Body Radiotherapy for up to Five Prostate Cancer Oligometastases: Interim Outcomes of a Prospective Clinical Trial. *Int. J. Cancer* **2020**, *146*, 161–168. [CrossRef] [PubMed]
14. D'Amico, A.V.; Whittington, R.; Malkowicz, S.B.; Schultz, D.; Blank, K.; Broderick, G.A.; Tomaszewski, J.E.; Renshaw, A.A.; Kaplan, I.; Beard, C.J.; et al. Biochemical Outcome after Radical Prostatectomy, External Beam Radiation Therapy, or Interstitial Radiation Therapy for Clinically Localized Prostate Cancer. *JAMA* **1998**, *280*, 969–974. [CrossRef] [PubMed]
15. Mano, R.; Eastham, J.; Yossepowitch, O. The Very-High-Risk Prostate Cancer: A Contemporary Update. *Prostate Cancer Prostatic Dis.* **2016**, *19*, 340–348. [CrossRef] [PubMed]
16. Spahn, M.; Joniau, S.; Gontero, P.; Fieuws, S.; Marchioro, G.; Tombal, B.; Kneitz, B.; Hsu, C.Y.; Van Der Eeckt, K.; Bader, P.; et al. Outcome Predictors of Radical Prostatectomy in Patients with Prostate-Specific Antigen Greater Than 20 Ng/Ml: A European Multi-Institutional Study of 712 Patients. *Eur. Urol.* **2010**, *58*, 1–7. [CrossRef]
17. Walz, J.; Joniau, S.; Chun, F.K.; Isbarn, H.; Jeldres, C.; Yossepowitch, O.; Chao-Yu, H.; Klein, E.A.; Scardino, P.T.; Reuther, A.; et al. Pathological Results and Rates of Treatment Failure in High-Risk Prostate Cancer Patients after Radical Prostatectomy. *BJU Int.* **2011**, *107*, 765–770. [CrossRef]
18. Joniau, S.; Briganti, A.; Gontero, P.; Gandaglia, G.; Tosco, L.; Fieuws, S.; Tombal, B.; Marchioro, G.; Walz, J.; Kneitz, B.; et al. Stratification of High-Risk Prostate Cancer into Prognostic Categories: A European Multi-Institutional Study. *Eur. Urol.* **2015**, *67*, 157–164. [CrossRef]
19. Sundi, D.; Wang, V.; Pierorazio, P.M.; Han, M.; Partin, A.W.; Tran, P.T.; Ross, A.E.; Bivalacqua, T.J. Identification of Men with the Highest Risk of Early Disease Recurrence after Radical Prostatectomy. *Prostate* **2014**, *74*, 628–636. [CrossRef] [PubMed]
20. Mohler, J.L.; Antonarakis, E.S.; Armstrong, A.J.; D'Amico, A.V.; Davis, B.J.; Dorff, T.; Eastham, J.A.; Enke, C.A.; Farrington, T.A.; Higano, C.S.; et al. Prostate Cancer, Version 2.2019, Nccn Clinical Practice Guidelines in Oncology. *J. Natl. Compr. Canc. Netw.* **2019**, *17*, 479–505. [CrossRef]
21. Briganti, A.; Karnes, J.R.; Da Pozzo, L.F.; Cozzarini, C.; Gallina, A.; Suardi, N.; Bianchi, M.; Freschi, M.; Doglioni, C.; Fazio, F.; et al. Two Positive Nodes Represent a Significant Cut-Off Value for Cancer Specific Survival in Patients with Node Positive Prostate Cancer. A New Proposal Based on a Two-Institution Experience on 703 Consecutive N+ Patients Treated with Radical Prostatectomy, Extended Pelvic Lymph Node Dissection and Adjuvant Therapy. *Eur. Urol.* **2009**, *55*, 261–270.
22. Touijer, K.A.; Mazzola, C.R.; Sjoberg, D.D.; Scardino, P.T.; Eastham, J.A. Long-Term Outcomes of Patients with Lymph Node Metastasis Treated with Radical Prostatectomy without Adjuvant Androgen-Deprivation Therapy. *Eur. Urol.* **2014**, *65*, 20–25. [CrossRef]
23. Mottet, N.; van den Bergh, R.C.N.; Briers, E.; Van den Broeck, T.; Cumberbatch, M.G.; De Santis, M.; Fanti, S.; Fossati, N.; Gandaglia, G.; Gillessen, S.; et al. Eau-Eanm-Estro-Esur-Siog Guidelines on Prostate Cancer-2020 Update. Part 1: Screening, Diagnosis, and Local Treatment with Curative Intent. *Eur. Urol.* **2021**, *79*, 243–262. [CrossRef]
24. Somford, D.M.; Hamoen, E.H.; Fütterer, J.J.; van Basten, J.P.; Hulsbergen-van de Kaa, C.A.; Vreuls, W.; van Oort, I.M.; Vergunst, H.; Kiemeney, L.A.; Barentsz, J.O.; et al. The Predictive Value of Endorectal 3 Tesla Multiparametric Magnetic Resonance Imaging for Extraprostatic Extension in Patients with Low, Intermediate and High Risk Prostate Cancer. *J. Urol.* **2013**, *190*, 1728–1734. [CrossRef]
25. Zhang, F.; Liu, C.L.; Chen, Q.; Shao, S.C.; Chen, S.Q. Accuracy of Multiparametric Magnetic Resonance Imaging for Detecting Extracapsular Extension in Prostate Cancer: A Systematic Review and Meta-Analysis. *Br. J. Radiol.* **2019**, *92*, 20190480. [CrossRef] [PubMed]
26. Sanda, M.G.; Cadeddu, J.A.; Kirkby, E.; Chen, R.C.; Crispino, T.; Fontanarosa, J.; Freedland, S.J.; Greene, K.; Klotz, L.H.; Makarov, D.V.; et al. Clinically Localized Prostate Cancer: Aua/Astro/Suo Guideline. Part I: Risk Stratification, Shared Decision Making, and Care Options. *J. Urol.* **2018**, *199*, 683–690. [CrossRef] [PubMed]
27. Jang, T.L.; Patel, N.; Faiena, I.; Radadia, K.D.; Moore, D.F.; Elsamra, S.E.; Singer, E.A.; Stein, M.N.; Eastham, J.A.; Scardino, P.T.; et al. Comparative Effectiveness of Radical Prostatectomy with Adjuvant Radiotherapy Versus Radiotherapy Plus Androgen Deprivation Therapy for Men with Advanced Prostate Cancer. *Cancer* **2018**, *124*, 4010–4022. [CrossRef]
28. Feldman, A.S.; Meyer, C.P.; Sanchez, A.; Krasnova, A.; Reznor, G.; Menon, M.; Kibel, A.S.; Choueiri, T.K.; Lipsitz, S.R.; Sun, M.; et al. Morbidity and Mortality of Locally Advanced Prostate Cancer: A Population Based Analysis Comparing Radical Prostatectomy Versus External Beam Radiation. *J. Urol.* **2017**, *198*, 1061–1068. [CrossRef]
29. Moltzahn, F.; Karnes, J.; Gontero, P.; Kneitz, B.; Tombal, B.; Bader, P.; Briganti, A.; Montorsi, F.; Van Poppel, H.; Joniau, S.; et al. Predicting Prostate Cancer-Specific Outcome after Radical Prostatectomy among Men with Very High-Risk Ct3b/4 Pca: A Multi-Institutional Outcome Study of 266 Patients. *Prostate Cancer Prostatic. Dis.* **2015**, *18*, 31–37. [CrossRef]
30. Johnstone, P.A.; Ward, K.C.; Goodman, M.; Assikis, V.; Petros, J.A. Radical Prostatectomy for Clinical T4 Prostate Cancer. *Cancer* **2006**, *106*, 2603–2609. [CrossRef] [PubMed]
31. Wurnschimmel, C.; Wenzel, M.; Wang, N.; Tian, Z.; Karakiewicz, P.I.; Graefen, M.; Huland, H.; Tilki, D. Radical Prostatectomy for Localized Prostate Cancer: 20-Year Oncological Outcomes from a German High-Volume Center. *Urol. Oncol.* **2021**, in press.
32. Gandaglia, G.; De Lorenzis, E.; Novara, G.; Fossati, N.; De Groote, R.; Dovey, Z.; Suardi, N.; Montorsi, F.; Briganti, A.; Rocco, B.; et al. Robot-Assisted Radical Prostatectomy and Extended Pelvic Lymph Node Dissection in Patients with Locally-Advanced Prostate Cancer. *Eur. Urol.* **2017**, *71*, 249–256. [CrossRef] [PubMed]

33. Grimm, P.; Billiet, I.; Bostwick, D.; Dicker, A.P.; Frank, S.; Immerzeel, J.; Keyes, M.; Kupelian, P.; Lee, W.R.; Machtens, S.; et al. Comparative Analysis of Prostate-Specific Antigen Free Survival Outcomes for Patients with Low, Intermediate and High Risk Prostate Cancer Treatment by Radical Therapy. Results from the Prostate Cancer Results Study Group. *BJU Int.* **2012**, *109*, 22–29. [CrossRef] [PubMed]
34. Bolla, M.; Van Tienhoven, G.; Warde, P.; Dubois, J.B.; Mirimanoff, R.O.; Storme, G.; Bernier, J.; Kuten, A.; Sternberg, C.; Billiet, I.; et al. External Irradiation with or without Long-Term Androgen Suppression for Prostate Cancer with High Metastatic Risk: 10-Year Results of an Eortc Randomised Study. *Lancet Oncol.* **2010**, *11*, 1066–1073. [CrossRef]
35. Roach, M., 3rd; Bae, K.; Speight, J.; Wolkov, H.B.; Rubin, P.; Lee, R.J.; Lawton, C.; Valicenti, R.; Grignon, D.; Pilepich, M.V. Short-Term Neoadjuvant Androgen Deprivation Therapy and External-Beam Radiotherapy for Locally Advanced Prostate Cancer: Long-Term Results of Rtog 8610. *J. Clin. Oncol.* **2008**, *26*, 585–591. [CrossRef]
36. Horwitz, E.M.; Bae, K.; Hanks, G.E.; Porter, A.; Grignon, D.J.; Brereton, H.D.; Venkatesan, V.; Lawton, C.A.; Rosenthal, S.A.; Sandler, H.M.; et al. Ten-Year Follow-up of Radiation Therapy Oncology Group Protocol 92-02: A Phase Iii Trial of the Duration of Elective Androgen Deprivation in Locally Advanced Prostate Cancer. *J. Clin. Oncol.* **2008**, *26*, 2497–2504. [CrossRef]
37. Fossa, S.D.; Wiklund, F.; Klepp, O.; Angelsen, A.; Solberg, A.; Damber, J.E.; Hoyer, M.; Widmark, A.; The Scandinavian Prostate Cancer Group-7 Investigators. Ten-and 15-Yr Prostate Cancer-Specific Mortality in Patients with Nonmetastatic Locally Advanced or Aggressive Intermediate Prostate Cancer, Randomized to Lifelong Endocrine Treatment Alone or Combined with Radiotherapy: Final Results of the Scandinavian Prostate Cancer Group-7. *Eur. Urol.* **2016**, *70*, 684–691. [PubMed]
38. Zietman, A.L.; Nakfoor, B.M.; Prince, E.A.; Gerweck, L.E. The Effect of Androgen Deprivation and Radiation Therapy on an Androgen-Sensitive Murine Tumor: An in Vitro and in Vivo Study. *Cancer J. Sci. Am.* **1997**, *3*, 31–36. [PubMed]
39. Pollack, A.; Joon, D.L.; Wu, C.S.; Sikes, C.; Hasegawa, M.; Terry, N.H.; White, R.A.; Zagars, G.K.; Meistrich, M.L. Quiescence in R3327-G Rat Prostate Tumors after Androgen Ablation. *Cancer Res.* **1997**, *57*, 2493–2500.
40. Stock, R.G.; Stone, N.N.; Cesaretti, J.A.; Rosenstein, B.S. Biologically Effective Dose Values for Prostate Brachytherapy: Effects on Psa Failure and Posttreatment Biopsy Results. *Int. J. Radiat. Oncol. Biol. Phys.* **2006**, *64*, 527–533. [CrossRef]
41. Zaorsky, N.G.; Palmer, J.D.; Hurwitz, M.D.; Keith, S.W.; Dicker, A.P.; Den, R.B. What Is the Ideal Radiotherapy Dose to Treat Prostate Cancer? A Meta-Analysis of Biologically Equivalent Dose Escalation. *Radiother. Oncol.* **2015**, *115*, 295–300. [CrossRef]
42. Brenner, D.J.; Hall, E.J. Fractionation and Protraction for Radiotherapy of Prostate Carcinoma. *Int. J. Radiat. Oncol. Biol. Phys.* **1999**, *43*, 1095–1101. [CrossRef]
43. Brenner, D.J.; Martinez, A.A.; Edmundson, G.K.; Mitchell, C.; Thames, H.D.; Armour, E.P. Direct Evidence That Prostate Tumors Show High Sensitivity to Fractionation (Low Alpha/Beta Ratio), Similar to Late-Responding Normal Tissue. *Int. J. Radiat. Oncol. Biol. Phys.* **2002**, *52*, 6–13. [CrossRef]
44. Zelefsky, M.J.; Yamada, Y.; Kollmeier, M.A.; Shippy, A.M.; Nedelka, M.A. Long-Term Outcome Following Three-Dimensional Conformal/Intensity-Modulated External-Beam Radiotherapy for Clinical Stage T3 Prostate Cancer. *Eur. Urol.* **2008**, *53*, 1172–1179. [CrossRef] [PubMed]
45. Nguyen, Q.N.; Levy, L.B.; Lee, A.K.; Choi, S.S.; Frank, S.J.; Pugh, T.J.; McGuire, S.; Hoffman, K.; Kuban, D.A. Long-Term Outcomes for Men with High-Risk Prostate Cancer Treated Definitively with External Beam Radiotherapy with or without Androgen Deprivation. *Cancer* **2013**, *119*, 3265–3271. [CrossRef]
46. Arcangeli, G.; Saracino, B.; Arcangeli, S.; Gomellini, S.; Petrongari, M.G.; Sanguineti, G.; Strigari, L. Moderate Hypofractionation in High-Risk, Organ-Confined Prostate Cancer: Final Results of a Phase Iii Randomized Trial. *J. Clin. Oncol.* **2017**, *35*, 1891–1897. [CrossRef]
47. Sujenthiran, A.; Nossiter, J.; Charman, S.C.; Parry, M.; Dasgupta, P.; van der Meulen, J.; Cathcart, P.J.; Clarke, N.W.; Payne, H.; Aggarwal, A. National Population-Based Study Comparing Treatment-Related Toxicity in Men Who Received Intensity Modulated Versus 3-Dimensional Conformal Radical Radiation Therapy for Prostate Cancer. *Int. J. Radiat. Oncol. Biol. Phys.* **2017**, *99*, 1253–1260. [CrossRef] [PubMed]
48. Yu, T.; Zhang, Q.; Zheng, T.; Shi, H.; Liu, Y.; Feng, S.; Hao, M.; Ye, L.; Wu, X.; Yang, C. The Effectiveness of Intensity Modulated Radiation Therapy Versus Three-Dimensional Radiation Therapy in Prostate Cancer: A Meta-Analysis of the Literatures. *PLoS ONE* **2016**, *11*, e0154499. [CrossRef]
49. Sheets, N.C.; Goldin, G.H.; Meyer, A.M.; Wu, Y.; Chang, Y.; Stürmer, T.; Holmes, J.A.; Reeve, B.B.; Godley, P.A.; Carpenter, W.R.; et al. Intensity-Modulated Radiation Therapy, Proton Therapy, or Conformal Radiation Therapy and Morbidity and Disease Control in Localized Prostate Cancer. *JAMA* **2012**, *307*, 1611–1620.
50. Kalbasi, A.; Li, J.; Berman, A.; Swisher-McClure, S.; Smaldone, M.; Uzzo, R.G.; Small, D.S.; Mitra, N.; Bekelman, J.E. Dose-Escalated Irradiation and Overall Survival in Men with Nonmetastatic Prostate Cancer. *JAMA Oncol.* **2015**, *1*, 897–906. [CrossRef]
51. Mizowaki, T.; Norihisa, Y.; Takayama, K.; Ikeda, I.; Inokuchi, H.; Nakamura, K.; Kamba, T.; Inoue, T.; Kamoto, T.; Ogawa, O.; et al. Long-Term Outcomes of Intensity-Modulated Radiation Therapy Combined with Neoadjuvant Androgen Deprivation Therapy under an Early Salvage Policy for Patients with T3-T4n0 m0 Prostate Cancer. *Int. J. Clin. Oncol.* **2016**, *21*, 148–155. [CrossRef]
52. Wilcox, S.W.; Aherne, N.J.; McLachlan, C.S.; McKay, M.J.; Last, A.J.; Shakespeare, T.P. Is Modern External Beam Radiotherapy with Androgen Deprivation Therapy Still a Viable Alternative for Prostate Cancer in an Era of Robotic Surgery and Brachytherapy: A Comparison of Australian Series. *J. Med. Imaging Radiat. Oncol.* **2015**, *59*, 125–133. [CrossRef] [PubMed]

53. Goupy, F.; Supiot, S.; Pasquier, D.; Latorzeff, I.; Schick, U.; Monpetit, E.; Martinage, G.; Herve, C.; Le Proust, B.; Castelli, J.; et al. Intensity-Modulated Radiotherapy for Prostate Cancer with Seminal Vesicle Involvement (T3b): A Multicentric Retrospective Analysis. *PLoS ONE* **2019**, *14*, e0210514. [CrossRef] [PubMed]
54. Incrocci, L.; Wortel, R.C.; Alemayehu, W.G.; Aluwini, S.; Schimmel, E.; Krol, S.; van der Toorn, P.P.; Jager, H.; Heemsbergen, W.; Heijmen, B.; et al. Hypofractionated Versus Conventionally Fractionated Radiotherapy for Patients with Localised Prostate Cancer (Hypro): Final Efficacy Results from a Randomised, Multicentre, Open-Label, Phase 3 Trial. *Lancet Oncol.* **2016**, *17*, 1061–1069. [CrossRef]
55. Macchia, G.; Deodato, F.; Cilla, S.; Cammelli, S.; Guido, A.; Ferioli, M.; Siepe, G.; Valentini, V.; Morganti, A.G.; Ferrandina, G. Volumetric Modulated Arc Therapy for Treatment of Solid Tumors: Current Insights. *Oncol. Targets* **2017**, *10*, 3755–3772. [CrossRef]
56. Hegazy, M.W.; Mahmood, R.I.; Al Otaibi, M.F.; Khalil, E.M. Hypofractionated Volumetric Modulated Arc Radiotherapy with Simultaneous Elective Nodal Irradiation Is Feasible in Prostate Cancer Patients: A Single Institution Experience. *J. Egypt Natl. Canc. Inst.* **2016**, *28*, 101–110. [CrossRef] [PubMed]
57. Schmitt, D.; Blanck, O.; Gauer, T.; Fix, M.K.; Brunner, T.B.; Fleckenstein, J.; Loutfi-Krauss, B.; Manser, P.; Werner, R.; Wilhelm, M.L.; et al. Technological Quality Requirements for Stereotactic Radiotherapy: Expert Review Group Consensus from the Dgmp Working Group for Physics and Technology in Stereotactic Radiotherapy. *Strahlenther. Onkol.* **2020**, *196*, 421–443. [CrossRef]
58. Guckenberger, M.; Baus, W.W.; Blanck, O.; Combs, S.E.; Debus, J.; Engenhart-Cabillic, R.; Gauer, T.; Grosu, A.L.; Schmitt, D.; Tanadini-Lang, S.; et al. Definition and Quality Requirements for Stereotactic Radiotherapy: Consensus Statement from the Degro/Dgmp Working Group Stereotactic Radiotherapy and Radiosurgery. *Strahlenther. Onkol.* **2020**, *196*, 417–420. [CrossRef] [PubMed]
59. Widmark, A.; Gunnlaugsson, A.; Beckman, L.; Thellenberg-Karlsson, C.; Hoyer, M.; Lagerlund, M.; Kindblom, J.; Ginman, C.; Johansson, B.; Björnlinger, K.; et al. Ultra-Hypofractionated Versus Conventionally Fractionated Radiotherapy for Prostate Cancer: 5-Year Outcomes of the Hypo-Rt-Pc Randomised, Non-Inferiority, Phase 3 Trial. *Lancet* **2019**, *394*, 385–395. [CrossRef]
60. Jackson, W.C.; Silva, J.; Hartman, H.E.; Dess, R.T.; Kishan, A.U.; Beeler, W.H.; Gharzai, L.A.; Jaworski, E.M.; Mehra, R.; Hearn, J.W.D.; et al. Stereotactic Body Radiation Therapy for Localized Prostate Cancer: A Systematic Review and Meta-Analysis of over 6,000 Patients Treated on Prospective Studies. *Int. J. Radiat. Oncol. Biol. Phys.* **2019**, *104*, 778–789. [CrossRef]
61. Brand, D.H.; Tree, A.C.; Ostler, P.; van der Voet, H.; Loblaw, A.; Chu, W.; Ford, D.; Tolan, S.; Jain, S.; Martin, A.; et al. Intensity-Modulated Fractionated Radiotherapy Versus Stereotactic Body Radiotherapy for Prostate Cancer (Pace-B): Acute Toxicity Findings from an International, Randomised, Open-Label, Phase 3, Non-Inferiority Trial. *Lancet Oncol.* **2019**, *20*, 1531–1543. [CrossRef]
62. Foerster, R.; Zwahlen, D.R.; Buchali, A.; Tang, H.; Schroeder, C.; Windisch, P.; Vu, E.; Akbaba, S.; Bostel, T.; Sprave, T.; et al. Stereotactic Body Radiotherapy for High-Risk Prostate Cancer: A Systematic Review. *Cancers* **2021**, *13*, 759. [CrossRef] [PubMed]
63. Bolla, M.; Henry, A.; Mason, M.; Wiegel, T. The Role of Radiotherapy in Localised and Locally Advanced Prostate Cancer. *Asian J. Urol.* **2019**, *6*, 153–161. [CrossRef] [PubMed]
64. Chin, J.; Rumble, R.B.; Kollmeier, M.; Heath, E.; Efstathiou, J.; Dorff, T.; Berman, B.; Feifer, A.; Jacques, A.; Loblaw, D.A. Brachytherapy for Patients with Prostate Cancer: American Society of Clinical Oncology/Cancer Care Ontario Joint Guideline Update. *J. Clin. Oncol.* **2017**, *35*, 1737–1743. [CrossRef] [PubMed]
65. Zaorsky, N.G.; Davis, B.J.; Nguyen, P.L.; Showalter, T.N.; Hoskin, P.J.; Yoshioka, Y.; Morton, G.C.; Horwitz, E.M. The Evolution of Brachytherapy for Prostate Cancer. *Nat. Rev. Urol.* **2017**, *14*, 415–439. [CrossRef]
66. Okamoto, K.; Wada, A.; Kohno, N. High Biologically Effective Dose Radiation Therapy Using Brachytherapy in Combination with External Beam Radiotherapy for High-Risk Prostate Cancer. *J. Contemp. Brachytherapy* **2017**, *9*, 1–6. [CrossRef]
67. Konaka, H.; Egawa, S.; Saito, S.; Yorozu, A.; Takahashi, H.; Miyakoda, K.; Fukushima, M.; Dokiya, T.; Yamanaka, H.; Stone, N.N.; et al. Tri-Modality Therapy with I-125 Brachytherapy, External Beam Radiation Therapy, and Short- or Long-Term Hormone Therapy for High-Risk Localized Prostate Cancer (Trip): Study Protocol for a Phase Iii, Multicenter, Randomized, Controlled Trial. *BMC Cancer* **2012**, *12*, 110. [CrossRef]
68. King, C.R.; DiPetrillo, T.A.; Wazer, D.E. Optimal Radiotherapy for Prostate Cancer: Predictions for Conventional External Beam, Imrt, and Brachytherapy from Radiobiologic Models. *Int. J. Radiat. Oncol. Biol. Phys.* **2000**, *46*, 165–172. [CrossRef]
69. Makino, T.; Mizokami, A.; Namiki, M. Clinical Outcomes of Patients with Localized and Locally Advanced Prostate Cancer Undergoing High-Dose-Rate Brachytherapy with External-Beam Radiotherapy at Our Institute. *Anticancer. Res.* **2015**, *35*, 1723–1728.
70. Makino, T.; Nakashima, K.; Iijima, M.; Kawaguchi, S.; Nohara, T.; Shigehara, K.; Izumi, K.; Kadono, Y.; Kumano, T.; Mizokami, A. Health-Related Quality of Life and Toxicity after Single-Fraction High-Dose-Rate Brachytherapy with External Beam Radiotherapy for Localized and Locally Advanced Prostate Cancer. *Anticancer. Res.* **2019**, *39*, 477–486. [CrossRef]
71. Wedde, T.B.; Småstuen, M.C.; Brabrand, S.; Fosså, S.D.; Kaasa, S.; Tafjord, G.; Russnes, K.M.; Hellebust, T.P.; Lilleby, W. Ten-Year Survival after High-Dose-Rate Brachytherapy Combined with External Beam Radiation Therapy in High-Risk Prostate Cancer: A Comparison with the Norwegian Spcg-7 Cohort. *Radiother. Oncol.* **2019**, *132*, 211–217. [CrossRef]

72. Yamazaki, H.; Masui, K.; Suzuki, G.; Aibe, N.; Shimizu, D.; Kimoto, T.; Yamada, K.; Ueno, A.; Matsugasumi, T.; Yamada, Y.; et al. High-Dose-Rate Brachytherapy with External Beam Radiotherapy Versus Low-Dose-Rate Brachytherapy with or without External Beam Radiotherapy for Clinically Localized Prostate Cancer. *Sci. Rep.* **2021**, *11*, 6165. [CrossRef] [PubMed]
73. Yamazaki, H.; Suzuki, G.; Masui, K.; Aibe, N.; Shimizu, D.; Kimoto, T.; Yoshida, K.; Nakamura, S.; Okabe, H. Radiotherapy for Clinically Localized T3b or T4 Very-High-Risk Prostate Cancer-Role of Dose Escalation Using High-Dose-Rate Brachytherapy Boost or High Dose Intensity Modulated Radiotherapy. *Cancers* **2021**, *13*, 1856. [CrossRef] [PubMed]
74. Kasahara, T.; Ishizaki, F.; Kazama, A.; Yuki, E.; Yamana, K.; Maruyama, R.; Oshikane, T.; Kaidu, M.; Aoyama, H.; Bilim, V.; et al. High-Dose-Rate Brachytherapy and Hypofractionated External Beam Radiotherapy Combined with Long-Term Androgen Deprivation Therapy for Very High-Risk Prostate Cancer. *Int. J. Urol.* **2020**, *27*, 800–806. [CrossRef] [PubMed]
75. Kishan, A.U.; Cook, R.R.; Ciezki, J.P.; Ross, A.E.; Pomerantz, M.M.; Nguyen, P.L.; Shaikh, T.; Tran, P.T.; Sandler, K.A.; Stock, R.G.; et al. Radical Prostatectomy, External Beam Radiotherapy, or External Beam Radiotherapy with Brachytherapy Boost and Disease Progression and Mortality in Patients with Gleason Score 9-10 Prostate Cancer. *JAMA* **2018**, *319*, 896–905. [CrossRef]
76. Zaorsky, N.G.; Doyle, L.A.; Yamoah, K.; Andrel, J.A.; Trabulsi, E.J.; Hurwitz, M.D.; Dicker, A.P.; Den, R.B. High Dose Rate Brachytherapy Boost for Prostate Cancer: A Systematic Review. *Cancer Treat. Rev.* **2014**, *40*, 414–425. [CrossRef]
77. Stone, N.N.; Potters, L.; Davis, B.J.; Ciezki, J.P.; Zelefsky, M.J.; Roach, M.; Shinohara, K.; Fearn, P.A.; Kattan, M.W.; Stock, R.G. Multicenter Analysis of Effect of High Biologic Effective Dose on Biochemical Failure and Survival Outcomes in Patients with Gleason Score 7-10 Prostate Cancer Treated with Permanent Prostate Brachytherapy. *Int. J. Radiat. Oncol. Biol. Phys.* **2009**, *73*, 341–346. [CrossRef]
78. Hellman, S.; Weichselbaum, R.R. Oligometastases. *J. Clin. Oncol.* **1995**, *13*, 8–10. [CrossRef]
79. Tabata, K.; Niibe, Y.; Satoh, T.; Tsumura, H.; Ikeda, M.; Minamida, S.; Fujita, T.; Ishii, D.; Iwamura, M.; Hayakawa, K.; et al. Radiotherapy for Oligometastases and Oligo-Recurrence of Bone in Prostate Cancer. *Pulm. Med.* **2012**, *2012*, 541656. [CrossRef]
80. Ahmed, K.A.; Barney, B.M.; Davis, B.J.; Park, S.S.; Kwon, E.D.; Olivier, K.R. Stereotactic Body Radiation Therapy in the Treatment of Oligometastatic Prostate Cancer. *Front. Oncol.* **2012**, *2*, 215. [CrossRef]
81. Berkovic, P.; De Meerleer, G.; Delrue, L.; Lambert, B.; Fonteyne, V.; Lumen, N.; Decaestecker, K.; Villeirs, G.; Vuye, P.; Ost, P. Salvage Stereotactic Body Radiotherapy for Patients with Limited Prostate Cancer Metastases: Deferring Androgen Deprivation Therapy. *Clin. Genitourin. Cancer* **2013**, *11*, 27–32. [CrossRef]
82. Schick, U.; Jorcano, S.; Nouet, P.; Rouzaud, M.; Vees, H.; Zilli, T.; Ratib, O.; Weber, D.C.; Miralbell, R. Androgen Deprivation and High-Dose Radiotherapy for Oligometastatic Prostate Cancer Patients with Less Than Five Regional and/or Distant Metastases. *Acta Oncol.* **2013**, *52*, 1622–1628. [CrossRef]
83. Decaestecker, K.; De Meerleer, G.; Lambert, B.; Delrue, L.; Fonteyne, V.; Claeys, T.; De Vos, F.; Huysse, W.; Hautekiet, A.; Maes, G.; et al. Repeated Stereotactic Body Radiotherapy for Oligometastatic Prostate Cancer Recurrence. *Radiat. Oncol.* **2014**, *9*, 135. [CrossRef]
84. Ost, P.; Jereczek-Fossa, B.A.; As, N.V.; Zilli, T.; Muacevic, A.; Olivier, K.; Henderson, D.; Casamassima, F.; Orecchia, R.; Surgo, A.; et al. Progression-Free Survival Following Stereotactic Body Radiotherapy for Oligometastatic Prostate Cancer Treatment-Naive Recurrence: A Multi-Institutional Analysis. *Eur. Urol.* **2016**, *69*, 9–12. [CrossRef] [PubMed]
85. Tosoian, J.J.; Gorin, M.A.; Ross, A.E.; Pienta, K.J.; Tran, P.T.; Schaeffer, E.M. Oligometastatic Prostate Cancer: Definitions, Clinical Outcomes, and Treatment Considerations. *Nat. Rev. Urol.* **2017**, *14*, 15–25. [CrossRef] [PubMed]
86. Shen, G.; Deng, H.; Hu, S.; Jia, Z. Comparison of Choline-Pet/Ct, Mri, Spect, and Bone Scintigraphy in the Diagnosis of Bone Metastases in Patients with Prostate Cancer: A Meta-Analysis. *Skelet. Radiol.* **2014**, *43*, 1503–1513. [CrossRef] [PubMed]
87. Maurer, T.; Eiber, M.; Schwaiger, M.; Gschwend, J.E. Current Use of Psma–Pet in Prostate Cancer Management. *Nat. Rev. Urol.* **2016**, *13*, 226. [CrossRef] [PubMed]
88. Fendler, W.P.; Schmidt, D.F.; Wenter, V.; Thierfelder, K.M.; Zach, C.; Stief, C.; Bartenstein, P.; Kirchner, T.; Gildehaus, F.J.; Gratzke, C.; et al. 68ga-Psma Pet/Ct Detects the Location and Extent of Primary Prostate Cancer. *J. Nucl. Med.* **2016**, *57*, 1720–1725. [CrossRef]
89. Maurer, T.; Gschwend, J.E.; Rauscher, I.; Souvatzoglou, M.; Haller, B.; Weirich, G.; Wester, H.J.; Heck, M.; Kubler, H.; Beer, A.J.; et al. Diagnostic Efficacy of (68)Gallium-Psma Positron Emission Tomography Compared to Conventional Imaging for Lymph Node Staging of 130 Consecutive Patients with Intermediate to High Risk Prostate Cancer. *J. Urol.* **2016**, *195*, 1436–1443. [CrossRef]
90. Perera, M.; Papa, N.; Christidis, D.; Wetherell, D.; Hofman, M.S.; Murphy, D.G.; Bolton, D.; Lawrentschuk, N. Sensitivity, Specificity, and Predictors of Positive (68)Ga-Prostate-Specific Membrane Antigen Positron Emission Tomography in Advanced Prostate Cancer: A Systematic Review and Meta-Analysis. *Eur. Urol.* **2016**, *70*, 926–937. [CrossRef]
91. Mole, R.H. Whole Body Irradiation—Radiobiology or Medicine? *Br. J. Radiol.* **1953**, *26*, 234–241. [CrossRef]
92. Resel Folkersma, L.; San Jose Manso, L.; Galante Romo, I.; Moreno Sierra, J.; Olivier Gomez, C. Prognostic Significance of Circulating Tumor Cell Count in Patients with Metastatic Hormone-Sensitive Prostate Cancer. *Urology* **2012**, *80*, 1328–1332. [CrossRef] [PubMed]
93. Nesseler, J.P.; Peiffert, D.; Vogin, G.; Nickers, P. Cancer, Radiotherapy and Immune System. *Cancer Radiother.* **2017**, *21*, 307–315. [CrossRef]

94. Sweeney, C.J.; Chen, Y.H.; Carducci, M.; Liu, G.; Jarrard, D.F.; Eisenberger, M.; Wong, Y.N.; Hahn, N.; Kohli, M.; Cooney, M.M.; et al. Chemohormonal Therapy in Metastatic Hormone-Sensitive Prostate Cancer. *N. Engl. J. Med.* **2015**, *373*, 737–746. [CrossRef] [PubMed]
95. Slaoui, A.; Albisinni, S.; Aoun, F.; Assenmacher, G.; Al Hajj Obeid, W.; Diamand, R.; Regragui, S.; Touzani, A.; Bakar, A.; Mesfioui, A.; et al. A Systematic Review of Contemporary Management of Oligometastatic Prostate Cancer: Fighting a Challenge or Tilting at Windmills? *World J. Urol.* **2019**, *37*, 2343–2353. [CrossRef] [PubMed]

MDPI
St. Alban-Anlage 66
4052 Basel
Switzerland
Tel. +41 61 683 77 34
Fax +41 61 302 89 18
www.mdpi.com

Cancers Editorial Office
E-mail: cancers@mdpi.com
www.mdpi.com/journal/cancers

www.ingramcontent.com/pod-product-compliance
Lightning Source LLC
Chambersburg PA
CBHW040818250926
51850CB00007BA/1205
9783036581682